Christian Paths to Health and Wellness

Peter Walters, PhD

Wheaton College

John Byl, PhD

Redeemer University College

EDITORS

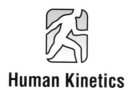

Human Kinetics

Library of Congress Cataloging-in-Publication Data

Christian paths to health and wellness / Peter Walters, John Byl, editors.
    p. cm.
    Includes bibliographical references and index.
    ISBN-13: 978-0-7360-6227-5 (soft cover)
    ISBN-10: 0-7360-6227-0 (soft cover)
    1. College students--Health and hygiene. 2. Health--Religious aspects--Christianity. I. Walters, Peter, 1959- II. Byl, John.
    RA777.3.C47 2008
    613--dc22

                          2007026835

ISBN-10: 0-7360-6227-0
ISBN-13: 978-0-7360-6227-5

Scripture quotations are taken, with exceptions noted, from the *Holy Bible,* New International Version. 1973, 1978, 1984 by International Bible Society. Colorado Springs, CO: Zondervan. Exception scripture quotations are taken from Peterson, E. 2003. *The message: The Bible in contemporary language.* Omaha, NE: Quickverse.

The Web addresses cited in this text were current as of August 9, 2007, unless otherwise noted.

Acquisitions Editor: Bonnie Pettifor Vreeman; **Developmental Editor:** Amy Stahl; **Assistant Editor:** Jackie Walker; **Copyeditor:** Holly Gilly; **Proofreader:** Darlene Rake; **Indexer:** Craig Brown; **Permission Manager:** Dalene Reeder; **Graphic Designer:** Fred Starbird; **Graphic Artist:** Dawn Sills; **Photo Manager:** Laura Fitch; **Photo Office Assistant:** Jason Allen; **Cover Designer:** Keith Blomberg; **Photographer (cover):** Scott Markewitz/Aurora Photos; **Photographer (interior):** © Peter Walters, unless otherwise noted; photos on pages 10, 17, 19, 148, 151, and 283 (top left and bottom right) © Human Kinetics; **Art Manager:** Kelly Hendren; **Associate Art Manager:** Alan L. Wilborn; **Illustrators:** Jason M. McAlexander, MFA (figures 6.9, 6.10, 6.12); Mic Greenberg (figures 4.1, 6.11a-b, 8.9, 9.8); all other illustrations by Argosy. **Printer:** Custom Color Graphics

Printed in the United States of America   10 9 8 7 6 5 4 3 2 1

Human Kinetics
Web site: www.HumanKinetics.com

United States: Human Kinetics
P.O. Box 5076
Champaign, IL 61825-5076
800-747-4457
e-mail: humank@hkusa.com

Canada: Human Kinetics
475 Devonshire Road Unit 100
Windsor, ON N8Y 2L5
800-465-7301 (in Canada only)
e-mail: orders@hkcanada.com

Europe: Human Kinetics
107 Bradford Road
Stanningley
Leeds LS28 6AT, United Kingdom
+44 (0) 113 255 5665
e-mail: hk@hkeurope.com

Australia: Human Kinetics
57A Price Avenue
Lower Mitcham, South Australia 5062
08 8372 0999
e-mail: info@hkaustralia.com

New Zealand: Human Kinetics
Division of Sports Distributors NZ Ltd.
P.O. Box 300 226 Albany
North Shore City
Auckland
0064 9 448 1207
e-mail: info@humankinetics.co.nz

Contents

Preface   vii

Acknowledgments   xi

Part I   Understanding Your Wellness and Mission — 1

Chapter 1   Valuing Wellness — 3
John Byl

Creation   5
Fall   6
Redemption   7
Fulfillment   9
Next Steps   11
Learning Tools   11

Chapter 2   God's Purpose and Your Life's Mission — 13
John Byl • Dianne E. Moroz

God's Mission   15
Making God's Purposes Your Purposes   15
Pressures That Shape Life's Mission   16
Your Mission Statement   17
Goals for the Journey   19
Next Steps   25
Learning Tools   26

Part II   Accepting and Caring for Your Body — 29

Chapter 3   Examining Body Image and Eating Disorders in Women and Men — 31
Heather Strong • John Byl

Introduction to Dieting, Weight Preoccupation, and Body Image   33
What Are Eating Disorders?   38

How Prevalent Are Eating Disorders?   41
What Causes Eating Disorders?   42
What God Wants for People   47
Recovery From an Eating Disorder   50
Next Steps   51
Learning Tools   51

Chapter 4   Weight Control - **59**
John Byl

Step 1: State the Goal   63
Step 2: Assess Your Present Lifestyle   65
Step 3: Design a Specific Plan   67
Step 4: Predict Obstacles   67
Step 5: Plan Intervention Strategies   67
Step 6: Assess Compliance With the Plan   69
Step 7: Assess Progress of Your Overall Goal   69
Next Steps   69
Learning Tools   69

Part III   Moving Your Body - - - - - - - - - - - - - - - - - - - **73**

Chapter 5   Cardiorespiratory Assessment and Training - - **75**
Peter Walters

Setting the Bar: Primary and Secondary Goals   76
Benefiting From Cardiorespiratory Exercise   77
Understanding the Three Energy Systems   80
Evaluating Cardiorespiratory Endurance   81
Discouraged After Your Aerobic Assessment? Consider This   83
Outlining an Aerobic Exercise Prescription   83
Sample Cardiorespiratory Fitness Programs   90
Next Steps   98
Learning Tools   98

Chapter 6   Muscular Strength Assessment and Training - - **105**
Peter Walters

Setting the Bar   106
Benefits of Strength Training   108
Assessing Muscular Strength   113
Strength: Encouragement and Possibilities   113

Basic Muscle Anatomy   115
Types of Strength Training   119
A Three-Phase Strength-Training Program   121
Safety in Strength Training   132
Next Steps   134
Learning Tools   134

Chapter 7   Flexibility Assessment and Training ‑ ‑ ‑ ‑ ‑ ‑ ‑ ‑ 143
Bob Weathers
What Is Flexibility?   144
Factors That Affect Flexibility   144
Importance of Flexibility   145
How Much Flexibility Is Enough?   147
Assessing Your Flexibility   147
Improving and Maintaining Your Flexibility   148
Next Steps   151
Learning Tools   152

Part IV   Understanding Your Behaviors ‑ ‑ ‑ ‑ ‑ 155

Chapter 8   Nutritional Health and Wellness ‑ ‑ ‑ ‑ ‑ ‑ ‑ ‑ 157
Peter Walters
The Digestive System   159
Six Major Nutrient Groups   162
Canadian Food Guide   183
Vegetarian Alternative   184
Next Steps   187
Learning Tools   188

Chapter 9   Emotional Health and Wellness ‑ ‑ ‑ ‑ ‑ ‑ ‑ ‑ 193
Peter Walters • Doug Needham • Bud Williams
Stress and the Mind–Body Connection   194
Pros and Cons of Stress   200
When Stress Turns Ugly   202
Depression   209
Happiness and Life Satisfaction   217
Next Steps   220
Learning Tools   222

Chapter **10**   **Sleep Habits and Wellness** - - - - - - - - - - **229**
Peter Walters

Chronic Sleep Deprivation   231
Sleep Thieves   231
Are You Sleep Deprived?   238
The Effects of Sleep Deprivation   240
The Architecture of Sleep   245
How Much Sleep Do You Need?   247
How to Sleep Like a Log   248
Next Steps   250
Learning Tools   251

Chapter **11**   **Personal Relationships and Wellness** - - - - - **255**
Peter Walters

Value of Relationships   256
Digging Deeper   257
Personality   258
Values   262
Spiritual Gifts   264
Your SHAPE   265
Healthy Relationships and Healthy Bodies   266
Next Steps   273
Learning Tools   273

Part **V**   **Conclusion** - - - - - - - - - - - - **281**

Chapter **12**   **Offering Your Life as a Living Sacrifice** - - - - - **283**
John Byl

Tools for Achieving Wellness   284
Seven Steps to Wellness   284
Next Steps   286
Learning Tools   286

Appendix A: Guide for Family and Friends of a Person With Food and Weight Problems   289

Appendix B: Questionnaires on Eating Behaviors   291

Appendix C: Strength-Training Program   295

Glossary   307

Index   315

About the Editors   323

About the Contributors   324

Preface

So God created man in his own image . . .

male and female he created them . . .

God saw all that he had made, and it was very good.

(Genesis 1:27, 31)

This textbook on personal physical wellness is about the woman who delights in mountain biking and the man who loves to run. It is about the people who struggle with body image. It is about the man who hesitates to join an aerobics class and the woman who resists starting a strength-training program, but who both overcome their fears and experience lifelong wellness. This book is about helping you "die young," as old as possible. It is about developing realistic and helpful resolutions about personal physical wellness and having the tools to accomplish the resolutions. This book is about knowing God and yourself and about how you can enjoy and care for the world God has placed you in; it's about knowing "that you yourselves are God's temple and that God's Spirit lives in you" (1 Corinthians 3:16). This text is about the pursuit of love, health, and happiness—and actually getting closer to them.

Purpose of This Book

This textbook is contextualized in narrative, supported and illustrated with current research findings, and filtered through the eyes of the Christian faith. It is a multiauthored resource, building on the strengths of a number of Christian academics who teach health and wellness. All the authors focus on assisting you to be positively engaged in personal physical wellness choices, exclaiming with God, after he created Adam and Eve, "It is very good!"

This book is geared toward first-year university or college students enrolled in an introductory course on health and wellness, specifically courses in Christian postsecondary institutions, but it will also benefit others interested in improving their physical wellness. It is an introductory text for those who are exploring and applying the concepts of health and wellness for the first time. A general understanding of health and wellness issues will benefit the general reader, and the comprehensive nature and unique perspective of this book will also make the material applicable and interesting to both the novice and the expert in the field of health and wellness.

Empowering you to take responsibility and initiative for your health and well-being is a main goal of this book. The book's content helps people, regardless of their interest in physical activity, learn about physical wellness and its importance to the whole person and apply the principles and concepts to daily living. The writers tried not to spoon-feed you, but to provide well-researched information in the context of narrative, challenging you to make discerning applications to your own lives. In essence this is a book of empowerment and healing. You will develop your awareness of physical wellness issues and develop a passion for proactive and permanent lifestyle changes.

The idea for this book was born out of a commitment to helping you embrace the concepts and lifestyle choices of health and well-being as part of the Christian life. Quick-fix solutions to negative lifestyle choices are not offered in this book. We aim to help you enter into constructive, positive, and realistic habit formation and transformation. The book provides hope, practical tools, and methods for change with a comprehensiveness that enables you to make gradual and significant permanent change through the wisdom of education and the power of the Holy Spirit.

Physical wellness is a unique topic that examines many facets of life experience. This textbook is specifically focused around four major themes: how God made people, how he made them to move, how he made them to be nourished, and how he made them to rest. Many professors at Christian universities were teaching from books that were not God centered, and they needed a text with a foundation that was God centered. That's why we wrote this book.

Structure of This Book

Part I, Understanding Your Wellness and Mission, looks at how scripture speaks about our body. Chapter 1, Valuing Wellness, explores a Biblical view of a person. Chapter 2, God's Purpose and Your Life's Mission, encourages you to live focused lives fixed on godly physical goals.

Part II, Accepting and Caring for Your Body, explores our body image and body composition. Chapter 3, Examining Body Image and Eating Disorders in Women and Men, deals with body image and the influence of cultural forces on attitudes toward it. The chapter also includes two powerful personal stories about how a woman and a man came to a positive body image. Chapter 4, Weight Control, examines how excess fat is often so easy to put on and so difficult to permanently remove. These two chapters concern us with the challenges of being too thin or too fat, or being too focused on displaying muscle.

Part III, Moving Your Body, addresses three common areas about how to help the body move. This part contains three chapters that help you understand how you can develop your cardiovascular endurance (chapter 5), muscular strength (chapter 6), and flexibility (chapter 7).

Part IV, Understanding Your Behaviors, focuses on behaviors. People need rhythmic patterns of activity and nutrition, of rest and leisure, and of time with friends and others. Chapter 8, Nutritional Health and Wellness, explores the key components of good nutrition, helping you develop positive and informed choices about your eating habits while fueling the physical body. Rhythmic patterns of rest and leisure greatly improve ability to function normally and to lower unhealthy stress levels. Chapter 9, Emotional Health and Wellness, clarifies the importance of allowing stress to motivate but not debilitate, and it gives guidance about how to work through depression. Chapter 10, Sleep Habits and Wellness, discusses the important healing effect of regular, sound sleep. Chapter 11, Personal Relationships and Wellness, talks about how to nurture all relationships to be positive, bringing wellness to all.

The concluding chapter encourages you to pull the whole book together and prepare or construct with a comprehensive strategy to maintain and develop personal wellness in a relationship with God. It provides a reflective meditation about the course and how it is up to you to choose to live well.

Features of This Book

Information in the chapters in this book is organized into sections, allowing for an easy-to-follow format:

- The objectives of each chapter are clearly identified in the beginning of each chapter and followed up with review questions at the end of each chapter.

- Specific information is often presented in concise, easy-to-read charts.

- New terms are highlighted in bold, defined, and listed in a glossary at the end of the book with a list of key terms appearing at the end of each chapter.

- One of the unique features of this book is that the text builds on personal stories, pertaining to the topic being covered. The main points of the chapter are explained through a logical narrative style, including some of the authors' personal stories, to foster the learning and practice of lifelong positive health and wellness choices. You will be drawn in by the stories and may find a personal connection to your own experience and that of others. Having been drawn into the stories, you will want to continue reading from one chapter to the next, discovering, understanding, questioning, laughing, wondering, and so on. Many of these stories are found in the "Real Life" sidebars, noted with the following icon:

- There are often two sides to a story, and the text includes point/counterpoint discussions with brief contrary positions on a topic, which demonstrate the impact ideas have on the way we live. These discussions are noted with the following icon:

- Personal wellness is often achieved through mental and physical discipline. However, it is also important for us to open ourselves to the power of God through the Holy Spirit. The Bible writes, "The fruit of the Spirit is love, joy, peace, patience, kindness, goodness, faithfulness, gentleness and self-control" (Galatians 5:22–23). Most chapters offer a brief vignette on the parts of the fruit of the Spirit, which demonstrates how the Spirit heals us and makes us well. These vignettes are noted with the following icon:

- The application activities at the end of each chapter help you reflect and make necessary applications to your own lives, often by writing your own positive and healing stories.
- A list of helpful print materials (Suggested Readings) and Internet resources (Suggested Web Sites) supports each chapter.

Personal physical wellness is an important topic to learn about. Because we're Christians, it is important that the questions posed, the solutions suggested, the actions considered, and the course followed fix "our eyes on Jesus, the author and perfecter of our faith, who for the joy set before him endured the cross, scorning its shame, and sat down at the right hand of the throne of God" (Hebrews 12:2). This same Jesus is preparing a place where "He will wipe away every tear from their eyes. There will be no more death or mourning or crying or pain. . ." (Revelation 21:4). Faculty and students can be a part of "making everything new" (Revelation 21:5).

This book is the first edition of a book with a Christian view of health and wellness. This textbook has a life of its own and can undoubtedly be strengthened. We want to continue to update this book so that it helps more people and brings a bigger smile to God's face. Your input about any concerns or suggestions you have is deeply valued. Please send your suggestions to byl@redeemer.ca or Peter.H.Walters@Wheaton.edu.

Acknowledgments

Writing this book required a community of people. The need for and structure of this text were developed by Christian academics that met at an annual conference hosted by the Christian Society for Kinesiology and Leisure Studies (CSKLS). To each person who helped us formulate this book, and for the prayers of many more, thanks.

CSKLS was founded and nurtured by Glen Van Andel. Without his formative work on CSKLS the need for this book would not have been so readily apparent, nor its development so speedy. Thanks, Glen, for your formative work with CSKLS and, consequently, the publication of this book.

Several writers shared their work with us. Thanks to Heather Strong, Dianne E. Moroz, Doug Needham, Bob Weathers, and Bud Williams for your valuable contributions. Sue Moen labored diligently on the nutrition chapter, as did Mar Magnuson on the strength chapter. Others, whose contributions we weren't able to include in the text, helped shape where we were going. To each of you, thanks. A special word of appreciation to Jesse Bjoraker for your thoughtful suggestions and careful editing of several chapters. Your ability to connect with young readers is remarkable.

We tested versions of this book during its various stages of development with students at Messiah College, Redeemer University College, Seattle Pacific University, and Wheaton College. Thank you, Jim Gustafson, Dianne E. Moroz, and Bob Weathers, for facilitating that work, and thanks to the students who contributed valuable advice and critiques.

Thanks to the wonderful folks at Human Kinetics for publishing this important text. Thanks especially to Bonnie Pettifor Vreeman for your confidence and for nudging the book through to acceptance. Amy Stahl was awesome in the way she kept us on our time lines, extended grace to us when we were late, and applied her precise and thoughtful editorial skills to sharpening the entire book. Amy, a huge thank-you!

Writing requires time, and those who sacrificed most because of the time we spent writing are Margery and Catherine and our children. Your love and support for us are amazing, and we are blessed by our families.

Thanks to God, who adopted us as his children. We are thankful to be part of his family. We trust this book is a blessing to all.

Peter Walters and John Byl

Understanding Your Wellness and Mission

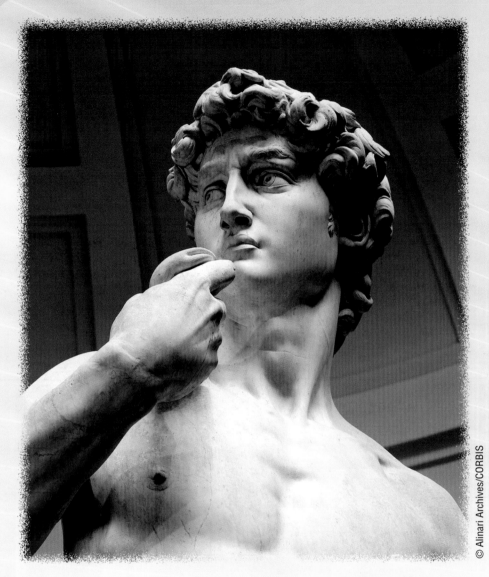

© Alinari Archives/CORBIS

Valuing Wellness

John Byl

After reading this chapter, you should be able to do the following:

❶ Understand a biblical view of the human body.

❷ Explain your view of the human body.

❸ Begin to think about how you should view and treat your body.

You've probably had days when you felt great and were happy to be alive and active. The purpose of this book is to encourage each person to bring honor to God by the way he or she lives. This is a book about enjoying, improving, and serving through physical wellness in relation to others.

I prepared to write this chapter by exploring the question "Does God really care about our physical being?" I found that people have very different perceptions of a person's value, particularly when they consider the value of their own bodies.

Think about how you view your body and how you believe God views your body. As you serve God, it is helpful to have a sense of his perspective and to remember how God created "male and female. . . [and] God saw all that He had made, and it was very good" (Genesis 1:27, 31).

This chapter explores a view of the body by looking at the implications of the Bible's teachings on creation, fall, redemption, and fulfillment. If you view the body like the fasting student and Plato do (see the sidebar on this page), then concern for physical wellness matters only insofar as you are

What Value Is Your Body?

Let's take a look at several personal views. Which best reflects your own? One student writes honestly about this topic:

> When I first fell in love with Jesus, I stopped loving my body. I thought that to be spiritual was to abstain from foods; fasting was a great door to a living relationship with God. However, my physical state became poor. Many of my friends alerted me to this, but I ignored them, seeing it as my way of becoming poor. (Byl, 1999, p. 73)

Socrates, coming from a similar perspective, constructs his argument as follows:

> When soul and body are both in the same place, nature teaches the one to serve and be subject, the other to rule and govern. In this relation which do you think most resembles the divine and which the mortal part? Don't you think it is the nature of the divine to rule and direct, and that of the mortal to be subject and serve?
>
> I do.
>
> Then which does the soul resemble?

Obviously, Socrates, soul resembles the divine, and the body the mortal (Socrates, 1954, p. 131).

Plato, also viewing a person's body negatively, argues that the soul is "marred by association with the body and other evils, but when she has regained that pure condition which the eye of reason can discern, you will then find her to be a far lovelier thing" (Plato, 1945, p. 345). The fasting student, Socrates, and Plato conclude that a person's body is something that "mars" the true person. Is that your view?

Another student writes about her body in a positive manner:

> I believe that I do love myself, but explaining that love is the hard part. You know, God has blessed me with so many things. I think that it would be like an insult to say that I did not love the me that God made. I love my sense of humor, my nose; yes, I love me. (Byl, 1999, p. 73)

Gabriel Marcel, a Christian existentialist, also appreciates people's physical selves, and argues, "I am my body. . . . I cannot validly say 'I and my body'" (Marcel, 1965, p. 18). The second student and Marcel view the body positively. Marcel goes even further by stating that he cannot talk about his body apart from who he is.

Think of the various statements you just read about the body. Did they make sense to you? Why or why not? Which student or philosopher seems to best reflect the Christian tenets regarding the view of who people are, particularly in the physical being?

able to let the good spirit control the evil body. On the other hand, if your view is more like the second student's (also mentioned in the sidebar on page 4), who viewed her body as "the me that God made," then concern for physical wellness matters.

Creation

As you know, the scriptures begin with God creating everything, including man and woman. God looked at all of **creation** and declared it was very good. God saw all of Adam and all of Eve—their emotions, their thoughts, their noses, their toes—and "it was very good" (Genesis 1:27–31).

This first chapter of the Bible teaches at least two important preliminary lessons. The first lesson is that God made all things. Other writers in the scriptures reemphasize this point (Psalm 33:9; 11:3; 147:15–20, and 2 Peter 3:5–7). The second lesson is that God created all things "very good." The first chapter in Genesis makes no distinction that some things of creation are very good, others are OK, and others are undesirable. God looked at all of creation at the very end and declared that all of it was "very good." In the New Testament, Paul reiterates this point: "For everything God created is good, and nothing is to be rejected" (1 Timothy 4:4). From the beginning to the end of the Bible a good creation, including good physical people, is a consistent theme.

Creation is about a personal God who walked in the garden with Adam and Eve and among everything he made. It is about a personal God who talks with his people. Creation is not about man and woman finding their origins in the impersonal process of time and chance that characterizes an **evolutionist** position on the origin of people.

God recognized and provided for the needs of this first man and woman. He knew of their need for food and provided plants to nourish them (Genesis 1:29). He knew of their need for emotional companionship and provided that in each other. Calvin Seerveld, an **aesthetician**, imagines Adam and Eve's first meeting as follows: "When Adam first discovered Eve and Eve saw Adam for the first time, I imagine they were amazed. Their skin rather tingled with anticipation. God was going to surprise them with something exciting, but they didn't know yet what it was. In the beginning, Adam and Eve probably smiled at one another, invitingly, a little bashfully" (Seerveld, 1976, p. 19).

But what does it mean to be created in the image of God? In the chapter titled "The Meaning of the Image" in his book *Man: The Image of God*, G.C. Berkouwer writes, "The image of God is something which concerns the whole man, his place in this world and his future, his likeness in his being a child of a Father, of this Father in heaven" (Berkouwer, 1962, p. 117). In other words, the image of God is not limited to a person's soul, body, or relationships; the image of God is potentially expressed through all aspects of a person, and in the garden the imaging was very good. Think about what kind of pictures Adam and Eve would put on their blogs and how they would finish the following sentence: "This past week we. . . ."

When you read Genesis 5, notice how the word *image* comes up: "When Adam had lived 130 years, he had a son in his own likeness, in his own image; and he named him Seth" (Genesis 5:3). Like parent, like child. People often comment on how much a newborn child looks like the father or mother. The comparison isn't surprising because indeed that is the child's origin.

The announcement that Seth was like Adam begins a list of many boys and girls born to Adam's descendants. Notice these words that precede the explanation of Seth in verse 3: "When God created man, He made him in the likeness of God. He created them male and female and blessed them" (Genesis 5:1–2). The equation is simple: Inasmuch as I am in the image of my father and mother, I am also in the image of God. In Genesis 1:26, God said, "Let us make man in our [my] image, in our [my] likeness." God made people in his image, and "crowned" humans "with glory and honor" (Psalm 8:5). People represent God wherever they go because they are in his image.

One aspect of being created in God's image is that God and people are "creators." All of Genesis 1 is about a God who creates, as opposed to Greek gods who came from creation. The Christian God is a creator God—a God who gets involved in the creative tasks. Jesus came into this world as a son of a carpenter and a homemaker. Genesis 2:15 says the Lord God took a man and woman and put them into the Garden of Eden, "to work it and to take care of it" and to extend that same care to animals (Genesis 1:26). One of God's commandments tells us to rest on the Sabbath day, but that follows six days of doing work (Exodus 20:8–11). Adam and Eve, their children, and all of us are created in the image of God, to be busy working in and caring for creation. People, created in God's image, are cultivators. Caring for your physical body is one of those creative tasks.

Not only did God create Adam and Eve, but he also provided for them so they could survive and

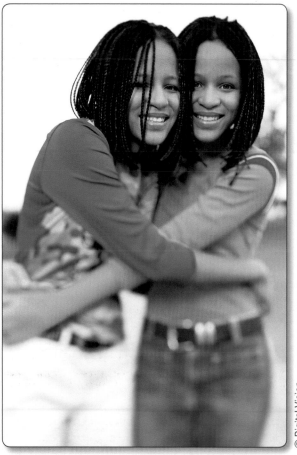

Children are made in the image of their parents and of God.

fully enjoy his creative goodness. Like Adam and Eve, you are created to be like God. The creation of you was also "very good," and you are called to care for and develop his creation, which includes your body.

Fall

Man and woman turned their backs on God in the Garden of Eden and ate the fruit God had declared off limits. Consequently, they broke their perfect relationship with God, with each other, and with all of creation. The painful reality of broken relationships soon became evident when Adam and Eve's son Cain killed his brother Abel (Genesis 4:8). The implications of Adam and Eve's **fall** are not limited to them. As the scripture points out: "We all, like sheep, have gone astray, each of us has turned to his own way" (Isaiah 53:6). Romans 3:23 adds: "All have sinned and fall short of the glory of God." The *fall* refers to a universal and

pervasive disposition of people to turn their backs on God. A result of the fall was that people would find gathering food and caring for themselves more difficult. In addition, people's decisions would be influenced by "conflicting spirits," or conflicting internal voices that influence toward what is good and toward what is bad.

Damaged Intimacy

The most intimate relationship in the world – the one between husband and wife – was also damaged as a result of the fall. Before the fall, Adam and Eve walked openly and unashamedly with each other and with God, and their relationship was great. After the fall they were more closed, ashamed, and quick to blame each other for wrongs. From that point on, maintaining good relationships would require hard work. Because of Adam and Eve's sin, even the closest relationships have discord, and will require effort for growth.

Desolate Creation

Creation itself experienced the fall. As Paul writes, "We know that the whole creation has been groaning as in the pains of childbirth right up to the present time" (Romans 8:22). This groaning, or response to pain and discomfort, is made worse by people's disobedience to God (Jeremiah 12:11). In other words, all of creation is hurting because of the fall and personal sin.

People still are inclined to reject God (to sin) even though sinning brings negative consequences. Consider the "seven deadly sins" (Proverbs 6:16–19). Think about their everyday meaning in your life and in the lives of those around you. Each of these sins adds brokenness to the world and to individuals' lives.

Pride

Pride goes before a fall. *Pride* is thinking you are the center of the world. You exhibit pride when you get upset and become impatient when stoplights turn red as you approach, when you're stuck in a traffic jam, or when your line for the bank teller is long.

Envy

To *envy* is to resent someone else's good fortune so much that you are tempted to destroy it or steal it from them. If your friend is doing well in a fitness program, you would exemplify envy if you sabotage the program so that you can gloat

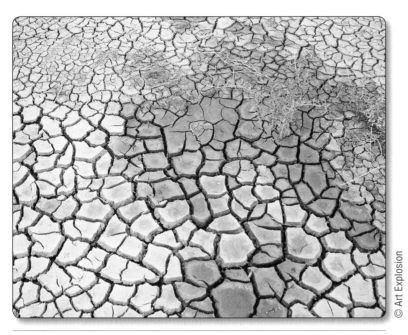

© Art Explosion

The whole of creation groans.

about his or her failure and your own success. The scripture teaches that "envy rots the bones" (Proverbs 14:30).

Anger

Experiencing *anger* means that you allow contempt for another to rule over you. A girl who is not loved by her father and turns to controlling food to vent her anger may find food controlling her life; a girl who is overweight and is heavily criticized by her father may overeat as a response to her anger and hurt over her father's remarks. The scripture teaches that uncontrolled "anger is cruel and fury overwhelming" (Proverbs 27:4).

Laziness and Apathy (Sloth)

The laziness in people may be part of why they dream of fitness but don't get off the couch to do anything about it. Scripture teaches that the lazy person wants to go but doesn't do anything to get anywhere (Proverbs 13:4). In other words, although the "couch potato" says he wants to be fit, his lack of action indicates he doesn't really want anything—and that's what he gets!

Greed and Materialism (Avarice)

Greed makes people want the best fitness equipment and finest fitness clubs to produce the finest body around, and they'll do anything to get it. The scriptures remind us: "Whoever trusts in his riches will fall" (Proverbs 11:28). If you count on money and material things, you will fail.

Overindulgence (Gluttony)

The *glutton* is captive to food because her thoughts are consumed by wanting more food or less food. The scripture says, "their god is their stomach" (Philippians 3:19).

Misguided or Sinful Desire (Lust)

People who let their bodies direct them into a lustful obsession to continually satisfy cravings for pleasure become captives of a vicious cycle, wanting more and more. Scripture describes the situation this way: "Having lost all sensitivity, they have given themselves over to sensuality so as to indulge in every kind of impurity, with a continual lust for more" (Ephesians 4:19). Addictions come from those kinds of cravings. One more drink or one more look at a sexy picture seems so innocent, but the taste or the look calls for one more, and another, and another. Those desires are like sponges that never become saturated.

Let's face it: Because Adam and Eve blew it, you are susceptible to doing your own thing, no matter the consequences. But that behavior ultimately

- damages your body,
- holds you in a prison of the things you crave, and
- leaves you dissatisfied and searching for what you're missing.

Falling into sin increases the suffering of this world and of your body.

Redemption

Rebellion against God causes people to be miserable, unhealthy, and unwell—but there is hope. Christ says, "I have come that they may have life, and have it to the full" (John 10:10). Christ died and rose again to bring life. God wants to change all things through Christ (Colossians 1:19–20). Through Christ's redemptive work, people are reconciled to God and are challenged to make all things as they were created and meant to be—very good. **Redemption** means that all things are made new in Christ.

At the beginning of this chapter, you read about a new Christian abstaining from food and not caring for his body as a way of worshipping the Lord. This new Christian may also have quoted from Proverbs 31:30: "Charm is deceptive, and beauty is fleeting." Or he could have quoted from Psalm 147:10–11: The Lord does not delight "in the legs of a man; the Lord delights in those who fear him." Is part of becoming reconciled to God doing what this new Christian did? I think the answer is no! The key part of each of these verses is the last one—the need to fear the Lord. Then, out of reverence for God, people need to glorify God in everything they do (1 Corinthians 10:31), because "everything God created is good" (1 Timothy 4:4) and needs to be redeemed, including the body.

Opposite of Sinning Causes Healing

The seven deadly sins cause much brokenness, but the opposite of each sin brings healing. Instead of feeling the pain caused by self-centered pride, give and receive love to feel healing. Instead of the rot caused by envy, experience the peace that gives life to the body (Proverbs 14:30). Instead of injury through furious, irrational anger, experience healing through gentle, irrational forgiveness, as God forgave you (Matthew 6:12; Ephesians 4:32). Instead of experiencing obesity caused by laziness, experience the promise of fullness in Proverbs 13:4: "The desires of the diligent are fully satisfied." Instead of being greedy for self-serving riches, live simply. Trust the scripture that says, "God will meet all your needs according to his glorious riches in Christ Jesus" (Philippians 4:19). Instead of being a captive to food, "eagerly await a Savior from [Heaven], the Lord Jesus Christ, who, by the power that enables him to bring everything under his control, will transform our lowly bodies so that they will be like his glorious body" (Philippians 3:20–21). Instead of being a captive to lust, follow the scripture that teaches: "Do not offer the parts of your body to sin, as instruments of wickedness, but rather offer yourselves to God" (Romans 6:13).

Even in falling into sin, you are still created in God's image. Moses asks this rhetorical question: "Is he [God] not your Father, your Creator, who made you and formed you?" (Deuteronomy 32:6) Elders praise God before his throne, saying, "You are worthy, our Lord and God, to receive glory and honor and power, for you created all things, and by your will they were created and have their being" (Revelation 4:11). Fallen? Yes! But you are created by God, held in his loving embrace, and asked to join God in caring for and developing creation. Amazing!

Even though you are created in God's image and you rebel against God, he still wants you to renew all things, including your physical wellness and your body (which is created in his image). Paul states, "God was reconciling the world to himself in Christ. . . . And he has committed to us the message of reconciliation. We are therefore Christ's ambassadors, as though God were making his appeal through us" (2 Corinthians 5:19–20). The Psalmist states this more forcefully: "You made [people] ruler over the works of your hands; you put everything under his feet" (Psalm 8:6). Through your body you are God's hands and feet in this world, created to do good.

God wants to renew the world—to reconcile it to him—and he wants you to be his ambassador on earth. Jesus said, "Go into all the world and preach the good news to all creation" (Mark 16:15). Notice that Jesus does not say "to all *people*," but "to all *creation*," every bit of it and of you. The good news of salvation found in Jesus Christ is important not only in your relationship to God and to each other, but also in your relationship to plants, animals, your body, and all of creation. Paul urges "in view of God's mercy, to offer your bodies as living sacrifices, holy and pleasing to God—this is your spiritual act of worship" (Romans 12:1–2).

Spiritual acts of worship are to be physical. When John the Baptist's disciples asked if Jesus was the Messiah, "Jesus replied, 'Go back and report to John what you hear and see: The blind receive sight, the lame walk, those who have leprosy are cured, the deaf hear, the dead are raised and the good news is preached to the poor'" (Matthew 11:4–5). Elsewhere the scripture says, "Be holy, because I, the Lord your God, am holy" (Leviticus 19:2; also Leviticus 11:44, 20:7). Did God intend for holiness to mean only sitting in temple courts, singing and praying? No! Examples of holiness in the Old Testament included honoring parents, taking a break from work, not turning to idols, not eating old meat, caring for the poor (Leviticus 19), not eating swarming things (Leviticus 11), and not hurting or killing children because other things had a higher value than they did (Leviticus 20:1–5). To be spiritual and holy today remains a physical act and includes patterns of sleeping, eating, and exercising.

Your body is so important to God that he refers to it as his temple. "Do you not know that your body is a temple of the Holy Spirit, who is in you, whom you have received from God? You are not your own; you were bought at a price. Therefore honor God with your body" (1 Corinthians 6:19–20). Take some time to read 1 Kings 6–7 for a description of the beauty of the temple—a place where people met God. God invites you to live in such a way that people see and meet him when they are in your physical presence (2 Corinthians 4:10–12).

God's Care for Your Body

God describes his **providence** for the body in Matthew 6:31–33: "Do not worry, saying 'What shall we eat?' or 'What shall we drink?' or 'What shall we wear?'. . . your Heavenly Father knows that you need them. But seek first his kingdom and his righteousness, and all these things will be given to you as well." Psalm 104:14–15 adds "He makes grass grow for the cattle, and plants for man to cultivate—bringing forth food from the earth: wine that gladdens the heart of man, oil to make his face shine, and bread that sustains his heart." God is a providential God. *Providence* is God's loving care and protection, and we can be confident in it.

God's concern for your body is also demonstrated through his many acts of healing (Exodus 15:26; Matthew 4:23, 8:16, 9:35, 10:8, 12:22, 21:14; Luke 22:51): "This healing was the sign of the reconciling and victorious Kingdom which in Him and with Him came to be" (Berkouwer, 1962, p. 230). His concern is also noted in laws to protect life. He commands: "You shall not murder" (Exodus 20:13). Why? "For in the image of God has God made man" (Genesis 9:6). God gives you the knowledge and power generally to keep you well and to make yourself well when you are ill; and from time to time he provides special healing.

God typically does not expect you to live an **ascetic** lifestyle that is austere, harshly self-disciplined, and devoid of material comforts. God "richly supplies us with everything for our enjoyment" (1 Timothy 6:17). Jesus came so that you "may have life, and have it to the full" (John 10:10). John prayed, "Dear friend, I pray that you may enjoy good health and that all may go well with you" (3 John 1:2). Preserving your physical wellness is a part of abundant living, of glorifying God with all that you are, and of redeeming this world for God.

Fulfillment

But what happens to people when they die? The scripture teaches: "Whoever believes in the Son has eternal life" (John 3:36). Notice the word *has.* The text does not say "will get," but "*has* eternal life." Today is a part of eternity. Death is only a passing from this life to the next. **Fulfillment** is God's honoring his promise that all things will be made new and that there will be an eternal "new heaven and a new earth" (Revelation 21:1).

So what does the future hold for people after death? Jesus said, "Do not let your hearts be troubled. Trust in God; trust also in me. In my Father's house are many rooms; if it were not so, I would have told you. I am going there to prepare a place for you. And if I go and prepare a place for you, I will come back and take you to be with me that you also may be where I am" (John 14:1–3).

The Apostles' Creed, written soon after the death of Christ, confesses, "I believe in the resurrection of the body, and life everlasting." The scriptures describe in 1 Corinthians 15:51–58 how people will be resurrected (see the passage on page 10).

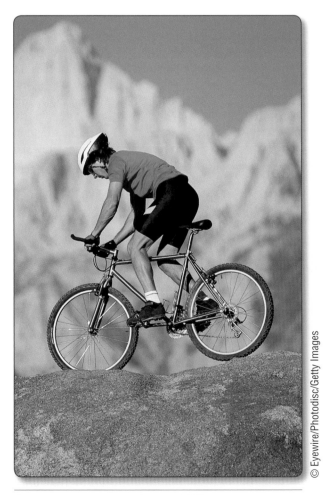

Jesus came so you can have a full life.

© Eyewire/Photodisc/Getty Images

Transition at Death

Listen, I tell you a mystery: We will not all sleep, but we will all be changed—in a flash, in the twinkling of an eye, at the last trumpet. For the trumpet will sound, the dead will be raised imperishable, and we will be changed. For the perishable must clothe itself with the imperishable, and the mortal with immortality. When the perishable has been clothed with the imperishable, and the mortal with immortality, then the saying that is written will come true: "Death has been swallowed up in victory." "Where, O death, is your victory? Where, O death, is your sting?" The sting of death is sin, and the power of sin is the law. But thanks be to God! He gives us the victory through our Lord Jesus Christ. Therefore, my dear brothers, stand firm. Let nothing move you. Always give yourselves fully to the work of the Lord, because you know that your labor in the Lord is not in vain. (1 Corinthians 15:51–58)

Jesus is living proof of the resurrection. After he rose from the dead he met with his disciples, ate with them, and let them touch him. His resurrection was physical (Luke 24:37–42). Jesus' resurrection is important because it assures us of our resurrection (1 Corinthians 15:16–19). Certainly, a living relationship with God gives purpose to our present life, but there is more to life than the present.

What are Christians being physically resurrected to? The scripture teaches that God "will create new heavens and a new earth" (Isaiah 65:17; see also 66:22 and 2 Peter 3:13). Biblical scholars do not know exactly what this new heaven and earth will be like, but the Bible shows glimpses. The writer of Revelation states that it will be a place where God "will wipe away every tear from their eyes. There will be no more death or mourning or crying or pain, for the old order of things has passed away" (Revelation 21:4). This new earth will be creation as it was meant to be—a place where resurrected Christians will be physically whole. Work on living a healthy life now, to be as you were created to be, and continue to experience wellness in eternity.

The Bible looks forward to a time when, in the New Jerusalem (i.e., heaven), "the city streets will be filled with boys and girls playing there" (Zechariah 8:5). We also read how the "infant will play near the hole of the cobra, and the young child put his hand into the viper's nest. They will

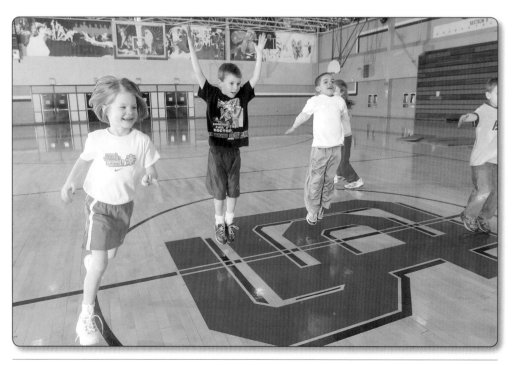

God enjoys active worship.

neither harm nor destroy on all my holy mountain" (Isaiah 11:8–9). The new heaven and new earth will be amazing. If God looks forward to seeing children playing and discovering his universe in heaven, he must certainly enjoy his children doing the same today.

A minister once told me that when he got to the new heaven and new earth he would like to become an astronaut. He was curious what all the planets looked like and wanted to explore them. Because he knew people live forever, he felt he had lots of time. Heaven for this minister was a continuation of what happens on earth. He wanted to glorify God by discovering more of his majesty as displayed in the planets, stars, and galaxies. After hearing the minister's story, I've decided that I want to play a lot more squash when I get to heaven. Can you imagine having forever to understand and develop your running speed or your ability to jump? To kick a ball? To throw? To catch? All this activity will be done simply for enjoyment and to praise the Maker, not to please anyone else. After the resurrection, Christians and God will together find delight in the physical body. Why not experience those delights in your life now, by healing brokenness, enjoying your wellness, and worshipping God actively?

Next Steps

Remember the two students who held different views of how to love God with their body? They wrote these words:

> When I first fell in love with Jesus, I stopped loving my body. I thought that to be spiritual was to abstain from foods; fasting was a great door to a living relationship with God. (Byl, 1999, p. 73)

> God has blessed me with so many things. I think that it would be like an insult to say that I did not love the me that God made. I love my sense of humor, my nose, yes; I love me. (Byl, 1999, p. 73)

How do you value your physical self and your relationships with others? How do you offer your life and body as a spiritual act of worship? Thoughtfully consider whether you agree or disagree with the Biblical arguments in this chapter. Talk about your thoughts with some other people. Ask yourself if you need to make some changes in the way you live so that what you do is consistent with what you say.

Key Terms

ascetic
aesthetician
creation
evolutionist

fall
fulfillment
providence
redemption

Review Questions

For each of these questions, choose at least two relevant scripture passages and explain how they support your position.

1. How does this chapter argue that creation affects who you are physically?

2. How does this chapter argue that the fall affects who you are physically?

3. How does this chapter argue that God's redemptive work affects who you are physically?

4. How does this chapter argue that God's ultimate fulfillment affects who you are physically?

Application Activities

Write your responses to the following questions in your journal:

1. How do you like yourself—all your parts?
2. How do you honor God with all of you, particularly with your physical body?
3. If you're a Christian, how do you hope to please and enjoy God when you pass on to the new heaven and new earth? Are you already doing some of that today?
4. Based on your answers to the previous three questions, do you need to make changes in your views of what it means to be a person and of who you are?

References

Berkouwer, G.C. (1962). *Man: The image of God.* Grand Rapids, MI: Wm. B. Eerdmans.

Byl, J. (1999). Spirituality and wellness: Student perspectives. In J. Byl & T. Visker (Eds.), *Physical education, sports, and wellness: Looking to God as we look at ourselves.* Sioux Center, IA: Dordt College Press.

Marcel, G. (1965). *Being and having.* London: Fontana Library.

Plato. (1945). *The republic of Plato.* Translated by Francis MacDonald Dornford. London: Oxford University Press.

Seerveld, C. (1976). Gallantry as a recreative moment in life. *Vanguard* (October): 19–21.

Socrates. (1954). Phaedo. *The last days of Socrates* (Hugh Tredennick trans.). Baltimore: Penguin.

Suggested Readings

Byl, J., & Visker, T. (Eds.). (1999). *Physical education, sports, and wellness: Looking to God as we look at ourselves.* **Sioux Center, IA: Dordt College Press.**

For readings on various Christian views of the body, read two chapters in this book:

Chapter 1: The Bible and the Body: A Biblical Perspective on Health and Physical Education, by John Cooper.

Chapter 2: The Incarnation and the Flesh, by Bud B. Williams.

Wolters, A. (1988). *Creation regained.* **Grand Rapids: Eerdmans.**

This is a book about using all created things in a way that pleases God.

Suggested Web Sites

www.gospelcom.net

This is a great Web site that helps you explore the Bible.

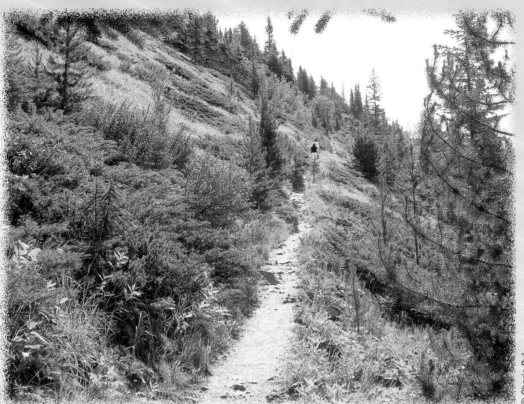

© Charis Byl

God's Purpose and Your Life's Mission

John Byl • Dianne E. Moroz

After reading this chapter, you should be able to do the following:

1 Understand how life choices and practices are affected by external pressures.

2 Understand how to live all areas of your life with your own choices.

3 Write a personal mission statement.

4 Understand how to methodically change certain aspects of your lifestyle through goal setting.

Alice Goes Nowhere in Particular

When people are "on a mission," they know exactly where they're going and are focused on getting there. Alice, in *Alice's Adventures in Wonderland,* exemplifies a lack of focus:

> Alice . . . went on. "Would you tell me, please, which way I ought to go from here?"
>
> "That depends a good deal on where you want to get to," said the Cat.
>
> "I don't much care where—" said Alice.
>
> "Then it doesn't matter which way you go," said the Cat.
>
> "—so long as I get somewhere," Alice added.

"Oh, you're sure to do that," said the Cat, "if you only walk long enough." (Carroll, 1960, p. 62)

Alice will get somewhere, but clearly she is not on a well-considered mission. She may make positive choices and end up in good places, or she may make bad choices and end up in bad places. The story of the race between the hare and the tortoise makes the same point. As slowly as the tortoise goes, all its energies were focused on crossing the finish line. The question for you is this: How do you develop a mission for your life and develop goals to accomplish it? That's the question we address in this chapter.

The process of answering important questions helps you discover the direction you want your life to go. For example, are you influenced by the "bigger is better" ideal? To what extent is materialistic gain important? David Myers (2006), a well-known writer on psychology, argues that as affluence has increased, depression has skyrocketed in North America: More than ever we have big houses and broken homes, high incomes, and low morale.

Robert Putnam (2000) asks in his penetrating book *Bowling Alone* why people watch the TV show "Friends" instead of having friends. Researchers reporting in the *American Sociological Review* made some important observations. Comparing survey responses in 1985 and 2004, the researchers found that the "number of people saying there is no one with whom they discuss important matters nearly tripled" (McPherson, Smith-Lovin, & Brashears, 2006, p. 353); and on average the number of people with whom they discussed important matters decreased from approximately three to two people during those 20 years. To what extent is this true in your life? How does your place of affluence and spiritual hunger affect your wellness choices? Ask yourself, What do I do to contribute to peace or to brokenness for myself, those around me, and the creation I need to care for?

Scripture speaks to Christians who, like Alice, lack focus. Have you ever been tossed around by big waves in the ocean or a lake? The Bible warns its readers against being tossed around like that, moving from one fad to another, but encourages people to lovingly stand firmly with God (Ephesians 4:14–15). The focus of this book is to give you tools so you can respond in a Biblically rooted, scientifically validated manner to Paul's urging in Romans 12:1–2 to "offer our bodies as living sacrifices, holy and pleasing to God." The purpose of this chapter is to help you be more intentional in your walk with God.

As you go through this text discovering how activity, nutrition, and life's rhythms can be used in ways to offer your body to God, we ask you to do two things. First, be committed to deliberately writing and living your own story. Map out your life so that you plan to go to great places more often. In other words, don't travel through life aimlessly as Alice did, and don't let your life be swayed by every wind of teaching. Second, read this text and other literature with **discernment** because you need to "continue to work out your salvation with fear and trembling, for it is God who works in you to will and to act according to his good purpose" (Philippians 2:12–13).

In this chapter you will begin mapping where you wish to travel. We ask you a lot of questions to help you look at the pressures that shape your choices. Next, we help you consider God's mission for people. Finally, you will work through steps that help you articulate your personal life's mission and your physical wellness goals.

God's Mission

I am certain God has a plan for all people. For example, God creates and preserves his creation. He does not decide to go one way one day and a completely different way another day. Scripture confirms that God has a plan for his people; it is a plan of hope and a plan with a future (Jeremiah 29:11). God has a mission. What images do you see in God's mission described by Isaiah in chapter 9 (see the sidebar on this page)? The words I see in God's mission have to do with light, joy, harvest, shattered yokes, wonderful counsel, peace, and eternity. These concepts are part of God's mission, and each leads to wellness.

Part of God's Mission

The people walking in darkness have seen a great light; on those living in the land of the shadow of death, a light has dawned. You have enlarged the nation and increased their joy; they rejoice before you as people rejoice at the harvest, as men rejoice when dividing the plunder. For as in the day of Midian's defeat, you have shattered the yoke that burdens them, the bar across their shoulders, the rod of their oppressor. Every warrior's boot used in battle and every garment rolled in blood will be destined for burning, will be fuel for the fire. For to us a child is born, to us a son is given, and the government will be on his shoulders. And he will be called Wonderful Counselor, Mighty God, Everlasting Father, Prince of Peace. Of the increase of his government and peace there will be no end. He will reign on David's throne and over his kingdom, establishing and upholding it with justice and righteousness from that time on and forever. The zeal of the Lord Almighty will accomplish this. (Isaiah 9:2–7)

Jesus' purpose on earth wasn't just to walk aimlessly around for a while and live with humanity. He had a mission. He did walk among people, but he came for a specific purpose. Luke states that purpose by recording Jesus' words: "The Spirit of the Lord is on me, because he has anointed me to preach good news to the poor. He has sent me to proclaim freedom for the prisoners and recovery of sight for the blind, to release the oppressed, to proclaim the year of the Lord's favor" (Luke 4:18–19). Jesus had a healthy and healing mission that directed everything he did.

Making God's Purposes Your Purposes

If God has a mission, then it is helpful for his people to have a mission. If you want to honor God, then your mission needs to be consistent with God's and empowered by him. A mission needs to be something that resonates deep within you, not something superficial that you devise quickly. Steven Covey argues that "the power of transcendent vision is greater than the power of the scripting deep inside the human personality and subordinates it, submerges it, until the whole personality is reorganized in the accomplishment of that vision" (Covey, Merrill, & Merrill, 1994, p. 106). A Christian's mission needs to be transcendent and thoroughly connected to God's vision.

Here are some questions to help you discover your mission: What are the biggest areas of suffering that touch my life? What can God's mission bring to that suffering? What role can I play as an agent of God? Or think about your part in the Lord's prayer: "Your kingdom come, your will be done on earth as it is in heaven" (Matthew 6:10). What role do you play in helping God's kingdom to come "on earth as it is in heaven"?

Scripture encourages people to "throw off everything that hinders and the sin that so easily entangles, and let us run with perseverance the race marked out for us" (Hebrews 12:1). Do you have that kind of focus in your life?

Do you have the kind of focus that allows you to interpret your daily choices against what is considered cool by culture and what God thinks? Think this through very practically: Are your choices about these things directly determined by Biblical principles—where you shop, the clothes you wear, how or where to vacation, what you drive, the way you spend your time, the way you spend money, where you go out with friends, and

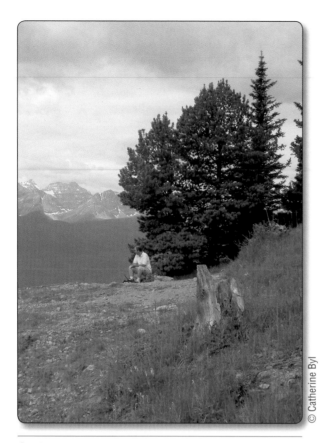

Goal-oriented living.

the way you care for your body? As you read the following verses, think about how they speak to your lifestyle in those areas.

> Do not be afraid, little flock, for your Father has been pleased to give you the kingdom. Sell your possessions and give to the poor. Provide purses for yourselves that will not wear out, a treasure in heaven that will not be exhausted, where no thief comes near and no moth destroys. For where your treasure is, there your heart will be also. (Luke 12:32–34)

> For we are God's workmanship, created in Christ Jesus to do good works, which God prepared in advance for us to do. (Ephesians 2:10)

What do you really treasure? Where is your heart? You are created to do good. Do the things you treasure encourage you to do good? Don't just pay lip service to these questions, because they form the basis of your life and of this textbook. If your heart is focused on acquiring more and more things, you won't take the time to care for your body. If your heart is focused on pleasing God, you will take the appropriate time to care

for your physical health because you are in the image of God.

Pressures That Shape Life's Mission

Many influences shape desires, judgments, and ultimately even goals. Some of these influences contribute to wellness and others take away from wellness. Two major influences are peer pressure and mass media. Think about how those two influences shape your answers to the questions you answered about your daily choices. If you were to create a collage of pictures from magazines or newspapers about what is cool, what would it look like? Do the violence, alcohol, and promiscuity in some corporate advertising, television shows, magazines, movies, and video games affect your sense of what is cool?

Peer Pressure

Peer pressure can both help and hinder health and wellness. When students were asked what the greatest victories in their lives were, one student responded this way: "The biggest victory in my life was to leave my old life behind. I was dating an alcoholic non-Christian. . . . I did things and have been to the wrong places. I knew my life was going downhill. . . . God took me out of that life and brought be back to him" (Byl & Visker, 1999, p. 74). Another student shared how "through a friend at school, God began the process of freeing me from the bondage in my life" (Byl & Visker, 1999, p. 74). Friends had a huge influence in both of these stories. The influence in the first story was negative; in the second story it was positive. You can look at your own life and see how friends kept you accountable to do good or how they took you down unhealthy paths. Ultimately you make the choices to follow or not, but the pressure to follow is often enormous.

Mass Media

Mass media have a powerful influence in shaping values and opinions. Some media products deal with significant issues and encourage people to live whole and healthy lives. However, as William D. Romanowski writes in his penetrating look at popular culture in the United States, "We need to be more aware of self-interest and self-reliance, a lust for power, violent resolutions to problems, materialism stereotypes. . . and even a humanistic outlook. American values? Perhaps, but definitely

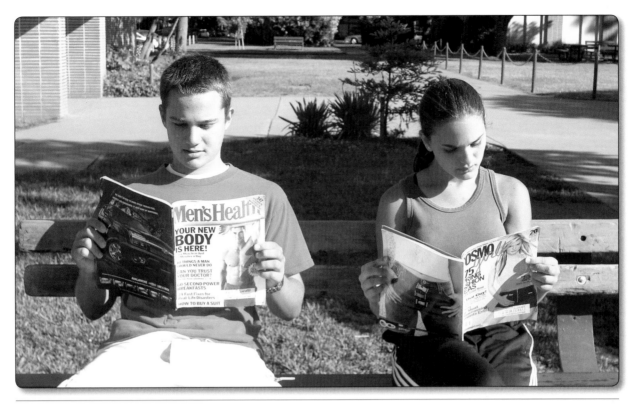

What shapes our view of what's cool?

not Christian values" (Romanowski, 2004, p. 134). How much do media, particularly television and movies, shape the way you think about yourself and the way you live?

Your Mission Statement*

*Adapted from Byl, 2002.

You've learned so far in this chapter what some of God's purposes are, how difficult it is to change, and how important it is to live with direction. Now it's time to clearly develop your personal **mission statement** that will direct your life and wellness. There are seven steps.

Step 1: Begin With a Central Theme

Think of a statement that describes the central theme of your mission. The statement should explain who you are, what you stand for, and why you exist. This statement is the focus of your life. Complete the four steps requested in the sidebar on page 18.

Here's how I've described how I can redeem things for God.

I know my life passions and gifts include sport, health, fun, and games. In the big picture I know God loves the world and is deeply grieved by its brokenness. I want to love the world as he wants me to and to be a healing influence. In the world of health I see and delight in people who actively walk, run, jump, and skip with smiling faces and healthy bodies. I love the feeling of a long, hard cycle on a warm day. I also see and grieve for people who are inactive, sad, and in poor health, and I'm unhappy with my own increased body fat and stressed lifestyle. I am really bothered when people don't get along and there is conflict. I totally enjoy watching and being a part of a group of people who are having fun with each other. I want all of us to be happy. I want to build myself, my city, my country, and this world in a way that pleases God.

Step 2: Write the Mission Statement

Begin to write your mission statement. Be realistic, though. The mission statement should push you to new and positive roads, but roads that are within reach. Don't worry if you can't get it just right at first or if you ramble a bit. Getting something down on paper gets you closer to a more specific mission statement. Here's an example of how I might

Making a Godly Difference

1. Answer this question: How does God want me to make a difference in this world?

   a. Think about the following passage. What does it say about God's leading? "Many are the plans in a man's heart, but it is the Lord's purpose that prevails" (Proverbs 19:21).

   b. Jesus is referred to as a shepherd. It is interesting that shepherds do not stand still but are usually on the move. What does it mean for your mission statement that you follow a dynamic God?

2. Find stillness to discern God's will. Listen to God's voice from your past; through scripture, prayer, the needs of others, your gifts and talents, your dreams, your broken places, and your imagination; and by picturing new possibilities (Sine & Sine, 2002). How does each of these situations help you focus your life?

3. Determine some practical ways to make a difference and list some scripture passages that speak to you about your purpose.

   a. Think about the following two passages. What do they say about God's love for people and the world?

      i. "For God was pleased to have all his fullness dwell in him, and through him to reconcile to himself all things, whether things on earth or things in heaven, by making peace through his blood, shed on the cross" (Colossians 1:19–20).

      ii. "For God so loved the world that he gave his one and only Son" (John 3:16).

   b. Listen to Bruce Cockburn's song "Laughter." He sings about people wanting to make a New Jerusalem and end up with New York. Look at the full lyrics at http://cockburnproject. net/songs&music/l.html. To what extent are our priorities laughable?

4. Find and describe positive ways you can redeem things for God. It's important that the mission statement be about you, not about someone else. Remain true to yourself.

---

start: "Because I'm in God's image, I want to joyfully and gently walk with God in my whole being and to share that encouraging walk with my wife, children, students, readers, and others, especially the marginalized and oppressed. I want to live more simply so that others may simply live. Stated briefly, I want to walk joyfully and gently with God and to encourage others to do the same."

Step 3: Refine Your Mission Statement

Refine the statement by keeping it short and simple so you can live by it in your daily life, because "faith by itself, if it is not accompanied by action, is dead" (James 2:17). The statement now should be one sentence long—two at the most. Maybe a Bible verse works as the framework for your mission statement. A colleague chose Jesus' words found in Mark 12:30: "Love the Lord your God with all your heart and with all your soul and with all your mind and with all your strength." I simplified my previous statement this way: "I want to joyfully and gently walk with myself, God, and others."

Step 4: Build Excitement and Inspire Action

Choose words for your mission statement that build excitement and inspire action. Your mission statement should not be a weight that hangs around your neck, but rather wings that help you soar. Use inspiring and strong verbs and adverbs to communicate your mission. My own statement began weakly with "I want to." I realized I needed to make a decision to *do* it, so I deleted "I want to." The terms *joyfully* and *gently* sounded too wimpy, so I changed them to *joy* and *gentleness*. *Running* is a more inspiring word than *walking,* but I don't want to run through life. I did change *walking* to *walk.* Finally, "myself, God, and others" was still a mouthful, so I changed that phrase to *companions,* but then decided to assume my walking included us all! My statement at this point: "Walk with joy and gentleness."

Step 5: Get Others' Input on Your Mission Statement

Talk to other people about their mission in life. Live prayerfully and listen to the Lord's leading. Study scripture to give you focus for your mission. Close friends that love you will remind you when you're focused too much or too little on yourself and your own well-being. They will also remind you when you are trying to be someone you're not or when your actions are consistent with your abilities and interests. Listen to your heart and what others say as you decide on the best route to take.

Step 6: Make Your Mission Statement Visible

Post copies of your mission statement in your room, put a copy in your wallet, or write it on your calendar. A bathroom mirror is both a personal and somewhat public space to remind you of your mission statement every day. The screen saver on your computer is another good place to put it.

Step 7: Revisit and Evaluate Your Mission Statement

Evaluation is key to the success of any plan. You need to evaluate your mission statement from time to time and adjust it as necessary, either to improve the statement or to reflect more closely on your life's purpose. Be open to the leading of the Holy Spirit. Don't go through life as Alice did, blown around by every fad (Ephesians 4:14), but focus on God (Hebrews 12:2) and run his race (Hebrews 12:1; see also 1 Corinthians 9:24 and Galatians 5:7).

Goals for the Journey

We've given you tools to establish a mission statement. Someone once told me that a mission statement is the place God calls us, the place where our deep gladness and the world's deep sadness meet. We've also explained how God created people good, in his image, and that the body is his temple. Throughout the rest of this book we explore more thoroughly the concept of the body as God's temple, the holy of holies, and how the Holy Spirit provides power to heal. An old gospel song says, "Little by little He is changing me." Your developing a mission statement and setting and achieving health and wellness goals are part of the process of sanctification and of becoming more like God.

You will refine your mission statement and develop more specific Christian paths to your health and wellness goals through the rest of this book. It's sometimes necessary to make permanent changes to your lifestyle or attitudes to achieve the goals you put in your mission statement. For example, you may wish to quit smoking, start an exercise program, or become more sociable. Changes that are permanent usually begin slowly. Psychological perceptions change first, sometimes years before actual behavior change is made. Prochaska, Norcross, and DiClemente (1994) developed the Transtheoretical Model of Stages of

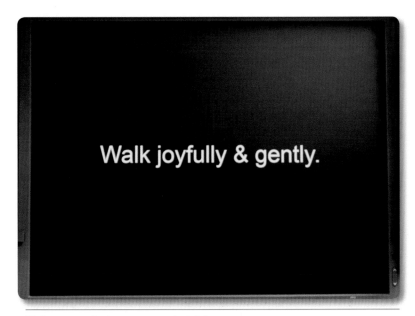

Make your mission statement visible.

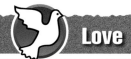

Love, as a fruit of the spirit, is that unconditional commitment to care for others in a way that only God truly can, and it brings healing. I remember having felt betrayed by someone. It was three years before I could go to that person so we could put the incident and negative feelings behind us. I couldn't do it earlier, despite the fact that I felt a constant pit in my stomach. It took three years of hiking before I took the final step on top of that mountain of forgiveness. I was ready for that last step. In some ways it was the same as the thousand steps before it. But when I made it, I knew it was done. The scenery on top was beautiful. The pit in my stomach was gone. The bounce in my step was restored. I learned again that we ought to forgive as God forgave us and that love binds people together and builds people up (Colossians 3:12–14; 1 Corinthians 8:1).

Love of self, God, others, and creation ought in some way be part of a mission statement; it certainly needs to be at the core of how to live. Love goes beyond the moment and is meant for a lifetime. If it is meant for a lifetime, build it into part of your journey plans, part of your mission. Let's take a more detailed look at a biblical view of love.

Think about God's love. The heavenly Father is so committed to caring for the entire world "that He gave His one and only Son" so that we could gain eternal life (John 3:16). Jesus died because he loved everyone, even though he knew dying on a cross would bring excruciating pain. In his high priestly prayer, Jesus begged people to obey God's commands and, through obedience, remain in God's love. Jesus ended the prayer by saying, "Love each other as I have loved you. Greater love has no one than this, that he lay down his life for his friends" (John 15:12–13). Jesus showed that kind of love.

God gives the ability to love, like Jesus, through the power of the Holy Spirit (Romans 5:5; 2 Thessalonians 2:13). Jesus said the greatest thing you can do with this gift is to "Love the Lord your God with all your heart and with all your soul and with all your mind.

. . [and] your neighbor as yourself" (Matthew 22:37–39). This gift is at the very core of living; it guides all actions and is the distinguishing mark of Christians (Schaeffer, 1970). This love makes you able to care for those who are easy to love as well as for your enemies (Matthew 22:39; Matthew 5:43). Think of the healing there could be within people, between them and others, and even among nations if people would love that way.

Because of the emphasis given to love in 1 Corinthians 13, it's no surprise that love is listed as the first fruit of the spirit. We know there will be no more "mourning or crying or pain" (Revelation 21:4) in the new world (heaven), because it is filled with love. God also gives the opportunity in the present world to experience the healing power of love. "With love the power of the future age already breaks into the present form of the world" (Kittel, 1972, 1:51).

People can experience great healing when they know that God loves them and that Jesus died on the cross to pay for their sin; when they can give and receive forgiveness, a caring handshake, and a hug; when their love finds expression in living obediently with God; and when they are committed to lovingly building others up and they get the same in return. Does your mission include letting God's love flow through you? Can people see that in your actions?

Love: Do you love yourself from the top of your head to the bottom of your feet? In a few sentences, describe what you love about yourself and what you have trouble loving about yourself.

_____

_____

_____

_____

_____

_____

Table 2.1   Transtheoretical Model of Stages of Change

Precontemplation	You are unaware of any need for behavior change. Others may suggest a change in your behavior but you are unconvinced.
Contemplation	You recognize that a behaviour change would be beneficial and decide to implement a change sometime in the distant future. No firm commitment is made, but you make a sort of "mental note" that it would be a good idea sometime.
Preparation	You prepare to make a change. For example, if your goal is fitness, you may gather information about benefits of exercise, cycle with friends once in a while, and buy running shoes. You prepare yourself mentally and physically before committing to a regular exercise program.
Action	A plan is established and implemented. This is the most difficult stage and relapse into the previous stage occurs frequently. This stage is only complete once the plan of action has been maintained for six months.
Maintenance	The behavior is maintained for about five years but requires compliance with a specific program. Assessment of the plan and of compliance to it are still necessary and there is a threat of relapse to previous stages.
Termination	The termination stage is defined when the behavior has been consistently maintained for five years. The behavior is now incorporated into your life and has become part of your identity. For example, you see yourself as a fit individual who runs four times per week. You no longer require self-monitoring, and relapse is unlikely (although possible) even when the program faces obstacles.

Adapted from Prochaska, Norcross, and DiClement, 1994.

Change (shown in table 2.1), which identifies six interactive stages in developing and implementing any behavior.

After you have committed to making a change in your behavior, you need to develop a plan of action. It is most valuable to write this plan in a booklet so it's concrete and provides a document for future reference.

Designing a Plan for a Permanent Lifestyle Change

The following seven steps will help you design a personal program that takes needs, goals, and lifestyle into consideration. It's essential to make very concrete decisions to reach your life mission; these concrete decisions are what we refer to as **goals.**

Step 1: State the Goal

Simply but specifically state your objective. Sometimes goals concern lifestyle changes, like developing healthier sleep patterns. Sometimes they concern a specific event, like qualifying for the Boston Marathon. Both require changing regular habits and behaviors. Be sure to write the goals down so that you are accountable—if only on paper. It's easy to be careless and to forget goals or to thoughtlessly change goals that are difficult to achieve if you don't write them down. It's also

important to develop a positive mindset about life's challenges, and setting positive goals is one way of doing that. Instead of writing something like, "I will stop eating fast foods," you might write, "I will eat balanced and healthy meals three times a day, seven days a week."

Also, be detailed and precise, using operationally defined standards of success. Specificity helps to focus effort and provides a way to measure success. Goals have four components:

1. doing
2. something
3. specifically
4. under special conditions.

Let's go back to the eating goal, for example. You can see how it uses the four components:

1. I will eat (doing)
2. meals, (something)
3. balanced and nutritious, (specifically)
4. three times a day, seven days a week (under special conditions).

It's easier to measure success toward a goal when it's written precisely.

Also, be realistic in establishing goals. Don't set them so high that they are unattainable or so low that they are achieved without effort. Set goals for your own situation; don't try to set goals by other people's standards and programs because each situation is unique. Setting a goal that is "your very best effort" is also unrealistic. Balancing one set of goals with all the other personal and vocational goals you have will require making trade-offs. Make your goals realistic in the overall context of your situation. For example, instead of saying, "I will do my best to get a good night's sleep," it is better to say, "I will get a good night of sleep, from 11 p.m. to 7 a.m., five times a week."

Step 2: Assess Your Present Lifestyle

It is very helpful to have a full understanding of the present behaviors and attitudes surrounding your goal before you develop a plan of action. Write down for a month things in your life that affect your goal. If you record activity for just a short time, like for a day, you may get a skewed impression of your daily activity or habits. Include specific information about the behavior you are planning to change. For example, if you plan to quit smoking, record specific information about where, when, and why you smoke. You may even include information about who you're with and how you feel when you smoke. A chart is an effective way to record information and assess it at a glance (see table 2.2).

Step 3: Design a Specific Plan

Use the assessment information to form a specific plan. The more specific the plan, the more

likely you are to achieve your goal. The plan must include measurable, concrete actions that specify what you will do, when, where, and how. For example, a plan like this is too general: "I plan to run two hours per week." It may leave you slapping your forehead on Saturday night when you realize you are out of time and didn't run. In contrast, this is much more specific: "I plan to run around my neighborhood for 30 minutes, from 7:00 to 7:30 p.m., Monday, Wednesday, Friday, and Saturday." When 7:30 p.m. on Monday rolls around, you can immediately judge if you implemented your plan. If you didn't, you can act accordingly by rescheduling the run or by examining the difficulty and readjusting. When you write a specific plan it's easy to monitor your compliance and moderate it when necessary.

Sometimes the drive toward immediate gratification forces people to set unrealistic goals. Break your goal down into small, achievable, measurable steps. For example, if your plan to quit smoking "cold turkey" doesn't work and you keep sneaking a cigarette during the day, your plan isn't effective for you. Redesign it by breaking your goal into small, easily achievable steps. Use the behavior assessment (step 2) to rank the cigarettes you smoke in a day from favorite to least favorite. Maybe you could start by eliminating the least favorite cigarettes once every three days. If at some point you find that a cigarette you've eliminated leaves you craving to the point where you give in and smoke, then select another cigarette to

Table 2.2 Daily Activity and Barriers to Daily Activity

	Monday	Tuesday	Wednesday	Thursday	Friday	Saturday	Sunday
Week 1	Squash at noon	Take a break	Golfed	Need to finish assignments	Tired at the end of the week	Need to do homework and shopping	Walked for 1 hour
Week 2	Meeting at noon	Scheduled break	Golfed	Need to get to work. I got behind because of golfing	Tired at the end of the week	Need to do homework and shopping	Rained. Stayed inside
Week 3	Squash at noon	Rained. Stayed inside	Too wet to golf	Went for a walk with a friend	Too cold to go outside	Too cold to go outside	Too cold to go outside
Week 4	Meeting at noon	Too tired to walk	Partners could not golf	Played a game of squash	Tired at the end of the week	Need to do homework and shopping	Walked for 1 hour

eliminate. You may even continue without eliminating anymore until you feel you're ready. At this point, you will already have eliminated some cigarettes, which is progress. Time is on your side when you're trying to change behaviors or attitudes. Because you're working on a *permanent* lifestyle change, the several months it may take to implement a plan is inconsequential if, ultimately, the behavior change improves health and wellness in the long run.

Step 4: Predict Obstacles

You will inevitably encounter obstacles as you work through your program, including illness, exams, financial problems, stress, and unforeseen demands on your time. Predict some of the most likely obstacles and decide ahead of time how you'll overcome them. This serves two purposes. First, it prepares you for predictable obstacles. Second, it gives you the confidence that your plan can survive other obstacles when they come up. It helps you to realize that the plan is a work in progress, requiring modification as you advance through it. Table 2.3 shows you how six barriers can affect a plan and how you can overcome them.

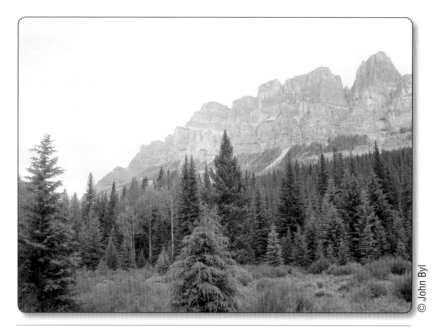

© John Byl

Too big an obstacle to overcome at once.

Implementing a Permanent Lifestyle Change

So far, you've developed a mission statement and analyzed and assessed your past. Steps 5 through 7 support gradual but significant life changes. Do not underestimate the difficulty in making changes. I have sometimes asked my students to move from their normal seat to sit on the opposite side of the classroom. They say that they feel strange, weird, or odd. Students don't like staying in their new seats, and they go back to their "normal" seating position the next time they come to class. If something as inconsequential as taking a different seat is challenging, how much more challenging it is to make a significant lifestyle change.

Step 5: Plan Intervention Strategies

Making a permanent lifestyle change requires a great deal of time, motivation, and commitment.

A relapse is a real risk, especially in the beginning. Design strategies to keep you compliant and to act as motivators. Here are six strategies that can help:

1. **Write a behavior contract.** This contract is a written promise to another person that you will complete activities according to plan. It usually includes a statement of the goal and the steps you will take to achieve it. Sign it and ask the person to whom you are accountable to sign it as a witness.

2. **Use positive and negative reinforcements.** It is important to reinforce success. Let's say, for example, that you follow your plan of cycling for three weeks. You could reward yourself by buying some cycling shorts or bike tools (positive reinforcement). On the other hand, if you didn't follow your plan, you might stay in on a Friday night instead of going out with friends (negative reinforcement).

3. **Get a support group.** This group may be a formal group, such as those for substance abusers, or just a group of friends you exercise with. The purpose of such a group is to keep you focused on your goals and to provide you with structure in your plan. It also indicates your commitment publicly and provides accountability to your goal.

Table 2.3 Barriers To Change

Barrier	Effect	Solution
Procrastination	Rather than jump into action, you may believe that your life is busy and the timing for a new action will be better later.	Ask yourself why you are waiting. Assess the relative importance of the behavior so you can assign appropriate priority.
Success or failure attitude	Belief that if you don't complete the plan as outlined, you have failed and change is impossible.	Recognize that there is no failure. If you cannot comply with your plan, the plan must be revised, not abandoned.
Education	People tend to feel invincible unless they understand the significance of lifestyle to disease prevention and wellness.	Devastating diseases such as cancer and heart disease are processes that begin as early as adolescence. The earlier you begin a healthy lifestyle, the greater the quality and quantity of life.
Instant gratification	Society has a mindset toward instant gratification. People would rather purchase quick-fix gimmicks to improve wellness than work hard.	Wellness is a lifelong process that is achieved and maintained only through frequent evaluation and action. Gratification is long-term, not instant.
Nonindividualized plan	You may turn to programs for diet or exercise that are not consistent with your lifestyle and enjoyment. A program that emphasizes activities you dislike has little value.	Individualize a plan so that you have selected the kinds of specific activities that are suited to your lifestyle and preferences.
Short-term change vs. permanent change	People tend to assume an intense exercise program until goals such as weight loss are met, only to return to unhealthy eating and the sedentary lifestyle that contributed to their desire to change in the first place.	Recognize that you are trying to make a permanent change in order to maintain a level of health and wellness. Slow, progressive change is permanent. Temporary change doesn't even guarantee temporary wellness, as in the case of restrictive diets that are unhealthy.

4. **Use behavior shaping.** In **behavior shaping,** you modify situations or behavior to be consistent with your plan. If you have planned to study and the dorm is too noisy, for example, move to the library each night for your study time. Shape your behavior by making certain areas study areas and other areas play areas, rather than confusing the two. Many students now try to combine homework with text messaging. Try to separate the two. Concentrate on homework, then do messaging at another time. **Behavior substitution** is when you replace an undesirable behavior with a healthy one. For example, instead of having coffee and a cigarette after dinner, take a brisk walk. Remember, though: Don't replace a bad habit with another bad habit. A common example of doing this is smoking to avoid overeating.

5. **Keep a journal or diary.** If developing a healthy sleep habit is your goal, for example, write a brief journal entry about how many hours of sleep you got, your bedtime and rising time, and your habits before sleep. With busy school demands, some students find they no longer spend enough time in devotions and prayer. If that's you, you could use a journal to formalize time spent with God by writing about prayers, devotions, or thoughts about scripture.

6. **Graph or chart your results.** Use a chart or graph to record compliance with your plan. For example, you could chart servings of each food group consumed per day, miles run, or hours of sleep. Charts and graphs

provide information about progress and compliance with your plan at a glance. Take pride in your accomplishments.

Step 6: Assess Compliance With the Plan

Use the charts, graphs, or records you developed in step 5 to assess whether you are compliant with your program. These may be the same as those used as intervention strategies. If you find you are not compliant with the plan, then reassess the plan. You may wish to go back to the previous step in your plan until you are ready to progress further. Never give up! If you don't manage to achieve your goal, your plan probably isn't appropriate for you at this time. Adjust your plan so that there are small, *easily achievable* steps that lead to the final goal. The only failure is abandoning the plan. If you continue to be noncompliant with plans despite several adjustments, you may not be truly committed to the plan. Go back to your mission statement and make sure that the goal you have set is one that you value in your walk with God. If the goal is set for poor reasons, it simply may not be valuable enough to you to justify the work and dedication it takes to make a permanent change.

Step 7: Assess Progress of Your Overall Goal

In addition to assessing compliance with your plan, evaluate whether your plan is helping you achieve your overall goal. For example, you may be compliant with your weight-loss program by reducing dairy and meat servings, but if you are substituting those foods with high-calorie items, the plan may not be reducing your body mass. Measure body mass (weight) periodically to ensure you are meeting your goals, but do it infrequently to avoid discouragement. For example, if your goal is weight loss, measure body weight weekly, rather than daily, because the common, day-to-day fluctuations can be disheartening and tempt you to abandon your program.

Next Steps

Paul offers a partial mission statement in his letter to the Romans when he urges Christians to "offer your bodies as living sacrifices, holy and pleasing to God—this is your spiritual act of worship. Do not conform any longer to the pattern of this world, but be transformed by the renewing of your mind. Then you will be able to test and approve what God's will is—his good, pleasing and perfect will" (Romans 12:1–2). You should now have a mission that will help you become very deliberate in running your race, running your life, and running in a deliberate way in conformity with God's will. The rest of this book will help you develop specific goals for your health and wellness based on your mission statement.

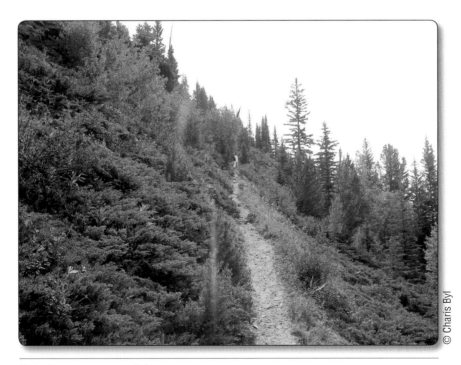

Enjoying a step toward the top.

© Charis Byl

Key Terms

behavior shaping

behavior substitution

discernment

goals

love

mission statement

Review Questions

1. List several external factors that shape the way you think and live.

2. What are some characteristics of God's mission?

3. What are the seven steps in preparing an effective mission statement?

4. What are the seven steps in preparing goals to make permanent lifestyle changes?

Application Activities

1. Reflect on the song "Today." You can find the lyrics for the song at www.briandoerksen. com/music/pdf/charts/today.pdf. Do you agree with the lyrics of the song? Does your life agree with the lyrics of the song? Is your whole life, including your physical health and wellness, focused on serving and living for God?

2. Imagine that you are 70 years old and are reflecting on the most important things that happened in your life as you write a letter to someone you love. What are those things?

3. Write your personal mission statement (in subsequent chapters we will revisit the mission statement and ask you to set specific goals for the different areas of your life, such as muscular strength, nutrition, and sleep):

    a. Write your central theme.

        1. How does God want you to make a difference in this world?

        2. Take quiet time to discern your answer.

        3. List three scripture passages and explain how they help you, in practical ways, to understand your place in this world.

        4. What are some positive steps you can take in redeeming some things for God?

    b. Write a realistic mission statement that is simple to remember and inspires you to action.

    c. What are some steps you can take or are taking to remind yourself of your mission statement?

4. Use the following examples (and the text provided in this chapter) to help you develop your goals and make a plan to achieve them. Pick one area of your life that you're concerned about, and develop a goal and a plan for achieving it.

    a. **Step 1:** State the goal. Write your overall goal in a sentence or two. You might write something like this: I would like to improve cardiorespiratory fitness by running 45 minutes three times per week.

    b. **Step 2:** Assess your present lifestyle. This is an example: I hate cycling, but I've tried running and liked that, so I will plan to run. I know that I get breathless quickly when I run, so I will start by walking and will work up to running. I work long days on Tuesdays and Thursdays and am too tired to work out on those days. Friday nights I play volleyball with my church group. I've checked my heart rate during the games, and I found that it doesn't fall within my target training heart rate zone of 142 to 175 beats per minute, so I can't really use that to improve fitness. I don't enjoy exercising in the morning and would prefer to work out in the evening. I think I would prefer to do my exercise alone, at least at first. Maybe later, when I'm more comfortable with my fitness, I'd enjoy exercising with others.

c. **Step 3:** Design a specific plan. Develop realistic, specific, measurable, and concrete steps. Goals should start out small to ensure some degree of success, and then proceed in easily achievable increments. Take a look at this example:

- *Week 1.* I will walk around the streets in my neighborhood on Monday, Wednesday, and Friday, from 7:00 p.m. to 7:30 p.m.

- *Week 2.* I will run for half of each exercise session.

- *Week 3.* I will try to run for the whole 30 minutes of each exercise session. I'll try to run fast enough to keep my heart rate within my target heart rate zone.

- *Weeks 4, 5, and 6.* I will increase the duration of those runs by 5 minutes a week, to a total of 45 minutes.

- *Weeks 7 and 8.* I will run the same route, but in only 40 minutes, to increase intensity. I'll check my heart rate to be sure I'm working harder.

- *Week 9.* I will run the same route in 37 minutes to increase intensity.

- *Week 10.* I will add more streets (or distance) to my route so that it takes 45 minutes to complete. I'll work at the midrange of my target heart rate zone.

Therefore, within only 10 weeks I will meet my goal of running 45 minutes on three days a week and within my target heart rate zone.

d. **Step 4:** Predict obstacles. Predict at least two obstacles and describe how you would overcome them. These are common obstacles and some ideas for overcoming them:

- *Illness:* If I am well enough to walk, I'll walk for only 20 minutes to 30 minutes so I stay in the routine of exercising. If I'm too sick to walk, I will plan to get back to my program as soon as I start attending classes again. I will reduce my intensity and duration when I resume exercising, and I'll build each day until I'm back to the place I was in my program before I got sick.

- *Exams:* During exam preparation I sleep less, have less time, and am more stressed. That is a time I should exercise to reduce stress and improve energy levels, but I always feel that I don't have enough time. To overcome this, I will exercise during exam weeks. I will decrease the duration if necessary, but I'll maintain the intensity. I can use the time exercising to review memory work for exams or to plan out an essay.

e. **Step 5:** Plan intervention strategies. Formulate intervention strategies to help you stick with your plan. For example, you might include some of these strategies:

- I will keep a logbook of my running to record the days, times, and how long I run and to record my heart rate.

- I will buy running clothes if I'm compliant for three weeks.

- If I miss a day of running, I'll make it up on Saturday.

- I will write a contract and ask a friend to ask me regularly about my training.

f. **Step 6:** Assess compliance with the plan. Evaluate how well you're sticking to your plan. Here's one way to do that: Weekly, I will examine my running log to see if I've been compliant with my plan. If I find I haven't been following my plan, I'll adjust it accordingly. For example, if I see that I can't seem to get out on Wednesdays, I'll plan to switch my exercise to another day or time. If the intensity is too hard and I'm walking more than running during my exercise sessions, I'll alter the plan so that the intensity is easier. I could try alternating five minutes of walking with five minutes of running and slowly increasing my running time until running for longer stretches is more comfortable.

g. **Step 7:** Assess progress of your overall goal. Here's an example of how you can plan to measure your progress: To determine whether I am achieving cardiorespiratory fitness, I'll take my resting heart rate every three weeks to see if it is decreasing. Before training and at the end of six weeks, I will use one of the walking or running tests to estimate aerobic power ($\dot{V}O_2$max) and see if it has improved.

5. **Love:** How do your actions show you know and experience the love of God, the love of and from others, and the love of yourself?

References

Byl, J. (2002). *Intramural recreation.* Champaign, IL: Human Kinetics.

Byl, J., & Visker, T. (Eds.) (1999). *Spirituality and wellness: Looking to God as we look at ourselves.* Sioux Center, IA: Dordt College Press.

Carroll, L. (1960). *Alice's adventures in Wonderland.* New York: New American Library.

Covey, S., Merrill, R., & Merrill, R. (1994). *First things first.* New York: Simon & Schuster.

Kittel, G. (Ed.). (1972). *Theological dictionary of the New Testament* (vol. 1). Grand Rapids, MI: Eerdmans.

McPherson, M., Smith-Lovin, L., & Brashears, M.E. (2006). Social isolation in America: Changes in core discussion networks over two decades. *American Sociological Review, 71*(3): 353-375.

Myers, D.G. (2006). Wealth, well-being, and the new American dream. Retrieved April 2, 2007, from www.davidmyers.org/Brix?pageID=49.

Prochaska, J.O., Norcross, J.C., & DiClemente, C.C. (1994). *Changing for good.* New York: Morrow.

Putnam, R.D. (2000). *Bowling alone: The collapse and revival of the American community.* New York: Simon & Schuster.

Romanowski, W.D. (2004). *Eyes wide open: Looking for God in popular culture.* Grand Rapids, MI: Brazos Press.

Schaeffer, F. (1970). *The mark of the Christian.* Downers Grove, IL: InterVarsity Press.

Sine, C., & Sine, T. (2002). *Living on purpose.* Grand Rapids, MI: Baker Book House.

Suggested Readings

Sine, C., & Sine, T. (2002). *Living on purpose.* **Grand Rapids, MI: Baker Book House.**

This is a helpful book that further promotes the ideas of living with a mission or purpose.

Romanowski, W.D. (2004). *Eyes wide open: Looking for God in popular culture.* **Grand Rapids, MI: Brazos Press.**

This is an award-winning and widely read book that discourages mindless acquiescence or blanket condemnation of popular culture but encourages thoughtful engagement and critique of mass media.

Suggested Web Sites

www.franklincovey.com/missionbuilder

The Franklin Covey organization shares an exercise to help you to create your own personal mission statement. Taking the time to seriously consider your answers to the questions will help you to define your values, principles, and priorities in your life.

www.leadertoleader.org/knowledgecenter/sat/mission.html

Leader to Leader Institution provides a great article with clearly laid-out steps and hints for success in developing your own mission statement.

www.mapnp.org/library/plan_dec/str_plan/stmnts.htm

The Free Management Library: Basics of Developing Mission, Vision and Values Statements site will help you develop your mission statement.

www.toolkit.cch.com/text/P03_4001.asp

The Business Owner's Toolkit: Developing a Mission Statement site will help you develop your mission statement.

www.things.org/music/bruce_cockburn/lyrics/further_adventures_of.html#laughter

Things.org is a personal Web site that also contains the lyrics of a number of Bruce Cockburn's songs.

PART

II

Accepting and Caring for Your Body

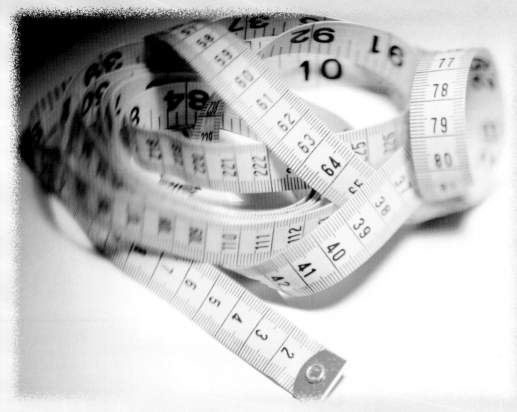

© Eyewire/Photodisc/Getty Images

Examining Body Image and Eating Disorders in Women and Men

Heather Strong • John Byl

After reading this chapter, you should be able to do the following:

1 Understand body image concerns and eating disorders in men and women.

2 Understand what causes eating disorders and how they can affect men and women.

3 Understand how eating disorders are treated, and gain information about seeking help and resources for those struggling with an eating disorder.

4 Understand how people distort a biblical view of themselves.

5 Appreciate God's love for people and their bodies.

You read in chapter 1 that you were created in God's image. You explored the biblical idea that God created people "very good"—short and tall, small framed and large framed. Some people agree with God's evaluation of them as "very good;" others skew this evaluation and view themselves as "very bad."

My Struggles With Eating

My name is Heather. During high school I was a straight-A student. I was on the school swim team, was in the concert band, and went to the youth group at our church. I always had a boyfriend and lots of other friends, but I never felt pretty or thin.

By the end of high school, life at home with my parents was tense, so I was looking forward to going away to a university, living on my own, and being able to be more independent. I was confident I would do well because I was a good student. However, my first year was a disaster. I failed most of my courses. I spent way too much time on my social life, and I gained a couple of extra pounds. I didn't realize at the time that I was struggling with low self-esteem and depression. I felt pretty awful about myself, and I thought that I would never go back to school. I decided I needed to take back some control of my life to prove to everyone that I was not stupid, even though I had convinced myself that I was.

I began exercising, and over the course of several months I began slowly taking control of my emotional state. I became very disciplined and structured with what I ate and how much I exercised. I dropped weight like crazy and got so many positive comments about my body that I felt I was finally doing something right. But there was a problem. I felt worse and worse inside every day. I couldn't hold myself together. I was sleeping more during the day and losing a lot of my motivation for life. Something inside me was eating me alive.

Eventually I decided to give the university a second try. I was still convinced I was ugly, stupid, and no good to society, but I thought that maybe it was time for a fresh start. My unhealthy, regimented eating and exercise patterns persisted, but I was adamant that I was merely an advocate for healthy living. I was really very unhealthy, though. I was teaching aerobics five times a week and was also hitting the weight room for cardio and weights every day. It looked to others like I was in control of my life, but for some reason I felt out of control. Something inside me was hurting and I could not figure it out.

When I woke up each morning I would be thinking about the food I would consume that day. Planning my meals and daily activity became a higher priority for me than planning when to study or do my class assignments. Even as I sat in class and shivered because I had very little body fat, all I could think about was what I would have for lunch. At that point my weight was pretty low. I hadn't had a menstrual period for almost eight months, and I wasn't feeding my body for the amount of activity I was doing. I was cold all the time, and I found it hard to concentrate in classes because my body was so tired.

Something inside me wasn't right. I hurt. I would sleep all the time during the day because I had trouble sleeping at night. I'd miss a lot of classes, and I couldn't understand my life. This was supposed to be my second chance, but I couldn't even get out of bed in the mornings.

One night I told my resident assistant (RA) that I needed to talk to her. I told her I couldn't stop thinking about food and that I found it difficult to get out of bed each morning. I had lost enthusiasm for life, and I was disappointed in myself for my lack of effort at school. My RA told me she thought I had an eating disorder. I laughed at that, because I was still eating. I was just really health conscious. I thought that to have an eating disorder you couldn't eat at all. Was I wrong! I searched the Internet for information about eating disorders. I could hardly believe my eyes. Every symptom I was experiencing was right there on the screen,

(continued)

(continued)

under the heading *anorexia nervosa*. I was shocked. I didn't know what to do.

It took me a few days to take in all I had just learned. I thought the next logical step was to talk to my parents and make an appointment with my family doctor. My doctor told me that I had obsessive–compulsive behaviors, depression, and an eating disorder. She described the many physical complications of an eating disorder, which scared me. I didn't know until then that people could die from an eating disorder, or ruin their chances of bearing children.

Soon after my visit with the doctor I began therapy with a psychologist. I started taking medicine, and I felt, finally, that I was improving. I learned from uncovering my pain that I was a perfectionist at heart. I had such high expectations for myself that I felt worthless when I failed during my first year at the university. I discovered I had placed my self-worth in things that were not dependable, like appearances, grades, boyfriends, and other friends. I discovered I wanted to go back to a time in life where things seemed "perfect," because I felt very guilty for failing in my first year at the university and for rebelling against my parents when I was a teenager.

Slowly (and let me emphasize the word slowly here) I began to learn to accept small things about myself. I struggled to confront the hurt and the pain I felt and to learn to love the person I was, inside and out. The most incredible thing I learned during my struggle was that, as a Christian, I could depend on God for support and unconditional love. I knew he wouldn't change and would love me no matter what. He had already proven to me that he was taking care of me; I just needed to accept it.

I learned to replace the terrible lies in my head—that I was worth nothing and that I was stupid—with the truth: God loves me. That was the spiritual awakening of my life. I had never needed to depend on God so much, or to face evil so directly. What it all came down to was acceptance.

I knew that God accepted me no matter what, but I had a hard time accepting me because I was not perfect according to society's standards, and society's standards had become my own. Unfortunately, I could never measure up to them.

I realized that society tells people a lot about how they need to live, what to wear, what to buy, and how to love. It became obvious to me that society's values rest on a superficial foundation. None of those values provided me with happiness. I could have the skinniest body in the world and still be unhappy. I could have a boyfriend, a closet full of clothes, and tons of friends. I could go to parties, I could have sex, but I could still be hurting inside.

A materialistic culture implies that those superficial things are fulfilling and bring happiness. People can rent that kind of happiness for a short period, but it won't fulfill their deepest needs. Those needs can be met in only one way, and that is through a relationship with Christ. He is the constant in a world filled with so many lies and inconsistencies.

Introduction to Dieting, Weight Preoccupation, and Body Image

Western culture has seen a dramatic increase in the number of young women and men suffering from **weight preoccupation** in the last 25 years (Cash, Winstead, & Janda, 1986; Braun et al., 1999; Polivy & Herman, 2002). The term *weight preoccupation* encompasses a wide variety of topics in this chapter, including dieting, body image, eating disorders, and other obsession tendencies with weight and food.

Women and men alike are experiencing more dissatisfaction with their bodies than ever before. Americans spend an estimated $50 billion a year on diets or diet-related products (Berg, 1997; Fraser, 1997). Researchers have reported that half of American women are on a diet (Cash & Henry, 1995; Smolak, 1996), 25 percent of men are on a diet (Smolak, 1996), 91 percent of women on a college campus had dieted (Kurth et al., 1995), and half

My name is Tom. I was pretty shy as a kid, and I didn't get involved in too many sports. My family always went to church together. My parents split up when I was young, and I always felt really bad about it. I was very angry at God for breaking up my family.

I was also teased a lot for being skinny when I was young, which made me feel really bad about myself. I didn't want to join any school sports teams, and I ended up avoiding friends and keeping to myself. By the time I reached high school I had grown taller and had a few friends, but I was still pretty skinny. I still didn't have a girlfriend. I remember like it was yesterday the day I decided I would try working out to get bigger. I thought I would definitely get a girlfriend if I worked out and had bigger muscles.

I started working out at our local gym and spent almost three hours a day, seven days a week in the gym. I was after that V-shaped upper body that supposedly drives girls crazy. I was pretty tired and sore at the end of most workouts, but I believed the "no pain, no gain" philosophy. When I looked at muscle magazines in stores, I used to envy the guys in them and wish I had a chest as developed as those weightlifters. I remember thinking I would do almost anything to get that kind of shape.

I started working out with a few new friends at the gym, and we became such good friends that we rarely spent time with anyone else. When I wasn't working out, I was thinking about which exercises I was going to focus on at my next workout. The weight training was making significant changes to my body, but I still wanted to get bigger. Some of the guys suggested I take a variety of nutritional supplements to develop my muscles even more. I tried about five kinds of supplements and kept working out. The changes became even more pronounced. By the end of a year I had tried every program out there. I was taking protein supplements and fat burners and trying the latest training programs to get the edge I needed to get bigger. I was getting amazing results.

I was in amazing shape by the time I went to the university. I had put on about 26 pounds (12 kilograms) of pure muscle. It was great, because for the first time in my life I was the cool guy. I felt other guys looked up to me, and lots of girls wanted to hang out with me.

I kept working out like crazy and taking crazy amounts of supplements until they just stopped working. I then decided I needed to look for a new product that would take me to the next level. One day (I remember this day so clearly) I overheard some of the guys in the changing room talking about some steroids they were using. I decided immediately that steroids were the key to getting the best results and helping me get even bigger.

I had heard in my health class about some negative side effects of steroids, but I ignored the information. I thought, If these guys are taking them and getting huge, and the steroids aren't hurting them, why shouldn't I take them? So I tried the steroids. After about a month, my upper body was awesome. I had huge arms and pecs, and my abs looked like the abs on the guys in the muscle magazines.

Soon after I started to take the steroids I began to have massive mood swings and got really bad acne. I was freaking out on my girlfriend and family all the time and was completely obsessed with working out. It didn't matter if it was Christmas day or my girlfriend's birthday—my first priority was to hit the gym for three hours to get my workout in.

Everyone close to me started to worry about me. They told me that my obsession with my body was taking over my life. My girlfriend dumped me because she said I wasn't making her a priority. My mom and sister wanted me to see a doctor because they knew I was on some kind of drug. I knew I needed to change some parts of my life, but I didn't want to give up my new body and the rush I felt from working out. I felt trapped.

My mom and sister love me and are always there for me, but my dad has not been a big part of my life. I remember wishing from a really young age that he was closer to me, but I never

(continued)

(continued)

knew how to make that happen. When I was working out so much I didn't have time or make time for my relationship with God. I don't think God was happy with my taking drugs, but I felt amazing and I was getting so many great comments about my body.

Since my family confronted me I have seen my family doctor and a couple of therapists. I don't take the steroids anymore, but I am still in the gym two to three hours a day. At this point it is hard for me to accept the changes I need to make, because I might have to change my body. I know I have a long way to go, but I am learning new things every day. I'm much better than I was a year ago. I've started reading my Bible again and discovering new insights into what God wants me to believe about my body and who I am. This has been the hardest experience of my life, but I know it is worth it.

of 9- and 10-year-old girls claim they would feel better if they lost some weight (Gustafson-Larson & Terry, 1992).

According to the National Eating Disorder Information Centre (NEDIC), **dieting** is a futile, often harmful, process of restrictive eating, usually caused by body dissatisfaction, preoccupation with thinness, and the false belief that self-worth is dependent on body size (Bear, 2000). Unlike healthy eating, which involves eating well-balanced snacks and meals from a variety of foods that give you energy to carry out your daily activities, dieting creates a physiologically driven preoccupation with food and can have devastating results, such as eating disorders, weight-loss surgery, and even suicide. Most people who diet do not understand or believe that healthy people come in all shapes and sizes (Bear, 2000).

The effects of dieting include a preoccupation with food, irritability, depression, and social withdrawal, as well as lowered self-esteem when diets fail (Bear, 2000). In cultures where acceptance and self-esteem are often linked to physical appearance, people seem increasingly to be judged by the way they look. Information everywhere tells people they can shape their lives by shaping their appearance. This reshaping usually starts with dieting and maybe a new exercise program. People who feel unloved, ineffective, out of control, or unlovable may try to take back control by controlling their physical appearance (Bear, 2000).

Bear, 2000; information adapted by permission from NEDIC: National Eating Disorder Information Centre, www.nedic.ca/knowthefacts/dietingfacts.shtml.

When people continually diet, they are attempting to alter their body or their physical appearance. They are also trying to alter the image they have of their body. **Body image** is a multidimensional construct and is defined as the picture you hold in your mind of your own body (Thompson et al., 1999). Body image encompasses four dimensions: cognitive, affective, perceptual, and behavioral. The cognitive component is what you *think* about your body (e.g., I think my hips are too wide). The affective component includes the *feelings* that you have about your body (e.g., I feel ugly or fat). The perceptual component includes how you *visualize* your body in your mind (e.g., I see myself as having wide hips). Finally, the behavioral component includes the things you *do* to try to change your body (e.g., exercising, dieting).

The concept of body image can be measured along a continuum. Some people may like the way their bodies look. Those positive thoughts have been linked to increased self-esteem, self-confidence, success in business, and success with interpersonal relationships (Thompson et

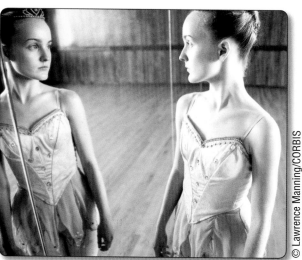

© Lawrence Manning/CORBIS

Our body image includes how we think, feel, and act toward our body shape and size.

Facts About Dieting and Weight Loss

- Anyone who goes on a restrictive diet will initially lose weight.

- An initial weight loss often makes people feel better about themselves because they experience a sense of control.

- Over time bodies on a restrictive diet become malnourished and begin to conserve energy, and dieters reach a weight plateau.

- The restrictive behavior makes people feel deprived of a normal existence and robs them of enjoyable meal times. Being malnourished brings mood swings and a desire to binge.

- The diet fails and dieters begin to regain the lost weight.

- The initial problems are still there and are compounded by feelings of failure from not losing enough weight or not keeping it off.

- Dieting can lead to lowered self-esteem, which is bad for health.

- Dieting can lead to increased weight through lowered basal metabolic rate.

- Dieting can lead to **bingeing** and eating disorders.

- Dieting can cause depression, mood swings, reduced sexual interest, and impaired concentration and judgment. Severe weight loss can bring heart disorders, elevated cholesterol, anemia, higher risk of infertility, hair loss, loss of muscle tissue, changes in liver function, and other complications.

- The risk of dying from heart disease is 70 percent higher in those with fluctuating weights than in those whose weight remains stable, regardless of initial weight, blood pressure, smoking habits, cholesterol level, or level of physical activity.

Adapted, by permission, from Bear, 2000, *Dieting and weight loss facts and fiction* (Toronto, Canada: National Eating Disorder). www.nedic.ca/knowthefacts/dietingfacts.shtml.

al., 1999). On the other hand, a negative body image may induce negative thoughts, which may lead to depression, excessive dieting and exercise, steroid abuse, and substance abuse (Thompson et al., 1999).

Every person has a body image—an idea of what he looks like. However, a distorted body image or an unhealthy emphasis on physical appearance may influence how a person thinks and feels about his body and what he decides to do about it.

Causes of Body Image Concerns for Men and Women

Many factors, such as puberty, peer pressure, family influences, the media, and gender differences, contribute to the development of body image concerns for both men and women. You'll learn about puberty and peer pressure briefly in this section, and you'll read about family, media, and gender differences when we talk about the

causes of eating disorders later in the chapter.

North American Cultural Ideals

For women in North America the currently accepted ideal body shape is a thin and lean physique that is very difficult for most women to attain (Garner, 1997; Wiseman et al., 1992). The cultural pressure to be thin may be transmitted to young women directly through parents or peers encouraging their daughter or friend to diet, or indirectly, through advertisements promoting the beauty and weight-loss industry. Research has found that perceived pressure for girls to be thin (either direct or indirect) was related to increases in their body dissatisfaction (Field et al., 2001; Stice & Whitenton, 2002).

Cultural pressures to attain an ideal physique also contribute to body dissatisfaction for men. However, the culturally accepted ideal physique for men is the V-shaped, lean and muscular body type (Olivardia, 2002). As for women, these cultural ideals are transmitted to men both directly

and indirectly. One study found that young men who perceived their parents and their friends were pressuring them to be a certain body size and shape were more likely to engage in strategies to alter their body size and shape (i.e., working out, taking supplements) (McCabe & Ricciardelli, 2003). In addition, another study (Field et al., 2001) found that parents who were concerned about their personal weight gain influenced the weight concerns that their adolescent boys experienced. Research has also found that young boys who claimed to try and alter their body size and shape to look like same-sex models and actors in the media were more likely to develop weight concerns and engage in negative dieting behaviors (Field et al., 2001).

Value Placed on Cultural Ideals

The body dissatisfaction and weight concerns that many young men and women experience can come from how much they internalize the culturally accepted ideals for their gender. For example, one study found that adolescent males who scored high on drive for *muscularity* (high value placed on looking muscular) were more likely to have low self-esteem and to engage in strategies to increase their body size (McCreary & Sasse, 2000; Smolak, Levine, & Thompson, 2001). Other research has found that male adolescent football players were more dissatisfied with their body shape and size than adolescent cross country runners. This finding was potentially due to the cross country runner's body shapes more closely resembling the culturally accepted ideal male body type (Parks & Read, 1997).

Similar results have also been found for women. For example, one research study found that women who placed greater value on the culturally accepted ideal body type experienced increases in body dissatisfaction (Stice & Bearman, 2001). Other research has found that adolescent and college-aged women who placed a greater emphasis and commitment on appearance ideals experienced greater body dissatisfaction (Cusumano & Thompson, 2000; Jones, Vigfusdottir, & Lee, 2004; Smolak et al., 2001; Stice et al., 1994).

Puberty

Puberty is one major contributor to the onset of body image concerns. Young adolescents' bodies start to develop and change during puberty in ways they are unfamiliar with. Many young girls feel threatened by the natural weight gain and the physiological changes that come during this period of development. As they try to control their feelings about their new bodies, young women may develop negative thoughts about their bodies. These young women may end up in a cycle that begins with dieting to control their new images and that leads to further dissatisfaction with the body (DeCastro & Goldstein, 1995).

Peer Pressure

Peer pressure is another contributing factor to body image and the subsequent need for societal approval. Appearances are intensely important for adolescents, especially adolescent girls. Young girls will often compare themselves to others and talk about their bodies, how much they weigh, and what they do to stay in shape. Research has demonstrated that adolescents who are a part of friendship groups have similar levels of body image concerns, are similarly preoccupied with thinness, and are on the same diet (Levine & Smolak, 2002).

We cover some of the other factors that play a role in the development of a negative body image later in this chapter. Some of them are avoidable and some aren't. However, some ideas and attitudes may need to be challenged to prevent or recover from a negative body image and to cultivate a healthy body image.

How to Deal With a Negative Body Image

There are several ways to overcome the negative thoughts and feelings a person may feel about the body. Martha Homme's (1999) Turning Point workbook, *Seeing Yourself in God's Image*, is an excellent resource with a step-by-step guide to help people overcome a negative body image and eating disorders. The workbook outlines several useful steps, and they are summarized in the paragraphs that follow.

First, as hard as it may be, it is necessary to "accept that bodies come in a variety of shapes and sizes" (Homme, 1999, p. 33). It is also important to not let your physical body or physical appearances define who you are (2 Corinthians 5:1). Society's definition of beauty is very narrow and constantly changing, but God's definition of beauty never changes. For example, 1 Peter 3:3–4 states, "Your beauty should not come from outward adornment, such as braided hair and the wearing of gold jewelry and fine clothes. Instead it should be that of your inner self, the unfading beauty of a gentle and quiet spirit, which is of great worth in God's sight."

People are often their own worst critics, and pick apart every aspect of themselves or others to make themselves feel better. Instead of picking yourself apart, try looking for the qualities about your appearance you do like, and focus on those. After all, all people were created unique by an amazing designer.

Second, recognize that your weight and shape will change at various times in your life. You probably experienced this when you went through puberty and perhaps during your first year at a university. There are other times when bodies commonly change: when women have children; when starting a new, sedentary desk job; and during aging. You can do things now to make those transition periods easier, such as eating a balanced, healthy diet; getting enough sleep; and figuring out what kind of exercise you like to do and doing it. Research has shown that a moderate amount of exercise is one of the most effective (and enjoyable) ways you can improve your body image (Hausenblas & Fallon, 2006; Martin & Lichtenberger, 2002).

Third, explore who you are and who you were created to be, and take a good look at your "internal self—emotionally, spiritually, and as a growing human being" (Homme, 1999, p. 33). When you do, you will decide where you want to spend your energy. Do you want to focus on pursuing the "perfect image," or on your spiritual growth and personal needs?

Finally, remember that attractiveness comes from within, and thinness or beauty does not always equal happiness. Feeling positive about yourself will affect how others view you, and you will always benefit from treating your body with the respect it deserves. Maybe respecting your body means taking up a new exercise program, spending some time in nature learning to relax, and rediscovering your relationship with God. Maybe it means hanging out with a different group of friends who respect you for who you are and not for what you look like. On a final note, make sure you "are aware of your own weight prejudice and what you think about people who don't fit the 'perfect image'" (Homme, 1999, p. 33), and realize that maybe your definition of beauty needs to change.

What Are Eating Disorders?

A person who feels very dissatisfied or unhappy with his or her body may take extreme measures to try to alter body size and shape. According to the American Psychiatric Association (2000), one of the key defining features of people with eating disorders is extreme dissatisfaction with body image.

Eating disorders are classified into three categories according to the *Diagnostic and Statistical Manual of Mental Disorders* (American Psychological Association, 2004): anorexia nervosa (AN), bulimia nervosa (BN), and eating disorders not otherwise specified (EDNOS). Binge eating disorder is classified under the EDNOS category. Other identified disorders that are related to eating disorders include anorexia athletica, female athlete triad syndrome, body dysmorphic disorder, and muscle dysmorphia. We explore each of these disorders further in the following sections.

Anorexia Nervosa

Anorexia nervosa is characterized by a person's refusal to maintain a minimal body weight, an intense fear of gaining weight, significant disturbance in the perception of the shape or size of his or her body, and, in females, no menstrual period (American Psychological Association, 2004). These are signs of anorexia:

- Dramatic weight loss
- Preoccupation with weight, food, calories, fat content, and dieting
- A refusal to eat certain foods

Individuals with anorexia will frequently comment about feeling "fat" or overweight, despite their weight loss, and experience anxiety about gaining weight or being "fat." Often these individuals will develop food and exercise rituals, find consistent excuses to avoid mealtimes or situations involving food, and withdraw from spending time with friends or participating in usual activities.

Bulimia Nervosa

Bulimia nervosa is characterized by repeated episodes of **bingeing** (eating an abnormally large amount of food at one time) followed by behaviors designed to eliminate food from the body (e.g., self-induced vomiting, fasting, or excessive exercise) (American Psychological Association, 2004). The warning signs of bulimia include evidence of binge eating, like disappearance of large amounts of food in short periods of time, as well as **purging** behaviors. People with bulimia will frequently make trips to the bathroom after meals, use laxatives or diuretics, or follow excessively rigid exercise regimens. People with bulimia are usually at a normal weight but, like those with anorexia, are obsessed with food and weight. Individuals with bulimia may also have cuts or calluses on the back of the hands and knuckles (caused by teeth scraping the hand during purging), discolored teeth, and damage to the esophagus.

Eating Disorders Not Otherwise Specified

Eating disorders not otherwise specified (EDNOS) is a broad category that encompasses binge eating disorder (BED), compulsive exercising (e.g., anorexia athletica, female athlete triad syndrome), and other symptoms of **disordered eating** behaviors that cannot be classified into either the anorexic or bulimic categories (American Psychological Association, 2004).

Binge Eating Disorder

Binge eating disorder is a recognized eating disorder that is characterized by frequent episodes of uncontrolled overeating (American Psychological Association, 2004). Researchers are just beginning to understand the causes and health consequences of binge eating disorder. These are warning signs of binge eating disorder:

- Eating frequently in large quantities
- Feeling out of control and unable to stop eating
- Feeling uncomfortably full after eating
- Feeling guilty and ashamed of binge eating

Individuals with binge eating disorder may also have failed at every diet they have tried; will most likely be overweight or obese; and typically eat for comfort, to avoid uncomfortable situations, and to deal with their feelings.

Anorexia Athletica

Anorexia athletica (compulsive exercising) is not a recognized diagnosis in the same way that anorexia, bulimia, and binge eating disorder are. However, many people who are preoccupied with food and weight exercise compulsively to control weight in a misguided attempt to gain a sense of power, control, and self-respect. There are several warning signs of anorexia athletica, including exercising beyond the requirements

for good health and having a fanatical obsession about weight and diet. People may also miss work or school and may withdraw from relationships to exercise. Those who struggle with compulsive exercising typically focus on exercise as a challenge and forget that physical activity can be fun. They define their self-worth in terms of their performance and are rarely satisfied with athletic achievements.

Information obtained from NEDIC, 1997.

Female Athlete Triad Syndrome

Female athlete triad syndrome is the combination of three interrelated conditions associated with athletic training: disordered eating, amenorrhea, and osteoporosis (Hobart & Smucker, 2000). It's hard to quantify the prevalence of the female athlete triad. Studies have reported disordered eating behavior in 15 to 62 percent of female college athletes. **Amenorrhea** is the absence of menses in two cases: when menarche (a female's first menstrual cycle) doesn't occur between the ages of 14 and 16 and normal sex characteristics don't develop, or when menstrual bleeding is absent for six months in a woman with regular menses. **Osteoporosis** is the loss of bone mineral density and the inadequate formation of bone, which can lead to increased bone fragility and risk of fracture. Premature osteoporosis puts athletes at risk for stress fractures as well as more devastating fractures of the hip or vertebral column. Lost bone density may be irreplaceable (Hobart & Smucker, 2000).

Warning signs of the female athlete triad syndrome are often seen in those who pursue sports and activities that emphasize low body weight and a lean physique, such as gymnastics, figure skating, ballet, long-distance running, diving, or swimming. Often individuals will feel fatigued, experience anemia (low iron), have electrolyte abnormalities, and have an increased number of fractures.

Body Dysmorphic Disorder

Body dysmorphic disorder (BDD), according to the American Psychiatric Association (American Psychiatric Association, 2000), is not an eating disorder per se, but has many characteristics or defining features related to eating disorders. BDD is defined as a preoccupation with an imagined or slight defect in appearance that causes clinically significant distress or impairment in functioning and is not better accounted for by another

Some of us are more vulnerable to getting an eating disorder because of our life circumstances. Following is a list of risk factors for various eating disorders. By reducing alterable risks, we reduce the likelihood of getting an eating disorder.

Risk Factors Contributing to Anorexia Nervosa

- Mean age of onset for anorexia is 17 years; peak years are between 13 and 18
- Perfectionist behavior
- Low self-esteem
- Preoccupation with becoming thin
- Dieting practices such as skipping meals
- Too much concern for body weight and appearance
- Participation in certain types of sports that emphasize maintaining a certain ideal body weight and shape, like figure skating, ballet, wrestling, rowing, running, or gymnastics

Risk Factors Contributing to Bulimia Nervosa

- Age of onset is usually adolescence to young adult
- Persons who have engaged in repeated dieting practices without success
- A strong need for social approval
- Conflict avoidance
- Inability to identify and assert personal needs
- Inadequate coping skills
- High distress levels
- Heavy emphasis on thinness in the family
- Lack of clear identities for two or more people in the family and difficulty distinguishing between their needs, feelings, opinions, and priorities

- Overprotective parents
- Lack of conflict resolution in the family

Risk Factors Contributing to Binge Eating Disorder

- Harmful dieting practices, such as avoiding eating during the day, restricting food intake to a low amount, and avoiding certain types of foods
- Low self-esteem
- Problems with assertiveness
- Mood swings
- Perfectionism
- All-or-nothing thinking
- High anxiety levels

Risk Factors Contributing to Female Athlete Triad

- Dieting at an early age
- Unsupervised dieting
- Restrictive diets and weight cycling in association with energy deprivation
- Reaching menarche before being emotionally prepared (weight associated with maturity decreases effective performance)
- Choosing a sport to participate in before the body matures or choosing a sport incompatible with body type

Risk Factors Contributing to Muscle Dysmorphia

- Being overweight as a child
- Early history of dieting practices
- Participation in a sport that demands thinness
- Having a job or profession that demands thinness (e.g., models, actors)

Adapted, by permission, from J.J. Robert-McComb, 2000, *Eating disorders in women and children: Prevention, stress, management, and treatment* (New York: Taylor and Francis).

disorder (e.g., anorexia nervosa). The following are signs and symptoms of body dysmorphic disorder:

- Frequently comparing one's appearance with others
- Repeatedly checking the appearance of the specific body part in mirrors
- Wearing excessive clothing, makeup, or hats to camouflage the perceived flaw

People with BDD often will have elaborate grooming rituals, excessively research the perceived defective body part, and usually seek surgery or other medical treatment despite medical recommendations against it. Those with BDD will avoid social situations in which the perceived flaw might be noticed and will feel anxious and self-conscious around others because of the imagined defect. People with severe body dysmorphic disorder may also drop out of school, quit their jobs, or avoid leaving their homes (American Psychological Association, 2000; Mayo Clinic, 2006).

Muscle Dysmorphia

Muscle dsymorphia is a preoccupation with the idea that one's body is insufficiently lean or muscular (Pope et al., 2005). Muscle dysmorphia is believed to be a subtype of the more general body dysmorphic disorder (Pope et al., 2005); and so, although it shares similar characteristics with eating disorders, it isn't a classified eating disorder. Generally speaking, muscle dysmorphia affects men more than women. Men with muscle dysmorphia view themselves as being "too small," when in reality they look normal or even incredibly muscular. As a result, they may neglect important social or occupational activities because of the way they believe they look or because they need to attend to a meticulous diet and regimented workout schedule (Kanayama et al., in press; Phillips, O'Sullivan, & Pope, 1997; Pope, Phillips, & Olivardia, 2000). A warning sign of muscle dysmorphia is a constant need for affirmation of physical appearance attributes (because the person with muscle dysmorphia sees himself as small). Individuals with muscle dysmorphia may be engaged in compulsive weightlifting or bodybuilding routines and may take steroids or other muscle-building drugs to get bigger.

How Prevalent Are Eating Disorders?

In the United States, conservative estimates suggest that *as many as 10 million females and 1 million males* are struggling with eating disorders such as anorexia or bulimia, and as many as *25 million more* people are struggling with binge eating disorder (Hoek & vanHoeken, 2003; Shisslak, Crago, & Estes, 1995). Although women are at higher risk for developing body image concerns and eating disorders, research has demonstrated that men are slowly becoming more and more at risk (Furnham & Calnan, 1998; Neumark-Sztainer et al., 1999).

Eating disorders affect both men and women, but they typically are expressed in very different ways. For example, women (like Heather) often strive to be thinner than they are, whereas men (like Tom) often want to be bigger, or at least more muscular and lean. But the most alarming statistic about eating disorders is that "according to the National Institute of Mental Health, one in ten anorexia cases ends in death from starvation, suicide, or medical complications like heart attack or kidney failure" (American Psychological Association, 2004).

Eating disorders typically develop during adolescence; the typical age of onset is between 13 and 18 years (Robert-McComb, 2001). On average, adolescents begin developing eating disorders at around age 17, which is usually their last year in high school or first year at a college or university.

Each year eating disorders increase on college campuses across North America. Many students are excited about leaving home, gaining independence, and pursuing their goals. However, students who feel the responsibility placed on them is too great may turn to inappropriate methods to hide or control their feelings of inadequacy or fear. It is often in these situations that college students develop eating disorders to help them cope with their new feelings. An article about college students and eating disorders reported the following:

When the pressures get to be too much, some [college students] may turn to anorexia as a way to block out what is happening. If they spend all of their time focusing on calories and their weight, they don't have time to think about anything else. Others might believe that the only way they will be accepted is if they are thin. If someone is having trouble in their courses and not getting the marks they wanted or expected to, they might also develop anorexia. As the scale goes down they start to believe that losing weight is the one thing they can succeed at and it makes them feel like they are accomplishing something. Others may turn to bulimia or compulsive eating as a way to deal with the pressures and all of the emotions they are experiencing. If they are feeling lonely, sad, tired, overwhelmed, depressed, scared, or confused, food can bring them a false sense of security and can also comfort them. When they binge, all their negative feelings disappear. When the bulimics purge, whether by vomiting or by compulsive exercising, it may help them to feel like they are releasing all of those feelings. Because food can only temporarily help deal with negative feelings, the binge–purge cycle will continue. (Thompson, 2000)

You might think that Christians are not affected by eating disorders. Research has indicated that assumption is false. A study by Cook and Reiley (1991) examined the prevalence of eating concerns among four college campuses for both women and men. Two campuses held an explicitly Christian world view and two campuses were nonsectarian. The results of the study suggested that eating concerns were more prevalent among women than among men and that there were no significant differences in eating concerns between the campuses with a Christian world view and the nonsectarian campuses.

Furthermore, the study reported that women on all four college campuses experienced significant eating and dieting concerns consistent with eating disordered behaviors, such as an intense fear of fat, persistent dieting, tendencies to overeat, abuse of laxatives, and purging. In the study, 52 percent of the women and 40 percent of the men identified themselves as overweight.

The study concluded that eating concerns are not exclusively a non-Christian or nonsectarian issue. The results from this study imply that eating concerns and eating disorders are prevalent on different kinds of college campuses, even those that espouse a Christian world view.

What Causes Eating Disorders?

Eating disorders are complex psychological disorders, and their onset may be influenced by sociocultural factors, psychological factors, biological influences, and conflict within the family (Epling & Pierce, 1988; Garfinkel, Garner, & Goldbloom, 1987; Sundgot-Borgen, 1994). Health professionals work to understand where eating disorders come from so they can attempt to explore and eventually change the way people think, feel, and act toward the body and their physical appearances.

Sociocultural Influences

Society in general has a very narrow definition of beauty, placing more emphasis on the outer appearance of an individual than on inner strengths and qualities. North American cultural pressures glorify thinness and place value on obtaining the "perfect" body. In general, people in these cultures think only men and women who are thin and shapely are beautiful (EDAP, 2000).

Western culture has confused and betrayed women and men by establishing unattainable ideals. Dick Moriarty, a professor at the University of Windsor, identified five sociocultural influences of eating disorders:

1. Cultural overemphasis on thinness
2. Glorification of youth
3. Changing roles of women and men in society
4. A fitness-crazed culture
5. Presence of the media

Moriarty & Moriarty, 1993.

Three examples of media that flood people with messages about the advantages of being thin are TV, movies, and magazines. Impressionable readers and viewers are told—sometimes directly and sometimes indirectly, by the choice of actors and models—that goodness, success, power, approval, popularity, admiration, intelligence, friends, and romantic relationships all require physical beauty in general, and thinness in particular. The corollary is also promoted: People who are not thin and beautiful are failures. They're portrayed as bad, morally lax, weak, out of control, stupid, laughable, lonely, disapproved of, and rejected.

Research has demonstrated that, for women, reading teen or fashion magazines and watch-

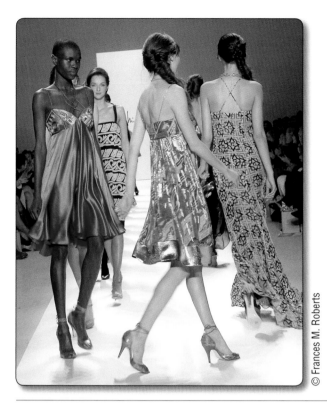

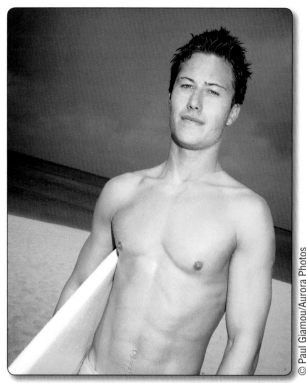

© Frances M. Roberts

© Paul Giamou/Aurora Photos

The North American ideal body shapes for women and men.

ing television are related to body dissatisfaction (Jones, Vigfusdottir, & Lee, 2004; Tiggemann, 2003), the perception of being overweight (McCreary & Sadava, 1999), and eating disorder symptoms (Harrison, 1997, 2000a, 2000b; Thomsen, Weber, & Brown, 2002). It's not hard to see where the dissatisfaction may come from. An article in *Health* magazine, for example, reviewed the body shapes and sizes of television network females and found that 32 percent of the women were underweight and only 3 percent were larger than the average girl. The numbers are actually flipped in the U.S. population at large. Fewer than 5 percent of the female viewers are underweight and about 25 percent are heavier than the average female (ANRED, 1999a).

Mary Pipher, author of *Reviving Ophelia*, states, "Girls compare their own bodies to our cultural ideals. They started developing eating disorders when our culture developed a standard of beauty that they couldn't obtain by being healthy. When unnatural thinness became the object of health, girls did unnatural things to be thin" (Pipher, 1994, p. 184).

A summary article of 25 experimental research studies provided more empirical data. The article reported that women in the United States had greater body dissatisfaction after they were exposed to media images of thin people than when they saw images of people who were average or plus sized. Women who were particularly vulnerable to body dissatisfaction after exposure to these media images included women who were younger than 19 years and who placed a lot of value on being thin (Groesz, Levine, & Murnen, 2002).

For men, research has shown that there are more exercise and weightlifting advertisements in North American male magazines or more emphasis on the muscular male than there were several years earlier (Anderson & Di Domenico, 1992). Studies have shown that North American media are using more male models that are bare chested, muscular, and have a marked V shape than they used in previous years (Parks & Read, 1997; Pope et al., 2001; Law & Labre, 2002). Studies have demonstrated that males are affected by visual signals. For that reason, media play a significant role in shaping the views of men (Barthel, 1992).

One media study, for example, created two 30-minute video segments. One contained appearance-loaded advertisements, and the other contained advertisements not related to appearance. The study revealed that "males exposed to appearance-related advertisements had significantly higher reports of muscle dissatisfaction.... Males who viewed the body image ideal advertisements became significantly more depressed following exposure" (Agliata & Tantleff-Dunn, 2004, p. 16).

A more recent study concluded that "participants who viewed advertisements with male models showed an increase in body dissatisfaction, while those who viewed only products demonstrated no change in body dissatisfaction. The importance of this finding is that the body dissatisfaction experienced through exposure to idealized images of men in the media is only the beginning of possible outcomes such as anabolic steroid use, eating disorders, and muscle dysmorphia" (Baird & Grieve, 2006, p. 115).

Magazines and other media vehicles focus more on muscularity, beauty, and thinness than on fitness or health. The advertising industry is a major culprit (Toro et al., 2005; Labre, 2005). Altered photographs in magazine advertisements enhance both the female and male physique, setting an unrealistic standard for body shapes most people can't attain.

On a positive note, the Dove skin care company launched the Campaign for Real Beauty in September 2004 to change the way women think about beauty. Dove uses real women in several commercials, posters, and magazine ads that challenge women's perceptions of beauty. We hope this campaign will serve as an effective, positive media tool to get women and men around the world to reframe their definitions of what real beauty is.

Psychological Influences

Many psychological and interpersonal factors contribute to the development of an eating disorder:

- Distorted body image (discussed previously)
- Depression
- Perfectionism
- Low self-esteem

Hinrichsen, Waller, & van Gerko, 2004; Lunner et al., 2000; Robert-McComb, 2001.

Thirty to fifty percent of people with anorexia also have mood disorders such as depression or anxiety (Mullen, 1999). Research has demonstrated that eating disorders may cause depression. For example, Stice and colleagues (2000) found that symptoms of eating disorders and dietary restraint predicted subsequent depression in initially non-depressed individuals.

Because eating disorders and mood disorders both involve chemical imbalances in the brain, the mind is altered and becomes flooded with negative thoughts. Antidepressants can correct the imbalance and restore normal mood and thought control. When the obsessive thoughts stop, the person can relax about weight and begin to resume normal eating patterns. People with these disorders need to receive counseling because the disorders come with significant emotional issues (Mullen, 1999).

According to Dr. Mullen, emotions are one of the three fundamental, God-given building blocks of human personality. The others are intelligence and will. People must be healthy in all three areas to function at the level of wholeness God intends. If a person's emotions are damaged, he or she will not function at the level that intelligence or will would permit. Success in life depends on emotional health, whether or not people acknowledge that (Mullen, 1999).

Perfectionism also contributes to the development of an eating disorder (Hasse & Clopton, 2001). Perfectionists develop exceptionally high and unrealistic standards for themselves on achievement tasks. You can see some characteristics of a perfectionist in Heather's story at the beginning of the chapter. Her world collapsed when she failed in her first year at the university. She didn't reveal, though, that even though she was struggling with depression at the time, she failed only two courses. Even in her depression her standards were so high for herself that she couldn't fathom why she could let herself fail. Failing, to Heather, meant her world was falling apart and she was worthless.

Related to perfectionism is the persistence of obsessive thoughts and tendencies. People with eating disorders commonly spend a substantial amount of their time obsessing about food: what they will eat, how much they weigh, and how they can change their shape (Gleaves et al., 2000; Polivy & Herman, 2002). A research study in the United States demonstrated that approximately 74 percent of individuals with eating disorders spent more than three hours a day thinking obsessively about food and weight. As many as 42 percent spent more than eight hours a day thinking about food, weight, and shape. Sixty-two percent of those with eating disorders in the study had fewer than three hours a day entirely free of such obsessive thoughts, and 37 percent had no free hours at all (Sunday, Halmi, & Einhorn, 1995).

These statistics are alarming and demonstrate that eating disorders are all-consuming. Average people quantifying where they spend their energy would say they spend less than 5 percent of their time thinking about food and weight. An individual with an eating disorder, on the other hand, thinks about food and weight all the time. It isn't surprising, then, that people with eating disorders struggle with working productively, going to classes, and maintaining friendships.

Self-esteem also plays a role in the development of eating disorders and body dissatisfaction. Some people argue that body dissatisfaction causes low self-esteem, but the converse may also be true: Low self-esteem may cause body dissatisfaction (Furnham, Badmin, & Sneade, 2002). Most women and men have body types that don't match their ideal. Striving for that unreasonable standard can contribute to lower self-esteem and depression in both women and men (Pope, Phillips, & Olivardia, 2000). People's wholeness is compromised as they use unwholesome ways to achieve the ideal they aspire to. Healthy self-esteem should come from a personal relationship with God, not because a person compares favorably with a digitally enhanced image.

Biological Influences

Eating disorders are typically characterized by and labeled with their most obvious features—a preoccupation with food and unhealthy behaviors surrounding appetite. Researchers have been curious about the biological basis of medical conditions where appetite is a central focus, as is the case with eating disorders (Polivy & Herman, 2002).

According to a review by Polivy and Herman (2002), studies of twins and families have provided evidence that eating disorders are transmitted genetically. Therefore, if a family member has had an eating disorder, you have a high risk of developing one, too. Family studies have also indicated that eating disorders appear to have a genetic line. In other words, certain families are more predisposed to eating disorders than other families (Spelt & Meyer, 1995).

Family Influences

Scientists have also found that, in addition to passing on genetic traits, families pass along concerns, fears, and preoccupations about weight (Klump, McGue, & Iacono, 2000). Parents who have eating disorders are more likely to have children with these deadly disorders. This happens through genetic transmission, as you just read, but environmental factors also come into play. For example, family members often praise individuals with eating disorders for their slenderness, and they envy the self-control and discipline required to achieve the thin physique (Branch & Eurman,

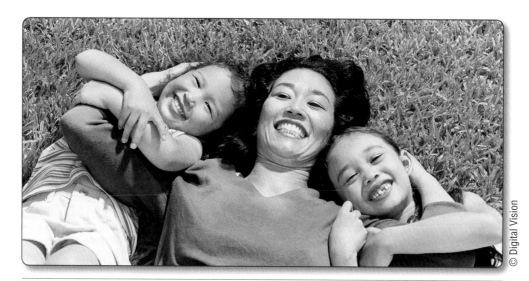

© Digital Vision

The family plays an important role in what we think and feel about our bodies.

1980). Unfortunately, family members may be blind to their relative's eating disorder, and they may continue to praise and reinforce the weight loss even when the person becomes severely ill (Polivy & Herman, 2002).

Family dynamics have also been implicated in a person's developing and maintaining an eating disorder (Minuchin, Rosman, & Baker, 1978; Haworth-Hoeppner, 2000). An individual with an eating disorder will often describe family members as intrusive, hostile, disrespectful of emotional needs (Minuchin, Rosman, & Baker, 1978), and overprotective (Shoebridge & Gowers, 2000). People with eating disorders may come from a critical and intimidating family environment (Haworth-Hoeppner, 2000).

Mothers may also play a significant role in young girls' developing eating disorders. Many mothers who think their daughters should lose more weight say so, and they describe their daughters to others as being less attractive than the ideal (Hill & Franklin, 1998; Pike & Rodin, 1991). Research has found that direct comments from a mother about the weight and shape of her daughter influence the daughter more powerfully than when a mother only models weight and shape concerns through dieting or extreme exercising (Ogden & Steward, 2000; Smolak, Levine, & Schermer, 1999). That's not to say modeling has an insignificant role. In a study of young elementary school children, Smolak, Levine, and Schermer (1999) found that the behaviors and attitudes a mother models to her young child do affect the child's weight- and shape-related attitudes and behaviors. Other research found that mothers' critical comments prospectively predicted eating disordered outcomes for their daughters (Vanfurth et al., 1996).

Mothers who have an eating disorder or an extreme preoccupation with food and weight negatively influence their children's attitudes and behaviors. Polivy and Herman (2002) showed that mothers with eating disorders tend to feed their children irregularly, use food for rewards and punishments, and express concern about their daughters' weight when the girls are as young as two years. Research by Agras, Hammer, and McNicholas (1999) demonstrated that by the time these children reach kindergarten, they exhibit more negative moods and are at serious risk for developing eating disorders. In sum, the family environment—especially the mother's role—has a significant influence on how children think and

feel about their bodies and physical appearance. This is especially true for daughters.

Differences Between Men and Women

Men and women express body image concerns and eating disorders differently (Cumella, 2003; Anderson, 1992; Anderson, 1998). Typically, women want only to get thinner and leaner. For example, one study indicated that 69 percent of girls wanted to lose weight (Furnham, Badmin, & Sneade, 2002). Men, on the other hand, generally want to get leaner or more muscular (Furnham, Badmin, & Sneade, 2002; Anderson & Di Domenico, 1992).

When using healthy standards of weight, women tend to view themselves as too heavy and men tend to view themselves as too light (Furnham & Calnan, 1998; Cash, Winstead, & Janda, 1986). One study discovered that men thought they would be more attractive to women if they had about 30 pounds (14 kg) more muscle, but that women actually preferred more average-looking men (Pope et al., 2000). Women, on the other hand, thought their most attractive weight was lower than their current weight, but men preferred women heavier than the women's preference (Fallon & Rozin, 1985; Grieve et al., 2005). Another study demonstrated that almost 47 percent of males wanted to become bigger, compared to fewer that 4.5 percent of females (Silberstein et al., 1988).

Although men and women differ in what they want their bodies to look like, the motivation behind why they want to change their bodies is often the same. Both genders struggle with how they view their bodies and how they accept who they are. Although the way they go about trying to alter their bodies may look different, the goal for men and women is the same: to try to control feelings by controlling the body and physical appearance; to gain approval and acceptance from others; and to cope with or manage stress, anxiety, and heavy emotions.

In summary, eating disorders are caused by many factors, and not all of them will be present in each person. No two people are exactly the same, so an eating disorder may show up in different ways. The information in this section provided a comprehensive overview of some of the more common causes of eating disorders. Eating disorders are serious issues with serious physical complications. Table 3.1 provides a short overview of physical signs and complications associated with each disorder we talked about in this chapter.

Table 3.1 Physical Complications of Eating Disorders

Anorexia nervosa	• Abnormally slow heart rate and low blood pressure, which means that the heart muscle is changing. The risk for heart failure rises as the heart rate and blood pressure levels lower. • Reduction of bone density (osteoporosis), which results in dry, brittle bones • Muscle loss and weakness • Severe dehydration, which can result in kidney failure • Fainting, fatigue, and overall weakness • Dry hair and skin; hair loss is common. • Growth of lanugo (downy hair) all over the body in an effort to keep the body warm
Bulimia nervosa	• Electrolyte imbalances that can lead to irregular heart beats and possibly heart failure and death. Electrolyte imbalance is caused by dehydration and loss of potassium and sodium from the body, and is a result of purging behaviors. • Potential for gastric rupture during periods of bingeing • Inflammation and possible rupture of the esophagus from frequent vomiting • Tooth decay and staining from stomach acids released during vomiting • Chronic, irregular bowel movements and constipation as a result of laxative abuse; peptic ulcers and pancreatitis
Binge eating disorder	• High blood pressure • High cholesterol levels • Heart disease as a result of elevated triglyceride levels • Secondary diabetes • Gallbladder disease
Muscle dysmorphia	• Side effects and complications from steroid use • Side effects from the overuse of protein supplements (e.g., kidney failure) • High risk for injury from long, exhaustive workouts
Female athlete triad/ anorexia athletica	• Abnormally slow heart rate • Bone fractures • Ammenorrhea (absence of menses) • Osteoporosis, and decreased bone density (which cannot be regained) • Fatigue that can inhibit athletic performance and increase risk of injury • Electrolyte abnormalities • Depression

Adapted from ANRED. Available: www.anred.com.

What God Wants for People

Genesis 1:26 confirms that God created each person in his image, with an identity that is both physical and spiritual. Ephesians 1:5 says that Christians have the special privilege of being adopted into God's family. God wants people to know the truth—him. John 8:32 states, "Then you will know the truth, and the truth will set you free." God's truth is that he loves all people unconditionally. He wants people to know that, even when they feel unlovable and worthless, they are worth so much in his eyes. This unconditional love, above everything, builds the foundation for the Christian's life. People who can't accept this love can't accept Christ, others, or themselves, because God is love (1 John 3:16).

Christ wants people to focus on him and to keep their eyes fixed on him. How can you be focused on him when you are anxious and concerned and obsessed with your body and with food? Society says that you need to be thin and beautiful to feel self-worth, but Christ has a different message. He is the source of self-worth; you don't need to find it in superficial, impermanent things. Your relationship with him, not the way you look or how much you weigh, should mean the most to you as a Christian. It's hard to live outside of society's standards! Christ never gave in to that pressure, though. He lived in the world, but he was not "of the world." Your aim is to live like Christ. The ultimate message he sends is that he loves you *unconditionally*, and he wants you to love yourself that way, too.

1 Corinthians 3:16 states, "Don't you know that you yourselves are God's temple and that God's Spirit lives in you?" Your body houses his spirit, so you need to be responsible and take care of your body, to make sure it is healthy enough to do his work. You are, in fact, "created in the image of God" (Genesis 1:27). Your image of a healthy body should be Christ's, not the world's. We don't mean that you should make your body an idol. Rather, with the attitude of Christ, replace the lies that the world tells (see Philippians 2:5–11).

The opening chapter of this book and of the Bible established that God's physical creation was very good. People get deceived, though, into thinking they are weak and ugly—not good. They look for a quick fix and end up like Eve in the Bible. She said to God after she took the forbidden fruit, "The serpent deceived me, and I ate" (Genesis 3:13). Paul warned people against thinking they're stronger or less gullible than Eve was: "I am afraid that just as Eve was deceived by the serpent's cunning, your minds may somehow be led astray from your sincere and pure devotion to Christ. For if someone comes to you and preaches a Jesus other than the Jesus we preached, or if you receive a different spirit from the one you received, or a different gospel from the one you accepted, you put up with it easily enough" (2 Corinthians 11:3–4). Maybe people put up too easily with

media's unrealistic and distorted views of what women and men should look like and become deceived, lose self-esteem, and try to be someone they're not.

Heed Paul's warning, then, in Romans 16:17–19: "I urge you, friends, to watch out for those who cause divisions and put obstacles in your way that are contrary to the teaching you have learned. Keep away from them. For such people are not serving our Lord Christ, but their own appetites. By smooth talk and flattery they deceive the minds of naive people. Everyone has heard about your obedience, so I am full of joy over you; but I want you to be wise about what is good, and innocent about what is evil." Paul says in his letter to Titus that imprisonment to evil should be a thing of the past. He writes: "At one time we too were foolish, disobedient, deceived and enslaved by all kinds of passions and pleasures. We lived in malice and envy, being hated and hating one another. . . . And I want you to stress these things, so that those who have trusted in God may be careful to devote yourself to doing what is good. These things are excellent and profitable for everyone" (Titus 3:3, 8). Take a hard look at how you allow media to shape and imprison your thoughts, emotions, actions, and lifestyle. Pray about how you can glorify God through your body, and take pleasure in his good gifts to you.

Peace

I remember my father describing the final minutes of his father's life. My grandfather died of cancer. Before his death, with his adult children surrounding his bed, he asked them to sing one of his favorite psalms. They sang with broken voices. As he passed from this life to the next, his parting words were that he could hear the angels singing. He died in peace.

To have **peace** is to live in harmony with God and others and to experience personal wellness within. The opposite of peace is to be at war; to be fighting; or to be at odds with God, with others, or within ourselves.

Sometimes things do trouble us and we cannot find peace. Joseph's brothers could not find peace when they were told to leave Benjamin behind. They were told "go back to your father in peace" (Genesis 44:17). They

could not, because they knew the anguish that would cause their father. We, too, may encounter situations when we are so totally disoriented about our future that we are disabled from acting. We feel like a wreck; we are not at peace.

The most profound way God gives us peace with him is by offering his son to us (Romans 5:1; Acts 10:36), the "Prince of Peace" (Isaiah 9:6-7; Micah 5:5), to live among us for a little while and understand our joys and struggles (John 1:14), to die for our sins (Colossians 1:20), and to ascend to the throne of God to intercede on our behalf (John 14:27). As the angels declared at Jesus' birth, "Glory to God in the highest, and on earth peace to men on whom his favor rests" (Luke 2:14; Matthew 2:10). May his favor rest upon us.

(continued)

(continued)

It is important to remember that Jesus does not offer peace as the world does. Christ says to the people during his triumphal entry into Jerusalem, "If you had only known on this day what would bring you peace" (Luke 19:42). It was not about international power but international service; it was not about taking life, but giving it.

How do we open ourselves to let the Spirit work God's peace in us? How do we prevent fear, uncertainty, and disorientation, from depriving us of peace? I remember waking from a nightmare as a child. The images in my mind were haunting, and trembling I went downstairs to waken my parents. They assured me everything was okay, it was just a dream, and they would watch over me and so would God. I went back to bed, with my mother watching over me and stroking my hair with her loving hands. I trusted her and fell asleep. We ought to have the same trust in the bigger arms and absolute love of our Heavenly Father, for he "who watches over you... will neither slumber nor sleep" (Psalms 121:3–4; 4:8—we are told five times in Psalm 121 that God watches over us). Through trusting God, we can find peace and rest.

God grants peace to those who love God's ways, as the psalmist David says, "Great peace have they who love your law, and nothing can make them stumble" (119:165) For those who live by his commandments, seeking God's holiness, God says "your peace would have been like a river" (Isaiah 48:18; 66:12).

We must live righteous lives that lead to peace (Romans 14:17–19; 1 Corinthians 7:15). We "must turn from evil and do good; [we] must seek peace and pursue it" (1 Peter 3:11). However, righteous living means a lot more than simply saying to those in need, "'Go in peace; keep warm; and eat your fill,' and yet you do not supply their bodily needs, what is the good of that?" (James 2:16; Romans 2:10). We find righteousness, purity, and peace by going beyond ourselves and being with criminals, getting our hands dirty with needy folks whose broken lives need God's peace.

The Israelites had peace offerings—or "fellowship offerings" as they are also called—and they provide an interesting lesson for wellness. God only accepted a peace offering when the people sought to live obedient and just lives. It is further interesting to note how the "fire must be kept burning on the altar continuously; it must not go out" (Leviticus 6:13)—like the eternal flame. If we are to offer our lives as peace offerings, we must be continually obedient and seeking justice. Obedient and just lives lead to peace among the nations, between friends, and within ourselves.

May we bless each other with peace as we come and go, not simply as a nice wish, but as a genuine gift. As trusting, obedient, justice-seeking children of God, we can experience peace—harmony and wellness—with God, others, and within ourselves. May peace govern us (Isaiah 60:17).

After Simeon saw the Christ child, he said, "Sovereign Lord, as you have promised, you now dismiss your servant in peace" (Luke 2:29). May God provide us with that peace, that wellness. May we receive the blessing that God instructed Aaron and his children to give to God's people: "The Lord bless you and keep you; the Lord make his face shine upon you and be gracious to you; the Lord turn his face toward you and give you peace" (Numbers 6:24–26).

Peace: During the next day look at yourself and others and try to bless everyone with God's peace. Blessing requires more than lip service. How did you bless people? What was the response?

_____

_____

_____

_____

_____

_____

_____

Recovery From an Eating Disorder

Because many factors contribute to the development of an eating disorder, and because every person's situation is different, the "best" treatment must be tailored to each individual. The process begins with evaluation by a physician or trained counselor.

Recovery is a difficult process that can take several months—even years. It takes more than abandoning starving. At minimum it involves

- maintaining a normal or near normal weight;
- in women, resuming normal menstrual periods (not triggered by medication);
- eating a well-balanced diet that includes a variety of foods; and
- reducing irrational fears about different types of food.

Recovering individuals need to work on relationships, too. They need to seek out age-appropriate relationships with family members and others. During recovery, they will begin to realize and become aware of unreasonable cultural demands for thinness; engage in fun activities that have nothing to do with food, weight, or appearance; gain a sense of self; and set realistic goals and plans for achieving them.

Information used with permission of ANRED: Anorexia Nervosa and Related Eating Disorders, Inc. www.anred.com.

Men struggling with body image concerns or eating disorders need to put in place a multidisciplined assessment and treatment plan like females do. Getting weight back to normal is a priority. Furthermore, destructive behaviors, such as bingeing, purging, using steroids, and being preoccupied with supplements, need to be reduced (Anderson & Holman, 1997). Developing muscle through a balanced weight-training program is also important. Emotionally, these men may be dealing with substance abuse, alcoholism, or shoplifting, which are some means of feeling good when physical needs are not being met. These men may also need help expressing emotions and exploring their relationships with their fathers (Cumella, 2003; Stein, 2005).

Recovery is a long, hard process. In the book *Eating Disorders in Women and Children*, Lewis refers to the recovery process as a spiritual quest: "It involves a rediscovery of one's connection with their inner-self, others, and nature. . . . Healthy spirituality is the process of learning how to live daily with the tension between our desire for perfection and the reality of our imperfection" (Lewis, 2001, p. 318).

These are some options for treating eating disorders (please refer to table 3.2 for specific treatment goals for the different eating disorders):

- Hospitalization to prevent death, suicide, and medical crisis

Table 3.2   Specific Treatment Goals for Different Eating Disorders

Anorexia nervosa	• Focus on restoring nutritional status, normalizing eating and exercise habits, and altering attitudes toward food and body size. • Concentrate on feelings about body image, weight gain, self-esteem, and identity development.
Bulimia nervosa	• Focus on interrupting the binge–purge cycle, normalizing eating patterns, and altering attitudes toward food and body size. • Understand emotional problems and conflicts that may have originally contributed to the bulimic behavior.
Binge eating disorder	• Focus on normalizing eating patterns and interrupting the bingeing cycle. • Change attitudes toward food and body size. • Understand emotional problems and conflicts that may have contributed to the bingeing behavior.
Female athlete triad syndrome	• Normalize eating patterns and exercise habits. • Alter attitudes toward food and body size. • Concentrate on feelings about body image, weight gain, self-esteem, and identity development.
Muscle dysmorphia	• Normalize eating patterns and exercise habits. • Become aware of cultural demands for unrealistic body ideals. • Engage in activities that have nothing to do with food, weight, or exercise.

Adapted, with permission, from ANRED. Available: www.anred.com.

- **Weight restoration** to improve health, mood, and cognitive functioning
- Medication to relieve depression and anxiety
- Dental work to repair damage and to minimize future problems
- Individual counseling to develop healthy ways of taking control
- Family counseling to change old patterns and create healthier new ones
- Group counseling to learn how to manage relationships effectively
- Nutrition counseling to expose food myths and design healthy meals
- Participation in support groups to break down isolation and alienation

Information adapted and used with permission of ANRED (ANRED, 1999c).

Next Steps

Eating disorders and weight preoccupation are serious and sometimes even life threatening. If you know someone struggling with an eating disorder, please review the Guide for Family and Friends of a Person With Food and Weight Problems in appendix A. You'll find two short questionnaires in appendix B. Complete them to understand more about your perceptions of food and weight and about some of your own behaviors. The questionnaires are not intended to be used for diagnostic purposes but for educational purposes only. If your answers to the questionnaires tell you to seek the advice of a counselor, pastor, teacher, or physician, please do so. Please remember to be true to yourself. If one or more points in this chapter fit you and your lifestyle, don't hesitate to seek out help.

Remember, facing these issues isn't easy. We find this quote from George Grinnell in his book titled *A Death on the Barrens* encouraging: "Enlightenment is not obtained through knowledge, but through a change in perspective" (Grinnell, 1996, p. 64).

Key Terms

amenorrhea

anorexia athletica

anorexia nervosa

binge eating disorder

bingeing

body dysmorphic disorder (BDD)

body image

bulimia nervosa

dieting

disordered eating

eating disorders not otherwise specified (EDNOS)

female athlete triad syndrome

muscle dysmorphia

osteoporosis

peace

purging

weight preoccupation

weight restoration

Review Questions

1. Identify five facts about dieting and describe why dieting is so harmful.

2. Identify and describe the four dimensions of body image.

3. Identify four ways to change a negative body image.

4. Identify and describe the three classified eating disorders and the five nonclassified disorders.

5. Describe three factors that can influence or cause eating disorders to develop.

6. How do men and women differ in experiencing body image concerns and eating disorders?

7. What are five of the identified risk factors (medical complications) associated with eating disorders in general?

8. What does God want people to believe about beauty and the body?

9. What are three treatment or recovery goals for a person struggling with each of the following: anorexia, bulimia, binge eating disorder, and muscle dysmorphia?

10. What can you do to help a friend or family member who is struggling with an eating disorder?

Application Activities

1. **Reflections on the body**

   Look up the verses in the following list and answer the questions about how they relate to body image.

   a. What does Western society say the body needs to look like?

   b. Read 1 Corinthians 6:19–20. To whom does your body belong and why?

   c. Look up Genesis 1:27. According to this verse, what should you see every time you look in the mirror?

   d. See Psalm 139:13–14. What does the psalmist acknowledge in these verses regarding the formation and nature of the body?

   e. If you have frequent negative thoughts about your body size and shape, write them down.

   Questions adapted from Homme's (1999) *Seeing Yourself in God's Image.*

2. **Gift assessment**

   Too often, we focus on negative perceptions of ourselves. Complete a gift assessment like the following on page 53 to explore your areas of strength and giftedness.

Spiritual Gift Inventory

I would like your opinion. I'd like to better understand how God has equipped me for service. One part of my discovery process involves getting feedback from a few people who know me reasonably well. Your thoughts about the way I relate to others will be very helpful. Please take a few minutes to complete the following assessment.

Observations about: _____

Provided by: _____

Relationship: _____

As you read the following descriptions please indicate to what degree each one describes me. Mark each letter with Y, S, N, or ?. When you're finished, try to decide which three are most descriptive. Indicate your top three choices by placing an (X) next to the appropriate letter.

Y – Yes, it very much describes me.

S – It somewhat or slightly describes me.

N – No, it doesn't describe me.

? – I'm not sure.

____ a. Developing strategies or plans to reach identified goals; organizing people, tasks, and events; helping organizations or groups become more efficient; creating order out of organizational chaos.

____ b. Pioneering new projects; serving in another country or community; adapting to different cultures and surroundings; being culturally aware and sensitive.

____ c. Working creatively with wood, cloth, metal, paints, glass, and so on; working with various kinds of tools; making things with practical uses; designing or building things; working with my hands.

____ d. Communicating with variety and creativity; developing and using particular artistic skills (art, drama, music, photography, etc.); finding new and fresh ways to communicate ideas to others.

____ e. Distinguishing between truth and error, good and evil; accurately judging character; seeing through phoniness or deceit; helping others to see what's right and wrong in situations.

____ f. Strengthening and reassuring troubled people; encouraging or challenging people; motivating others to grow; supporting people who need to take action.

____ g. Looking for opportunities to build relationships with people who don't believe in Christ; communicating openly and effectively about my faith; talking about spiritual matters with people who don't believe in Christ.

____ h. Trusting God to answer prayer and encouraging others to do so; having confidence in God's continuing presence and ability to help, even in difficult times; moving forward in spite of opposition.

____ i. Giving liberally and joyfully to people in financial need or to projects requiring support; managing money well to free more of it for giving.

____ j. Working behind the scenes to support the work of others; finding small things that need to be done and doing them without being asked; helping wherever needed, even with routine or mundane tasks.

From P. Walters and J. Byl, 2008, *Christian paths to health and wellness* (Champaign, IL: Human Kinetics). Adapted, by permission, from Bruce Bugbee and Don Cousins. *The Network Curriculum Participant Guide,* © 1994, 2005 by The Willow Creek Community Chruch and Bruce Bugbee and Don Cousins. (2005) The Zondervan Corporation. For additional resources, go to www.brucebugbee.com.

___ k. Meeting new people and helping them to feel welcome; entertaining guests; opening my home to others who need a safe, supportive environment; setting people at ease in unfamiliar surroundings.

___ l. Frequently offering to pray for others; expressing amazing trust in God's ability to provide; showing confidence in the Lord's protection; spending a lot of time praying.

___ m. Carefully studying and researching subjects I want to understand better; sharing my knowledge and insights with others when asked; sometimes gaining information that is not attainable by natural means.

___ n. Taking responsibility for directing groups; motivating and guiding others to reach important goals; managing people and resources well; influencing others to perform to the best of their abilities.

___ o. Empathizing with hurting people; patiently and compassionately supporting people through painful experiences; helping those generally regarded as undeserving or beyond help.

___ p. Speaking with conviction to bring change in other people's lives; exposing cultural trends, teachings, or events that are morally wrong or harmful; boldly speaking truth even in places where it may be unpopular.

___ q. Faithfully providing long-term support and nurture for a group of people; providing guidance for the whole person; patiently but firmly nurturing others in their development as believers.

___ r. Studying, understanding, and communicating biblical truth; developing appropriate teaching material and presenting it effectively; communicating in ways that motivate others to change.

___ s. Seeing simple, practical solutions in the midst of conflict or confusion; giving helpful advice to others who are facing complicated life situations; helping people take practical action to solve real problems.

Thank you for taking the time to complete this assessment. Your opinions are valuable to me in this process, and I deeply appreciate your help.

From P. Walters and J. Byl, 2008, *Christian paths to health and wellness* (Champaign, IL: Human Kinetics). Adapted, by permission, from Bruce Bugbee and Don Cousins. *The Network Curriculum Participant Guide,* © 1994, 2005 by The Willow Creek Community Chruch and Bruce Bugbee and Don Cousins. (2005) The Zondervan Corporation. For additional resources, go to www.brucebugbee.com.

References

Agliata, D., & Tantleff-Dunn, S. (2004). The impact of media exposure on males' body image. *Journal of Social and Clinical Psychology, 1*: 7-22.

Agras, S., Hammer, L., & McNicholas, F. (1999). A prospective study of the influence of eating-disordered mothers on their children. *International Journal of Eating Disorders, 25*: 253-62.

American Psychiatric Association. (2000). *Diagnostic and statistical manual of mental disorders* (5th ed.). Washington, DC: American Psychiatric Association.

American Psychological Association. (2004). Eating disorders: Psychotherapy's role in effective treatment. Retrieved June 28, 2007, from www.apahelpcenter.org/articles/article.php?id=50.

Anderson, A. (1992). Eating disorders in males: A special case? In K.D. Bromnell, J. Rodin, & J.H. Wilmore (Eds.). *Eating, body weight, and performance in athletes: Disorders of modern society* (pp. 172-188). Philadelphia: Lea and Febiger.

Anderson, A. (1998). Eating disorders in males: Critical questions. In R. Lemberg & L. Cohn (Eds.). *Eating disorders: A reference sourcebook* (pp. 73-79). Phoenix, AZ: Oryx.

Anderson, A., & Di Domenico, L. (1992). Diet vs. shape content of popular male and female magazines: A dose-response relationship to the incidence of eating disorders. *International Journal of Eating Disorders, 11*: 283-287.

Anderson, A.E., & Holman, J.E. (1997). Males with eating disorders: Challenges for treatment and research. *Psychopharmacology Bulletin, 33*(3): 391-397.

ANRED. (1999a). What causes eating disorders? Retrieved June 28, 2007, from www.anred.com/causes.html.

ANRED. (1999b). Muscle dysmorphic disorder. Retrieved June 28, 2007, from www.anred.com/musdys.html.

ANRED. (1999c). Treatment and recovery. Retrieved June 28, 2007, from www.anred.com/tx.html.

Baird, A.L., & Grieve, F.G. (2006). Exposure to male models in advertisements leads to a decrease in men's body satisfacton. *North American Journal of Psychology, 8*(1): 115-122.

Barthel, D. (1992). Men, media and the gender order when men put on appearances: Advertising and the social construction of masculinity. In S. Craig. *Men, masculinity, and the media: Research on men and masculinities.* Thousand Oaks, CA: Sage Publications.

Bear, M. (2000). Dieting and weight loss facts and fiction. National Eating Disorder Information Pamphlet, Toronto. Retrieved June 27, 2007, from www.nedic.ca/knowthefacts/dietingfacts.shtml.

Berg, F.M. (1997). *Afraid to eat: Children and teens in weight crises.* Hettinger, ND: Healthy Weight Publishing Network.

Branch, C.H., & Eurman, E.L. (1980). Social attitudes towards patients with anorexia nervosa. *American Journal of Psychiatry, 137*: 631-632.

Braun, D.L., Sunday, S.R., Huang, A., & Kalmi, K.A. (1999). More males seek treatment for eating disorders. *International Journal of Eating Disorders, 25*: 415-424.

Bugbee, B., Cousins, D., & Hybels, B. (1994). *Network: The right people . . . in the right places . . . for the right reasons: Understanding God's design for you in the church.* Grand Rapids, MI: Zondervan Publishing House.

Cash, T.E., & Henry, P. E. (1995). Women's body images: The results of a national survey in the U.S.A. *Sex Roles, 33*: 19-28.

Cash, T.F., Winstead, B.A., & Janda, L.H. (1986). The great American shape-up. *Psychology Today, 30*: 37.

Cook, K.V., & Reiley, K.L. (1991). Eating concerns on two Christian and two nonsectarian college campuses: A measure of sex and campus differences in attitudes towards eating. *Adolescence, 26*: 273-287.

Cumella, E.J. (2003). Examining eating disorders in males. *Behavioral Health Management, 23*(4): 38-41.

Cusumano, D.L., & Thompson, J.K. (2000). Media influence and body image in 8–11-year-old boys and girls: A preliminary report on the multidimensional media influence scale. *International Journal of Eating Disorders, 29*: 37–44.

DeCastro, J.M., & Goldstein, S.J. (1995). Eating attitudes and behaviors of pre- and post-pubertal females: Clues to the etiology of eating disorders. *Physiology and Behaviour, 58*: 15.

EDAP. (2000). Statistics: Eating disorders and their precursors. Retrieved June 28, 2007, from www.edap.org/p.asp?WebPage_ID=286&Profile_ID=41138.

Epling, W.F., & Pierce, W.D. (1988). Activity based anorexia nervosa. *International Journal of Eating Disorders, 7*: 475-485.

Fallon, A.E., & Rozin, P. (1985). Sex differences in perceptions of desirable body shape. *Journal of Abnormal Psychology, 94*: 102-105.

Field, A.E., Camargo, C.A., Jr., Taylor, C.B., Berkey, C.S., Roberts, S.B., & Colditz, G.A. (2001). Peer, parent, and media influences on the development of weight concerns and frequent dieting among preadolescent and adolescent girls and boys. *Pediatrics, 107*: 54-60.

Fraser, L. (1997). *Losing it: America's obsession with weight and the industry that feeds on it.* New York: Penguin Books.

Furnham, A., Badmin, N., & Sneade, I. (2002). Body image dissatisfaction: Gender differences in eating attitudes, self-esteem, and reasons for exercise. *Journal of Psychology, 136*(6): 581-596.

Furnham, A., & Calnan, A. (1998). Eating disturbances, self-esteem, reasons for exercising and body weight dissatisfactions in adolescent males. *European Eating Disorders Review, 6*: 58-72.

Garfinkel, P.E., Garner, D.M., & Goldbloom, D.S. (1987). Eating disorders: Implications for the 1990s. *Canadian Journal of Psychiatry, 32*: 624-631.

Garner, D.M. (1997). The 1997 body image survey results. *Psychology Today, 30*: 30-41.

Gleaves, D.H., Lowe, M.R., Snow, A.C., Green, B.A., & Murphy-Eberenz, K.P. (2000). Continuity and discontinuity models of bulimia nervosa: A taxometric investigation. *Journal of Abnormal Psychology, 109*: 56–68.

Grieve, F.G., Newton, C.C., Kelley, L., Miller, R.C., & Kerr, N. (2005). The preferred male body shapes of college men and women. *Individual Differences Research, 3*(3): 188-192.

Grinnell, G. (1996). *A death on the barrens.* Toronto: Northern Books.

Groesz, L.M., Levine, M.P., & Murnen, S.K. (2002). The effect of experimental presentation of thin media images on body satisfaction: A meta-analytic review. *International Journal of Eating Disorders, 31*: 1-16.

Gustafson-Larson, A.M., & Terry, R.D. (1992). Weight-related behaviors and concerns of fourth grade children. *Journal of American Dietetic Association, 92*: 822.

Harrison, K. (1997). Does interpersonal attraction to thin media personalities promote eating disorders? *Journal of Broadcasting and Electronic Media, 41*: 478-500.

Harrison, K. (2000a). Television viewing, fat stereotyping, body shape standards, and eating disorder symptomatology in grade school children. *Communication Research, 27*: 617-640.

Harrison, K. (2000b). The body electric: Thin ideal media and eating disorders in adolescents. *Journal of Communication, 50*: 119-143.

Hasse, H.L., & Clopton, J.R. (2001). Psychology of an eating disorder. In J.J. Robert-McComb (Ed.). *Eating disorders in women and children: Prevention, stress management and treatment.* Boca Raton, FL: CRC Press.

Hausenblas, H.A., & Fallon, E.A. (2006). Exercise and body image: A meta-analysis. *Psychology and Health, 21*: 33-47.

Haworth-Hoeppner, S. (2000). The critical shapes of body image: The role of culture and family in the production of eating disorders. *Journal of Marriage and Family, 62*: 212-27.

Hill, A.J., & Franklin, J.A. (1998). Mothers, daughters and dieting: Investigating the transmission of weight

control. *British Journal of Clinical Psychology, 37*: 3-13.

Hinrichsen, H., Waller, G., & van Gerko, K. (2004). Social anxiety and agoraphobia in the eating disorders: Associations with eating attitudes and behaviors. *Eating Behaviors, 5*: 285-291.

Hobart, J.A., & Smucker, D.R., (2000). The female athlete triad. *American Family Physician, 61*(11): 3357-3370.

Hoek, H.W., & van Hoeken, D. (2003). Review of the prevalence and incidence of eating disorders. *International Journal of Eating Disorders, 34*: 383-396.

Homme, M. (1999). *Seeing yourself in God's image: Overcoming anorexia and bulimia.* Chattanooga, TN: Turning Point.

Jones, D.C., Vigfusdottir, T.H., & Lee, Y. (2004). Body image and the appearance culture among adolescent girls and boys: An examination of friend conversations, peer criticism, appearance magazines and the internalization of appearance ideals. *Journal of Adolescent Research, 19*: 323-339.

Kanayama, G., Barry, S., Hudson, J.I., & Pope, H.G., Jr. (In press). Body image and attitudes towards male roles in anabolic-androgenic steroid users. *American Journal of Psychiatry, 163*: 697-703.

Klump K., McGue M., & Iacono, W.G. (2000). Age differences in genetic and environmental influences on eating attitudes and behaviors in preadolescent and adolescent female twins. *Journal of Abnormal Psychology, 109*: 239-51.

Kurth, C.L., Krahn, D.D., Nairn, K., & Drewnowski, A. (1995). The severity of dieting and bingeing behaviors in college women: Interview validation of survey data. *Journal of Psychiatric Research, 29*: 211-25.

Labre, M.P. (2005). Burn fat, build muscle: A content analysis of men's health and men's fitness. *International Journal of Men's Health, 4*(2): 187-200.

Law, C., & Labre, M.P. (2002). Cultural standards of attractiveness: A 30-year look at changes in male images in magazines. *Journalism & Mass Communication Quarterly, 79*(3): 697-711.

Levine, M.P., & Smolak, L. (2002). Body image development in adolescence. In T.F. Cash & T. Pruzinsky (Eds.). *Body image: A handbook of theory, research, and clinical practice.* New York: Guilford.

Lewis, L. (2001). Spirituality. In J.J. Robert-McComb (Ed.). *Eating disorders in women and children: Prevention, stress management and treatment.* Boca Raton, FL: CRC Press.

Lunner, K., Werthem, E.H., Thompson, J.K., Paxton, S.J., McDonald, F., & Halvaarson, K.S. (2000). A cross-cultural examination of weight-related teasing, body image, and eating disturbances in Swedish and Australian samples. *International Journal of Eating Disorders, 28*: 430-35.

Martin, K.A., & Lichtenberger, C.M. (2002). Fitness enhancement and changes in body image. In T.F. Cash & T. Pruzinsky (Eds.). *Body image: A handbook of theory, research, and clinical practice* (pp. 414-421). New York: Guilford.

Mayo Clinic. (2006). Body dysmorphic disorder. Retrieved June 28, 2007, from www.mayoclinic.com/health/body-dysmorphic-disorder/DS00559/DSECTION=2.

McCabe, M.P., & Ricciardelli, L.A. (2003). Socio-cultural influences on body image and body changes among adolescent boys and girls. *Journal of Social Psychology, 143*: 5-26.

McCreary, D.R., & Sadava, S.W. (1999). Television viewing and self-perceived health, weight, and physical fitness: Evidence for the cultivation hypothesis. *Journal of Applied Social Psychology, 29*: 2342–2361.

McCreary, D.R., & Sasse, D.K. (2000). An exploration of the drive for muscularity in adolescent boys and girls. *Journal of American College Health, 48*: 297–304.

Minuchin, S., Rosman, B.L., & Baker, L. (1978). *Psychosomatic families: Anorexia nervosa in context.* Cambridge, MA: Harvard University Press.

Moriarty, D., & Moriarty, M. (1993). Socio-cultural influences of eating disorders: Shape, superwoman, and sport. Paper presented at the Annual Meeting of the Canadian Association for Health, Physical Education, Recreation and Dance. Moncton, New Brunswick, Canada.

Mullen, G.W. (1999). *Why do I feel so down when my faith should lift me up?* Kent, England: Sovereign Work Ltd.

NEDIC. (1997). Know the facts: Definitions. Retrieved June 28, 2007, from www.nedic.ca/knowthefacts/definitions.shtml.

Neumark-Sztainer, D., Story, M., Falkner, N.H., Beuhring, T., & Resnick, M. (1999). Disordered eating among adolescents with chronic illness: Exploring the role of family and other social factors. *Archives of Pediatrics and Adolescent Medicine, 152*: 871-878.

Ogden J., & Steward, J. (2000). The role of the mother-daughter relationship in explaining weight concern. *International Journal of Eating Disorders, 28*: 78-83.

Olivardia, R. (2002). Body image and muscularity. In T.F. Cash, & T. Pruzinsky (Eds.). *Body image: A handbook of theory, research, and clinical practice* (pp. 211-218). New York: The Guilford Press.

Parks, P.S.M., & Read, M.H. (1997). Adolescent male athlete: Body image, diet, and exercise. *Adolescence, 32*: 593-603.

Phillips, K.A., O'Sullivan, R.L., & Pope, H.G. (1997). Muscle dysmorphia. *Journal of Clinical Psychiatry, 58*: 361.

Pike, K.M., & Rodin, J. (1991). Mothers, daughters, and disordered eating. *Journal of Abnormal Psychology, 100*: 198-204.

Pipher, M. (1994). *Reviving Ophelia: Saving the selves of adolescent girls.* New York: Ballantine.

Polivy, J., & Herman, C.P. (2002). Causes of eating disorders. *Annual Review of Psychology, 53*: 187-213.

Pope, C.G., Pope, H.G., Menarda, W., Faya, C., Olivardia, R., & Phillips, K.A. (2005). Clinical features of muscle dysmorphia among males with body dysmorphic disorder. *Body Image, 2*: 395-400.

Pope, H.G., Gruber, A.J., & Mangweth, B., Bureau, B., de Col, C., Jouvent, R., & Hudson, J. (2000). Body image perception among men in three countries. *American Journal of Psychiatry, 157*: 1297-1301.

Pope, H.G., Olivardia, R., Borowiecki, J.J., & Cohane, G.H. (2001). The growing commercial value of the male body: A longitudinal survey of advertising in women's magazines. *Psychotherapy and Psychosomatics, 70*: 189-192.

Pope, H.G., Phillips, K.A., & Olivardia, R. (2000). *The adonis complex: The secret crisis of male body obsession.* New York: The Free Press.

Robert-McComb, J.J. (Ed.). (2001). *Eating disorders in women and children: Prevention, stress management and treatment.* Boca Raton, FL: CRC Press.

Shisslak, C.M., Crago, M., & Estes, L.S. (1995). The spectrum of eating disturbances. *International Journal of Eating Disorders, 18*(3): 209-219.

Shoebridge P., & Gowers, S.G. (2000). Parental high concern and adolescent onset anorexia nervosa—A case control study to investigate direction of causality. *British Journal of Psychiatry, 176*: 132-37.

Silberstein, L.R., Striegel-Moore, R.H., Timko, C., & Rodin, J. (1988). Behavioral and psychological implications of body dissatisfaction: Do men and women differ? *Sex Roles, 19*: 219-232.

Smolak, L. (1996). *Next door neighbors: Eating disorders awareness and prevention puppet guide book.* Seattle: National Eating Disorders Association.

Smolak, L., Levine, M.P., & Schermer, F. (1999). Input and weight concerns among elementary school children. *International Journal of Eating Disorders, 25*: 263-71.

Smolak, L., Levine, M.P., & Thompson, J.K. (2001). The use of the socio-cultural attitudes towards appearance questionnaire with middle school boys and girls. *International Journal of Eating Disorders, 29*: 216-223.

Spelt, J., & Meyer, J.M. (1995). Genetics and eating disorders. In J.R. Turner, L.R. Cardon, & J.K. Hewitt (Eds.). *Behavior genetic approaches in behavioral medicine* (pp.167-85). New York: Plenum.

Stein, M. (2005). Managing weight across the spectrum of eating disorders. *Eating Disorders Review, 16*: 1-3.

Stice, E., & Bearman, S.K. (2001). Body-image and eating disturbances prospectively predict increases in depressive symptoms in adolescent girls: A growth curve analysis. *Developmental Psychology, 37*: 597-607.

Stice, E., Hayward, C., Cameron, R.P., Killen, J.D., & Taylor, C.B. (2000). Body image and eating disturbances predict onset of depression among female adolescents: A longitudinal study. *Journal of Abnormal Psychology, 109*: 438-444.

Stice, E., Schupak-Neuberg, E., Shaw, H.E., & Stein, R.I. (1994). Relation of media exposure to eating disorder symptomatology: An examination of mediating mechanisms. *Journal of Abnormal Psychology, 103*: 836-840.

Stice, E., & Whitenton, K. (2002). Risk factors for body dissatisfaction in adolescent girls: A longitudinal investigation. *Developmental Psychology, 38*: 669-678.

Sunday, S.R., Halmi, K.A., & Einhorn, A. (1995). The Yale-Brown-Cornell eating disorder scale: A new scale to assess eating disorder symptomatology. *International Journal of Eating Disorders, 18*: 237-245.

Sundgot-Borgen, J. (1994). Eating disorders in female athletes. *Sports Medicine, 17*: 176-188.

Thompson, C. (2000). College students and eating disorders. Retrieved June 28, 2007, from www.mirror-mirror.org/college.htm.

Thompson, J.K. (1990). *Body image disturbance: Assessment and treatment.* New York: Pergamom.

Thompson, J.K., Heinberg, L.J., Altabe, M., & Tantleff-Dunn, S. (1999). *Exacting beauty: Theory, assessment, and treatment of body image disturbance.* Washington, DC: American Psychological Association.

Thomsen, S.R., Weber, M.M., & Brown, B.L. (2002). The relationship between reading beauty and fashion magazines and the use of pathogenic dieting methods among adolescent females. *Adolescence, 37*: 1-18.

Tiggemann, M. (2003). Media exposue, body dissatisfaction and disordered eating: Television and magazines are not the same! *European Eating Disorders Review, 11*: 418-430.

Toro, J., Castro, J., Gila, A., & Pombo, C. (2005). Assessment of sociocultural influences on the body shape model in adolescent males with anorexia nervosa. *European Eating Disorders Review, 13*: 351-359.

Vanfurth, E.F., Vanstrien, D.C., Martina, L.M.L., Vanson, M.J.M., Hendrickx, J.J.P., & vanEngeland, H. (1996). Expressed emotion and the prediction of outcome in adolescent eating disorders. *International Journal of Eating Disorders, 20*: 19-31.

Wiseman, C.V., Gray, J.J., Mosimann, J.E., & Ahrens, A.H. (1992). Cultural expectations of thinness in women: An update. *International Journal of Eating Disorders, 11*(1): 85-89.

Suggested Readings

For books written by world leaders in the study of eating disorders, look up the following:

Homme, M. (1999). *Seeing yourself in God's image: Overcoming anorexia and bulimia.* **Chattanooga, TN: Turning Point.**

McGee, R. (1998). *The search for significance.* **Nashville, TN: Word.**

Mullen, G. (1999). *Why do I feel so down when my faith should lift me up?* **Kent, England: Sovereign Work Limited.**

Pipher, M. (1994). *Reviving Ophelia: Saving the selves of adolescent girls.* **New York: Ballantine.**

Pope, H.G., Phillips, K.A., & Olivardia, R. (2000). *The Adonis complex.* **New York: The Free Press.**

Robert-McComb, J.J. (Ed.) (2001). *Eating disorders in women and children: Prevention, stress management, and treatment.* **Boca Raton, FL: CRC Press.**

Wolfe, N. (1997). *The beauty myth.* **New York: Harper Collins.**

Zerbe, K. (1993). *The body betrayed.* **Carlsbad, CA: Gurze Books.**

Suggested Web Sites

www.anred.com

Helpful information and resources from Anorexia Nervosa and Related Eating Disorders, Inc.

www.campaignforrealbeauty.com

A Web site for the Dove Campaign for Real Beauty.

www.mirror-mirror.org

Helpful information about eating disorders.

www.nedic.ca

This Web site is for the National Eating Disorder Information Centre (NEDIC), a Toronto-based non-profit organization established in 1985 to provide information and resources about eating disorders and weight preoccupation. NEDIC is the result of the concerted efforts of a group of health care providers.

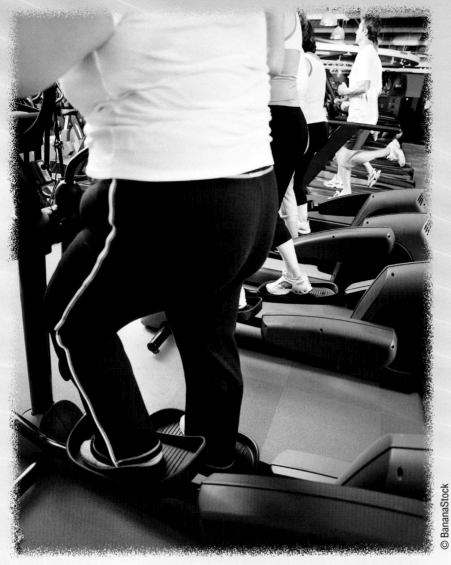

© BananaStock

Weight Control

John Byl

After reading this chapter, you should be able to do the following:

1. Understand that obesity creeps up on people slowly (more frequently in North America than in other parts of the world).
2. Be able to calculate and interpret your body mass index.
3. Learn to set a realistic fat-loss goal through making permanent lifestyle changes.

ew people in Canada and the United States live their entire lives without being concerned at some point with increased body weight. In the midst of global interest in poverty and malnourishment, North Americans need to consider why they eat so much. **Obesity** is **pandemic** in Canada and the United States. Widespread obesity occurs among all age groups, starting with childhood and affecting large numbers of people (especially males) between ages 45 and 60 (Central West Health Planning Information Network, 2004). Although a few percentage points of people in North America are underweight, more than half are too heavy for maximal health and well-being (Central West Health Planning

Quick Facts About Obesity

Obesity affects 300 million people world-wide.

Consider statistics about Canada:

- Overweight (BMI of 25 to 29.9 – BMI is explained later in this chapter) and obesity affects 50 percent of men and 30 percent of women.

- Prevalence of obesity doubled between 1985 and 1999.

- Obesity levels in adults increased 24 percent between 1995-1996 and 2000-2001.

- Women, aged 20 to 34, decreased obesity levels by 9 percent.

- The cost of dealing with obesity in 1997 was estimated at more than $1.8 billion

Compare statistics from the United States:

- An estimated 16 percent of children aged 6 to 19 are overweight.

- More than 65 percent of adults are overweight or obese.

- An estimated 300,000 deaths a year are attributable to obesity.

Adapted from Central West Health Planning Information Network (2004) and Department of Health and Human Services (2005).

Information Network, 2004). Research by Flegal and colleagues (2002) indicates that *two-thirds* of Americans are overweight or obese. In the future, obesity is expected to reverse the centuries-long trend of longer life expectancy (Olshansky et al., 2005). People's life expectancy in one part of the world is reduced because they have too little food, and people's life expectancy in another part of the world is reduced because they eat too much food. This chapter is about overeating, overweight, and obesity in North America.

When I was 20 years old, I weighed a healthy 180 pounds (81 kg). Over the next 30 years, I gained approximately one pound (0.5 kg) each year until I weighed 210 pounds (95 kg). A gradual increase in weight is called **creeping obesity**. Part of the increase may result from decreasing **metabolism,** a process that begins close to age thirty. At 210 pounds I was too heavy and decided to do something about it. My goal was to bike more and work off my extra weight by increasing time spent doing an activity I love. Things were going well until, a few weeks into my new routine, a driver who had consumed too much alcohol struck me off my bike. I was confined to a wheelchair for a month, used crutches for another month, and used a cane for a few more weeks. I began to slowly regain my mobility. I had double vision for half a year, so I was unable to do any sports. I was gaining almost a pound every two weeks during my recovery, and within six months I weighed 220 pounds (100 kg). I maintained that new weight for the next year and a half. Because of my injuries I was still unable to do vigorous activities and I slipped into a depression. The doctor prescribed antidepressant medications. Unfortunately, one of the side affects of my medicine was increased appetite. Within two months I had gained another 20 pounds (9 kg) and weighed in at 239.5 pounds (109 kg). The scale never did cross 240 pounds (110 kg), but I desperately needed to act.

My obesity crept up on me over 30 years and was accelerated by a catastrophic event in my life. I have a good friend who let obesity creep up on her during her university years. Early in her college career, she ate differently and reduced her activity level from when she was in high school. She gained only about a pound (0.5 kg) a month during the academic months. That added up to 8 pounds (4 kg) a year, and approximately 32 pounds (16 kg) over four years, though. The balance of energy input and output does not have to be off by much before, over a long period of

Costs of Obesity in the United States

"In the United States alone poor diet and physical inactivity are associated with 400,000 deaths per year, and obesity-related medical expenditures in 2003 approximated $75 billion. Obesity is also an emerging problem in middle- and low-income countries, where the health and fiscal costs are likely to be devastating" (Levine et al., 2005, p. 584). Diseases linked to obesity include heart disease, diabetes, and various forms of cancer.

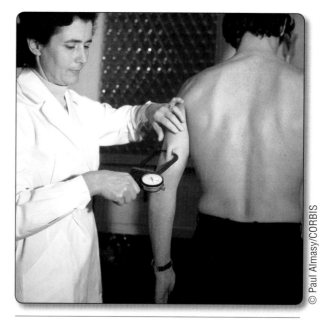

© Paul Almasy/CORBIS

Skinfold measurement devices are to be used by trained technicians.

time, a person gains or loses a lot of weight. Daily choices determine, in large part, long-term health and well-being.

The chapter about body image described how people can fool themselves by thinking they are fat when they're not. When people want to lose weight they are really interested in losing fat, not muscle. It's not always wise to use weight to determine fatness. I looked in the mirror and I knew I was fat. However, the best way to determine body fat is to go through **hydrostatic weighing**. Because fat floats and muscle sinks (think of soup with meatballs in it) people who are weighed in water get a very accurate determination of fat mass and muscle mass. However, this approach requires special equipment and takes considerable time to perform. Two simpler weighing methods correlate positively with hydrostatic weighing. One is **skinfold measurements**, in which a skilled technician measures skin folds at various points on the body. Another simpler method uses various **electrical impedance devices.** The devices measure the resistance of a small electrical charge that is run through the body. Fat has less water in it than muscle does and offers more resistance. By measuring this resistance, a technician can measure body fat. Check with your institution to see if one of these methods of accurately measuring body fat is available to you.

A simple way to get a fairly close estimate of your body fat is to calculate your body mass index (BMI) and compare yourself to established standards. The sidebar on page 62 shows how to calculate your BMI (or you can refer to table 4.1). When I calculated a BMI for my height (6'1", or 1.85 m), I was in the obese category. People with muscular bodies will end up with a higher BMI that suggests they have more fat than they actually do. See the Web sites for the Office of Nutrition Policy and Promotion (2003) and the Department of Health and Human Services (2006) for more information on the use of BMI. I think I have more muscle, but I still need to lose weight. I should weigh fewer than 186 pounds, or 85 kilograms, according to the BMI. My initial 40-pound (18-kg) weight loss goal was in the right range. How quickly I got there would depend on my determination and commitment to a healthy weight and lifestyle.

Table 4.1 Body Mass Index Guidelines

Formula = weight (kg) / [height (m)]^2

Underweight	Less than 18.5
Normal weight	18.5 – 24.9
Overweight	25 – 29.9
Obesity	Greater than 30

Information obtained from Department of Health and Human Services: Center for Disease Control and Prevention, 2006.

Calculating Your Body Mass Index (BMI)

Weight in pounds ÷ height in inches squared × 703 = BMI
or weight in kilograms ÷ height in meters squared = BMI

Here are some examples, using someone 6 feet, 1 inch tall (1.85 m).

Imperial Measurements

235 pounds ÷ (73 inches × 73 inches) × 703 = 31.00

210 pounds ÷ (73 inches × 73 inches) × 703 = 27.71

185 pounds ÷ (73 inches × 73 inches) × 703 = 24.40

Metric Measurements

107 kilograms ÷ (1.85 × 1.85) = 31.00

95 kilograms ÷ (1.85 × 1.85) = 27.76
84 kilograms ÷ (1.85 × 1.85) = 24.54

Standards for Men and Women

Underweight is a BMI less than 18.5.

Normal is a BMI 18.5 to 24.9.

Overweight is a BMI 25 to 29.9.

Obese is a BMI above 30.

Information obtained from Department of Health and Human Services: Center for Disease Control and Prevention (2006).

You can find a very helpful BMI calculator at www.hc-sc.gc.ca/fn-an/nutrition/weights-poids/guide-ld-adult/bmi_chart_java-graph_imc_java_e.html. It will automatically calculate your BMI when you type in your weight and height, and it will tell you if you are at an increased health risk.

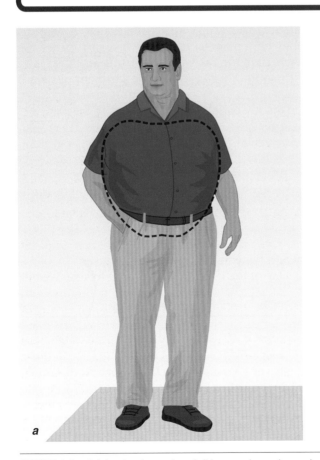

a

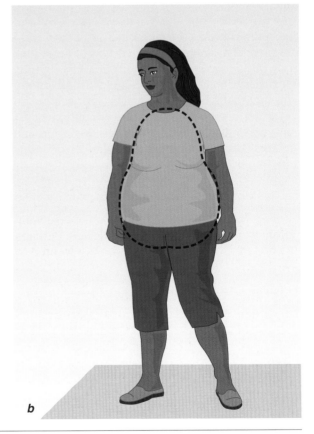

b

FIGURE 4.1   (a) Apple-shaped and (b) pear-shaped people.

Reprinted, by permission, from J. Wilmore and D. Costill, 2004, *Physiology of Sport and Exercise,* 3rd ed. (Champagin, IL: Human Kinetics), 679.

Another way to calculate your health risk from obesity is to see if you are shaped like an apple or a pear (see figure 4.1). People who store extra fat in the abdomen and chest are at a higher risk of developing health problems than those who store extra fat on the hips and thighs. To determine your shape you can calculate your waist-to-hip ratio (WHR). Measure your hip at the widest part and your waist at the smallest part, then divide your waist measurement by your hip measurement. This formula will work the same whether using imperial or metric measurements. For example, if your waist measures 75 centimeters and your hips measure 100 centimeters, divide 75 by 100 and you have a WHR of 0.75. The measurements work for inches as well. For example, if your waist is 30 inches around and your hips are 40 inches wide, you divide 30 by 40 and you have a WHR of 0.75. A WHR more than 0.8 for women or 1.0 for men signals an increased risk of developing weight-related health problems.

The implementation of permanent health lifestyle changes was discussed in chapter 2. Seven steps were identified for helping you achieve your goals. The remainder of this chapter provides content structured around meeting your weight-control goal.

Step 1: State the Goal

The first step in dealing with being overweight involves setting a personal goal to lose fat. My goal was to permanently change my lifestyle to lose about a pound (0.5 kg) a week over 50 weeks. A half kilogram, or one pound, of fat is about 3,500 calories, so I needed to create an imbalance in my **calorie** output and input. I needed to expend 500 calories more than I took in each day for a whole year. To burn 500 calories, I'd need to walk for 90 minutes, eat 7 fewer slices of bread, or do a combination of exercising more and eating less. Perhaps this wasn't a very practical plan, but I wanted to give it a shot. I knew I had an aggressive goal, and I wanted to complete it in a healthy manner. I know many of the diet plans out there work for some people, but they weren't for me. I mentioned my weight gain to my doctor when I went for a second visit regarding my medications. He said it simply, if somewhat unsympathetically: You gain weight by what you put in your mouth. I was putting too much into my mouth and I needed to reduce it. I also know that eating fewer than 1,000 calories a day isn't helpful for three reasons:

1. The first reason has to do with healthy sustainability.
2. The second reason has to do with viewing God's gifts.
3. The third reason has to do with efficient ways of cutting fat.

Healthy Sustainability

The first reason to avoid a drastic reduction in calories is that making small lifestyle changes is more sustainable. Eating fewer than 1,000 calories a day would be setting myself up for disaster; the change would be too drastic. I would probably have the will power to keep up a highly reduced calorie intake for a couple of weeks, but then it would all crash and I'd probably binge and gain back quickly all the weight I had lost, if not more. Lifestyle changes need to be small, incremental, and sustainable. I wanted not only to lose some weight but, more important, I wanted also to improve my lifestyle and make permanent changes.

What's the best weight-loss strategy—to exercise, to eat fewer calories, or to exercise and eat fewer calories? In one study, males were involved in a 12-week program. The men in the exercising group reduced body weight 0.3 percent. Those in the group that reduced calories lost 8.4 percent. The group that both reduced calories and exercised lost 11.4 percent. Results for females in a similar program were slightly less (Hagan et al., 1986; Wing et al., 1998). Researchers have determined that combining exercise and calorie reduction is the healthiest and most sustainable route to weight loss, probably because that approach is more achievable than drastically increasing exercise or decreasing calories (Jakicic & Otto, 2006). One of the keys to sustaining weight loss or maintaining a healthy weight appears to be physical activity—and that is totally apart from other health benefits of physical activity.

One of the reasons it is difficult to keep weight off is that a lighter body with less fat requires less energy to maintain. People who have lost weight need to maintain a diet with fewer calories and maintain levels of activity used during weight loss to maintain their body composition at the new, healthier levels (Fogelholm & Kukkoken-Harjula, 2000a; Leibel, Rosenbaum, & Hirsch, 1995). People often revert to previous eating and activity levels and consequently return to their previous weight levels, or they regain even more than they'd lost (Fogelholm, & Kukkoken-Harjula, 2000b).

Permanent lifestyle change comes from making small, positive changes.

Food Is God's Gift

A second reason to not cut food intake drastically is that to view food as an enemy does not seem a right view of God's good gifts. The Bible states, "For everything God created is good, and nothing is to be rejected if it is received with thanksgiving, because it is consecrated by the word of God and prayer" (1 Timothy 4:4–5). Why should I view as bad something God created as good?

Two diet approaches, the Atkins diet and the Ornish diet, approach weight loss from opposite extremes, but each requires the dieter to avoid or greatly limit some types of food. The **Atkins diet** is high in protein and saturated fat and restricts all carbohydrate. The strength of the Atkins diet is that one feels satiated, or feels full, quite quickly and so consumes fewer calories. However, the Atkins diet contains low levels of antioxidants and may promote osteoporosis and atherosclerosis (Bravata et al., 2003; Reddy et al., 2002). The **Ornish diet,** on the other hand, relies largely on carbohydrate and includes only minimal amounts of animal protein. Growing evidence suggests,

though, that a diet containing moderate amounts of beneficial fat and protein (skinless poultry, fish, eggs, and lean cuts of red meat with fat trimmed, cooked slowly with no or very little salt) is a part of a healthy diet (O'Keefe & Cordain, 2004). Not only does eating some meat once a day help a person from a nutritional perspective, but it also helps one feel satiated sooner.

Following an ancient hunter–gatherer diet may improve health, help maintain a healthy weight, and prevent cardiovascular diseases. The hunter–gatherer eating plan includes the following three items (O'Keefe & Cordain, 2004, p. 102):

1. Replacing saturated and trans fat with **monounsaturated fat** and **polyunsaturated fat**
2. Increasing consumption of omega-3 fat from either fish or plant sources such as nuts
3. Eating a diet high in various fruits, vegetables, nuts, and whole grains and avoiding foods with a high **glycemic** load (a large amount of quickly digestible carbohydrate)

The sidebar on this page provides helpful suggestions for following such an eating plan.

Fundamentals of the Hunter-Gatherer Diet and Lifestyle

- Eat whole, natural, fresh foods; avoid processed and high-glycemic-load foods.
- Consume a diet high in fruits, vegetables, nuts, and berries and low in refined grains and sugars. Nutrient-dense, low-glycemic-load fruits and vegetables such as berries, plums, citrus, apples, cantaloupe, spinach, tomatoes, broccoli, cauliflower, and avacados are best.
- Increase consumption of omega-3 fatty acids from fish, fish oil, and plant sources.
- Avoid trans fat entirely, and limit intake of saturated fat. This means eliminating fried foods, hard margarine, commercial baked goods, and most packaged and processed snack foods. Substitute mono-

unsaturated and polyunsaturated fat for saturated fat.
- Increase consumption of lean protein, such as skinless poultry, fish, and game meats and lean cuts of red meat. Cuts with the words *round* or *loin* in the name usually are lean. Avoid high-fat dairy and fatty, salty, processed meats such as bacon, sausage, and deli meats.
- Incorporate olive oil or non-trans-fatty-acid canola oil into your diet.
- Drink water.
- Participate in daily exercise from various activities (incorporating aerobic and strength training and stretching exercises). Outdoor activities are ideal.

Reprinted from O'Keefe & Cordain, 2004, p. 103.

Cutting Fat

My third reason for not limiting the calories I ate to fewer than 1,000 a day was that, although I was interested in losing weight, I was most interested in losing fat. I had already concluded that the best way to achieve my weight-loss goal would be through a combination of increasing exercise and reducing calories. Muscle tissue burns more calories in daily use than fat does. The more muscular you are, the more calories you burn even when resting. Daily physical exercise is a key to losing and maintaining weight (Wing, 1999).

Step 2: Assess Your Present Lifestyle

After a month of setting my weight-loss goal I hadn't lost much weight because I hadn't adequately considered the second step of goal setting, assessing my present situation (see page 22 in chapter 2). I needed to make my goals realistic in the overall context of my personal situation. I asked myself, aside from the medication, what was causing me to choose to eat too much. I was busy with some projects. It was the end of the semester. I was behind in my work. Things at home stressed me. I medicated my stress with trips to the cookie jar and peanut container. Eating food made me feel treated, cared for,

even pampered. I was determined to lose weight, but my lifestyle choices didn't help me. I had failed at my first goal, but I was still committed to improving my lifestyle, so I needed to refine my goal. I knew that the plan I was making was important because to continue getting fatter would be to increase my risks of cancer, heart disease, type 2 diabetes, high blood pressure, gall bladder disease, psychological problems, and physical limitations. I had to act with the interest of long-term goals in mind, and physical activity would need to play a role in reaching my long-term goals.

I set two new goals. The first was to accomplish the tasks before me without letting them stress me out, to minimize my involvement in outside projects, and to maintain my weight until I could get on top of things. I figured these three tasks would take about a month to accomplish. My second goal was to lose a pound (0.5 kg) every two weeks for 10 weeks following the period of trying to get my life back in control. I knew I would have trouble losing weight when I was under stress, but I did not want to get worse.

The semester came to a close, as did other responsibilities. I stopped my involvement in two organizations I was committed to. Guess what? Those organizations continued quite well without me! At the end of a month my weight was still the same and I was ready to begin the road of cutting weight and cutting fat.

Increased BMI and Sleep Deprivation

Losing weight is about a lifestyle change. For example, when I am stressed, I sleep less. Research has shown a relationship between sleep and body composition. The research indicates the fewer hours a person habitually sleeps, from approximately 7.7 hours a night, the higher the BMI score will be. Part of the explanation for increased BMI for short sleepers is that leptin, a hormone that suppresses appetite, is suppressed and gherlin, a hormone that stimulates appetite, is increased. The result of inadequate sleep is greater appetite. It was hypothesized in this study that "these hormone alterations may contribute to the BMI increase that occurs with sleep curtailment"

(Taheri et al., 2004, p. 214). In addition to a greater appetite, those who sleep less also have a preference to fatty and high-calorie foods (Dinges & Chugh, 1997).

On the other hand, the more hours a person habitually sleeps, from more than 7.7 hours a night, the higher the BMI score will be. At least two reasons for this increase in BMI scores may exist. Some people may have broken sleep and actually spend more time in bed. But the more likely reason is that when people are in bed they are expending less energy (Taheri et al., 2004). Long sleepers also exercise less (Ayas et al., 2003). For more benefits of sound sleep take a look at chapter 10.

Before I talk about more rigorous activity suggestions, though, it's time to get you into an active mindset. By that, I mean pursuing a daily lifestyle in which your every choice is the more active alternative. As you go about your day, stand more, walk more, and get outside more! Live with activity in mind. Burning just 100 more calories a day adds up to burning about 3,000 calories a month, or about eight pounds (eight kilograms) a year. Make the important lifestyle choices to seek activity, live by activity, and be nourished by activity. These 11 helpful tips can increase your daily exercise time by 30 to 45 minutes while barely changing your routine:

1. **Frequent flights:** Use stairs at every opportunity at home, school, dorms, or the mall. Welcome the challenge to enhance your fitness by pushing your heart, using your muscles, building your bones, and using extra calories.

2. **Knead some dough?** Try to prepare some of your own foods rather than ordering in. The cost is cheaper so you will save some "dough," the quality will be better, and you will use more calories as you prepare the food.

3. **Walk through writer's blocks.** When you are looking for some creative thoughts for writing, go for a walk. Take along a writing pad and pen or a pocket tape recorder. Let your mind wander, and as your mind comes up with ideas, stop to record them. If you are working on a group project, try walking with your group instead of meeting at the local doughnut shop. You will find the walking stimulating to the brain, and therefore academically productive. Your benefits will be in your grades and in your physical health.

4. **Be the fan of the game.** Be a boisterous, clapping, jumping-up-and-down, stamping, laughing cheerleader for your team. If you're at a soccer match, walk up and down the sidelines to cheer your team on.

The players will appreciate your encouragement, but the physical and emotional release will do even more good for you than for the team you are cheering.

5. **Walk and roll.** When driving somewhere, always bring along some walking shoes, inline skates, or jump ropes. If there is a traffic jam, pull off and release your frustrations with a 10-minute break to explore the area on foot or on skates.

6. **Think on your feet.** Occasionally, read a book while you are walking back and forth across a room.

7. **Walk the talk phone calls.** When you're on a phone call, walk the talk by talking and walking around the room. If you don't have a portable phone, get an extension cord for the phone or headset.

8. **Stretch your computer time.** Too much time at your computer becomes counterproductive. Take some time off and go for a walk, or at least do some occasional stretches.

9. **Add time during ad time.** When watching television, an advertisement is a signal to get up to do some laundry, make a "walk the talk" phone call, organize some papers, or do some other quick chore. Do not use this time to get a snack or eat. Get off your seat to change the channel instead of using the remote control.

10. **Start a walking bus.** You might not always feel safe walking from home to class or to the store, church, recreation center, or other places. But there is safety in numbers. Try to arrange trips with neighbors and walk together to these places.

11. **Parking lot walks.** Park as far from the building as is safe and reasonable. You'll get more of a walk to the building and back again to your car.

Adapted from Jeanie's Weight Loss Diet Now, 2007.

I knew the first bit of weight loss is the easiest, so I thought I'd set a 10-week time period and then reset my goals after that. I was determined to enjoy each morsel of food eaten during three (slightly smaller) balanced meals a day and three nutritious snacks a day, which would include lots of raw vegetables and whole fruits. (Turn to chapter 8, about nutrition, for more information on balanced eating.) To help me enjoy my food I would eat one peanut at a time instead of a handful at a time, and for dinner I would lay my utensil down for a while after every third bite.

I stopped eating on the run and took time to eat each of my meals and snacks, which helped me to reduce stress and enjoy my food. I also tried to avoid eating anything after 8:00 p.m. I committed myself to biking or walking a total of an hour a day to increase my physical activity. Biking benefits me by increasing my muscle mass, improving my cardiovascular system, using up calories, improving my meditative time with God, and reducing my stress. Increasing physical activity level is essential to losing weight and maintaining weight loss.

Walking is an inexpensive, safe, and technically easy activity for increasing activity level. Research by Fogelholm and Kukkoken-Harjula (2000a) found that 25 to 30 minutes of daily walking would improve health, while 35 to 45 minutes of walking each day should lead to further health improvements and also reduce body weight. Other researches claim each level should be about 25 minutes higher (Jakicic et al., 1999; Jakicic et al., 2003; Klem et al., 1997; Schoeller, Shay, & Kushner, 1997; U.S. Department of Health and Human Services & U.S. Department of Agriculture, 2005). Still other studies note that even though weight might not be significantly reduced by those levels of walking, the activity will improve body composition by decreasing fat and improving muscle mass (Bond et al., 2002; Fox et al., 1996; Irwin et al., 2003).

In one study, researchers measured the activity levels of people who did not include purposeful exercise into their daily lives. They recruited 10 lean and 10 mildly obese, sedentary volunteers and measured their daily movements two times a second for 10 days. Data analysis showed that the "obese participants were seated for 164 minutes longer per day than were lean participants" (Levine et al., 2005, p. 584). The difference in calories for this activity level was approximately 352 calories a day, the difference between leanness and obesity. This study underlines the importance of more activity throughout the day.

Step 3: Design a Specific Plan

Designing a specific plan is the third step in setting goals. I found my plan relatively easy to follow when I was at home, even though the people who lived with me had to wait longer for me to finish my meal. I tried to help by eating less, and eventually we came to a nice arrangement. Write out the specific components of your plan in a positive way and make them work. Revisit your plan from time to time to see where you're having difficulties. Revise your plan and you'll succeed.

Step 4: Predict Obstacles

Predicting obstacles means becoming more self-aware and accepting personal responsibility for actions (Claps, Katz, & Moore, 2005). Celebrations, trips, or other unusual food situations were obstacles for me. I needed to be more careful when I ate out and to order salads (without dressing) instead of fries. Eating more slowly and savoring each bite made eating more enjoyable, and I consumed fewer calories. If I had a celebration in the evening I would eat a light snack at mealtime so I didn't arrive at the celebration famished and want to eat everything in sight, putting away too many calories with too little pleasure. It's OK to occasionally use food to celebrate, but food is meant to nourish, not to satisfy unresolved psychological and emotional cravings.

Stress was another major obstacle to achieving my weight-loss goal. It helped knowing that the easy response to stress was for me to open a food container. When the stress came I tried other things, like taking a nap, exercising on my stationary bicycle for 30 minutes, praying, drinking a glass of water, or having a very small snack (and enjoying it). I also tried to let stressors have less effect on me. (The stress chapter later in this book provides information about how to deal with stress in healthy ways.)

Step 5: Plan Intervention Strategies

Making a permanent lifestyle change requires a great deal of time, motivation, and commitment. For that reason, relapse is a formidable risk, especially in the beginning. My fifth step was to design strategies to keep me compliant and to act as motivators toward my goal. I told my wife about my plan and invited her to join in with me, or at least to keep me accountable. The biggest motivator for me was my love for cycling. It felt great to get back on the bike. My extra weight had made climbing hills more difficult, and my heart rate went too high too quickly. Eating less and being more active helps me in my cycling. I'm a numbers person, and watching my heart rate on the heart monitor as I'd bike was motivation enough.

Being able to fit into my clothes again was another motivator. Because I had gained 20 pounds (9 kg) very quickly, I didn't fit into most of my clothes. Fortunately, it was summer and a couple pairs of shorts worked for most occasions. As motivation, I hung one pair of shorts that I used to fit into in my bedroom. I tried them on once a week. At the beginning I could hardly get them on. Six weeks into my plan I could get the shorts on, but I still needed to lose about an inch (2.5 cm) before the clasp would come together. I kept reminding myself I'd get there.

Making life changes isn't easy. Ecclesiastes 10:18 says, "If a man is lazy, the rafters sag; if his hands are idle, the house leaks." I guess the same could be said for caring for the body. The body sags when people are too lazy to care for it. People need to find ways that work for their specific situations as they try to become well. When you eat reasonable portions, more food is available to share with others. Your eating less lets you share more. The prophet Isaiah spoke about this when he wrote, "If you spend yourselves in behalf of the hungry. . . Your people will rebuild the ancient ruins and will raise up the age-old foundations; you will be called Repairer of Broken Walls, Restorer of Streets with Dwellings" (Isaiah 58:10, 12). Jesus makes this point even more strongly when he argues the people's question: "'Lord, when did we see you hungry or thirsty or a stranger or needing clothes or sick or in prison, and did not help you?' He will reply, 'I tell you the truth, whatever you did not do for one of the least of these, you did not do for me.' Then they will go away to eternal punishment, but the righteous to eternal life" (Matthew 25:44–46).

For your part, recognize that it's not easy to make permanent lifestyle changes. Avoid quick fixes for decreasing weight, such as smoking, dieting, vomiting, and laxatives. Going for the quick fix is tempting, but it will hurt your health more than help it (Paxton, Valois, & Drane, 2004; Lowry, Galuska, & Fulton, 2000; Tomeo, Field, & Berkey, 1999; Middleman, Vazquez, & Durant, 1998). Get to know yourself better, and learn what will work for you to make you well.

Reducing Repetitive Strain Injury and Building Activity Into Your Lifestyle

- The Office of Environmental Health and Safety at the University of Virginia offers eight quick and easy stretches you can do at your computer. Hold each stretch for 5 to 10 seconds. Go to http://keats.admin.virginia.edu/ergo/stretch.html for more information.

- "Workers who used computer software to remind them occasionally to assume good posture, take short breaks, and occasionally stretch do more accurate work and as a result are more productive, according to a new Cornell University study. 'We found that alerting computer users to take short rests and breaks improved work accuracy without any reductions in overall keystroke and mouse use,' says Alan Hedge, professor of design and environmental analysis at Cornell and director of Cornell's Human Factors and Ergonomics Laboratory. In his study, Hedge found that workers receiving the alerts were 13 percent more accurate on average in their work than coworkers who were not reminded. The more the workers typed, the better their accuracy: the fastest typist made almost 40 percent fewer errors than his counterpart who did not receive the computer alerts" (www.news.cornell.edu/releases/Sept99/computer.breaks.ssl.html).

Step 6: Assess Compliance With the Plan

The scale is the easiest measure for weight loss, so I use it once every couple weeks to get a sense of my progress. I had used graphs to plot my weight before, but when I got off the projected line I felt I had failed. Now I keep the numbers in my head and keep pushing toward my goal of being more fit for regular living. I focus on enjoying the changes I have made so far. Research indicates that the weight scale is still a useful accountability tool for those that are overweight and seeking to lose some weight (Klem et al., 1997; McGuire et al., 1999; Qi & Dennis, 2000; Byrne, Cooper, & Fairburn, 2003; O'Neil & Brown, 2005). One study concluded that people who weigh themselves more often than others weigh less and are more successful in losing weight (Jeffrey, 2004).

Weighing can be a problem, though, for those who are not overweight. The scale will encourage them to weigh less and less when they should be weighing more and more. Chapter 3 described how culture skews a person's view of himself or herself, and how the scale can become a weapon of bodily destruction, not an aid toward physical wellness.

Remember that the devil is a deceiver and wants people to live in bondage to the impossible standards of the magazine images. Trying to achieve those standards brings no satisfaction or joy. On the other hand, God created each person uniquely and offers a life of freedom, satisfaction, and joy. Decide daily which road of wellness to take.

Step 7: Assess Progress of Your Overall Goal

I know that weight fluctuates significantly from day to day, so I decided to reassess in 10 weeks how close I was to my goal weight. I was successful in my 10-week goal, so I celebrated! I then changed my goals to focus on maintaining my lifestyle changes and increasing my activity level. Occasionally I would get on the scale, and my weight decreased by about a pound (0.5 kg) a month. But, more important, I felt like I was getting back in control of my life, had more energy, felt happier, and enjoyed life a lot more. I decided to keep moving forward—to live a life that honors God by offering up my body as a living sacrifice of praise to him. With thanksgiving, I will enjoy each morsel of food he has provided. I will enjoy each crank of the pedal as I bike up hills more easily than before because I weight less and am fitter.

Next Steps

My next steps are to continue to make my goals a reality. The next step for you is to get a realistic assessment of your body composition. If you have a healthy body composition and weight, enjoy that and maintain it. If you are too lean and light, eat healthy and allow yourself to look a little fuller. If you are overweight then use the seven steps I used to help bring my weight down. More important than losing weight, though, is significantly improving the quality of your life by having a much healthier body composition and carrying around less excessive and unhealthy fat.

Key Terms

Atkins diet
calorie
creeping obesity
electrical impedance devices
glycemic
hydrostatic weighing
metabolism

monounsaturated fat
obesity
Ornish diet
pandemic
polyunsaturated fat
skinfold measurements

Review Questions

1. What is the typical pattern in which most people become overweight?

2. What is the difference between being overweight and having excess fat?

3. What are the seven steps you could take to permanently change your lifestyle to reduce your level of fat (if that's a change you need to make)?

Application Activities

1. Perform a BMI calculation or other procedure to determine your body fat. What is your level of body fat?

2. Develop a goal for your level of body fat, whether it's to lose fat, gain fat, or maintain your level of fatness:

    a. What is your mission statement? Is this the same as before? If it is different, what did you change and why?

    b. Write down your specific goal in a sentence or two.

    c. In a paragraph or two, assess the behavior and attitudes you are trying to change.

    d. Refine your goal with small, realistic, specific, measurable, and concrete steps.

    e. In a paragraph or two, predict and describe two significant obstacles that prevent you from achieving your goal and describe your plan to overcome those obstacles.

    f. What specific intervention strategies will you have in place to assist you in complying with your plan (the text suggests six strategies on pages 23-25 in chapter 2)?

    g. How will you evaluate your compliance with your plan?

    h. How will you measure progress in achieving your goal?

References

Ayas, N.T., White, D.P., Al-Delaimy, W.K., Manson, J.E., Stampfer, M.J., Speizer, F.E., Patel, S., & Hu, F.B. (2003). A prospective study of sleep duration and coronary heart disease in women. *Archives of Internal Medicine, 163*: 205-209.

Bond, B.J., Perry, A.C., Parker, L., Robinson, A., & Burnett, K. (2002). Dose-response effect of walking exercise on weight loss: How much is enough? *International Journal on Obesity, 26*(11): 1484-1493.

Bravata, D.M., Sanders, L., Huang, J., Krumholz, H.M., Olkin, I., Gardner, C.D., & Bravata, D.M. (2003). Efficacy and safety of low-carbohydrate high-protein diets: A systematic review. *Journal of the American Medical Association, 289*: 1837-1850.

Byrne S., Cooper, Z., & Fairburn, C. (2003). Weight maintenance and relapse in obesity: a qualitative study. *International Journal of Obesity, 27*: 955-962.

Central West Health Planning Information Network. (2004). Obesity in adolescents, adults and older adults in Ontario. Retrieved November 31, 2004, from www.healthinformation.on.ca/reports/Central%20West%20HIU/2004/Obesity%20Report.pdf.

Claps, J.B., Katz, A., & Moore, M. (2005). A comparison of wellness coaching and reality therapy. *International Journal of Reality Therapy, 24*(2): 39-41.

Department of Health and Human Services. (2005). Overweight and obesity. Retrieved June 28, 2007, from www.cdc.gov/nccdphp/dnpa/obesity.

Department of Health and Human Services. (2006). BMI—body mass index. Retrieved August 13, 2007, www.cdc.gov/nccdphp/dnpa/bmi/index.htm.

Dinges, D., & Chugh, D.K. (1997). Physiologic correlates of sleep deprivation. In J.M. Kinney, H.N. Tucker (Eds.). *Physiology, stress, and malnutrition: Functional correlates, nutritional intervention* (pp. 1-27). New York: Lippincott-Raven.

Flegal, K.M., Carroll, M.D., Ogden, C.L., & Johnson, C.L. (2002). Prevalence and trends in obesity among US adults, 1999-2000. *Journal of the American Medical Association, 288*: 1723-1727.

Fogelholm, M., &. Kukkonen-Harjula, K. (2000a). Does physical activity prevent weigh gain: A systematic review. *Obesity Review, 1*(2): 95-111.

Fogelholm M., & Kukkonen-Harjula, K. (2000b). Effects of walking training on weight maintenance after a very low-energy diet in premenopausal obese women: A randomized controlled trial. *Archives of Internal Medicine, 160*(14): 2177-2184.

Fox, A.A., Thompson, J.L., Butterfield, G.E., Gylfdottir, U., Moynihan, S., & Spiller, G. (1996). Effects of diet and exercise on common cardiovascular disease risk factors in moderately obese older women. *American Journal of Clinical Nutrition, 63*(2): 225-233.

Hagan, R.D., Upton, S.J., Wong, L, & Whittam, J. (1986). The effects of aerobic conditioning and/or calorie restriction in overweight men and women. *Medical Science in Sports and Exercise, 18*: 87-94.

Irwin, M.L., Yasui, Y., Ulrich, C.M., Bowen, D., Rudolph, R.E., Schwartz, R.S., Yukawa, M., Aiello, E., Potter, J.D., & McTiernan, A. (2003). Effect of exercise on total intra-abdominal body fat in postmenopausal women: A randomized controlled trial. *Journal of the American Medical Association, 289*(3): 1323-1330.

Jakicic, J.M., Marcus, B.H., Gallagher, K., Napolitano, M., & Lang, W. (2003). Effect of exercise duration and intensity on weight loss in overweight, sedentary women. A randomized trial. *Journal of the American Medical Association, 290*: 1323-1330.

Jakicic, J.M., & Otto, A.D. (2006). Treatment and prevention of obesity: What is the role of exercise? *Nutrition Reviews, 64*(2): S57-S61.

Jakicic, J.M., Winters, C., Lang, W., & Wing, R.R. (1999). Effects of intermittent exercise and use of home exercise equipment on adherence, weight loss, and fitness in overweight women: a randomized trial. *Journal of the American Medical Association, 282*: 1554-1560.

Jeanie's Weight Loss Diet Now. (2007). 11 clever ways to fit fitness into your day. Retrieved September 19, 2007, from http://groups.msn.com/Jeanie'sWeightLossDietNow/moveit.msnw.

Jeffrey, R.W. (2004). How can health behavior theory be made more useful for intervention research? *International Journal of Nutrition and Physical Activity*. Retrieved June 28, 2007, from www.pubmedcentral.nih.gov/articlerender.fcgi?artid=509286.

Klem, M.L., Wing, R.R., McGuire, M.T., Seagle, H.M., & Hill, J.O. (1997). A descriptive study of individuals successful at long-term maintenance of substantial weight loss. *American Journal of Clinical Nutrition, 66*: 239-246.

Leibel, R.L., Rosenbaum, M., & Hirsch, J. (1995). Changes in energy expenditure resulting from altered body weight. *New England Journal of Medicine, 332*(10): 621-628.

Levine, J., Lanningham-Foster, L.M., McCrady, S.K., Krizan, A.C., Olson, L.R., Kane, P.H., Jensen, M.D., & Clark, M.M. (2005). Interindividual variation in posture allocation: Possible role in human obesity. *Science, 307*(January 28): 584-586.

Lowry, R., Galuska, D.A., & Fulton, J.E. (2000). Physical activity, food choice, and weight management practices among US college students. *American Journal of Preventative Medicine, 18*: 18-27.

McGuire, M.T., Wing, R.R., Klem, M.L., & Hill, J.O. (1999). Behavioral strategies of individuals who have maintained long-term weight losses. *Obesity Research, 7*: 334-341.

Middleman, A.B., Vazquez, I., & Durant, R.H. (1998). Eating patterns, physical activity, and attempts to change weight among adolescents. *Journal of Adolescent Health, 22*(1): 37-42.

Office of Nutrition Policy and Promotion. (2003). Canadian guidelines for body weight classifications in adults. Retrieved June 28, 2007, from www.hc-sc.gc.ca/hpfb-dgpsa/onpp-bppn/qa_public_e.html.

O'Keefe, J.H., & Cordain, L. (2004). Cardiovascular disease resulting from a diet and lifestyle at odds with our paleolithic genome: How to become a 21st-century hunter-gatherer. *Mayo Clinical Proceedings, 79*: 101-108.

Olshansky, S.J., Passaro, D.J., Hershow, R.C., Layden, J., Carnes, B.A., Brody, J., Hayflick, L., Butler, R.N., Allison, D.B., & Ludwig, D.S. (2005). A potential decline in life expectancy in the United States in the 21st century. *New England Journal of Medicine, 352*: 1135-1137.

O'Neil, P.M., & Brown, J.D. (2005). Weighing the evidence: Benefits of regular weight monitoring for weight control. *Journal of Nutrition Education and Behavior, 37*(6): 319-322.

Paxton, R.J., Valois, R.F., & Drane, J.W. (2004). Correlates of body mass index, weight goals, and weight-management practices among adolescents. *Journal of School Health, 74*(4): 136-143.

Qi, B.B., & Dennis, K.E.. (2000). The adoption of eating behaviors conducive to weight loss. *Eating Behaviors, 1*: 23-31.

Reddy, S.T., Wang, C.Y., Sakhaee, K., Brinkley, L., & Pak, C.Y. (2002). Effects of low-carbohydrate high-protein diets on acid-base balance, stone-forming propensity, and calcium metabolism. *American Journal of Kidney Disease, 40*: 265-274.

Schoeller, D.A., Shay, K., & Kushner, R.F. (1997). How much physical activity is needed to minimize weight gain in previously obese women? *American Journal of Clinical Nutrition, 66*: 551-556.

Taheri, S., Lin, L., Austtin. D., Young, T., & Mignot, E. (2004). Short sleep duration is associated with reduced leptin, elevated ghrelin, and increased body mass index. *PLoS Medicine, 1*(3): 210-216.

Tomeo, C.A., Field, A.E., & Berkey, C.S. (1999). Weight concerns, weight control behaviors, and smoking initiation. *Pediatrics, 104*: 918-924.

U.S. Department of Health and Human Services, & U.S. Department of Agriculture. (2005). Dietary guidelines for Americans 2005. Retrieved September 8, 2006, from www.healthierus.gov/dietaryguidelines/.

Wing, R.R. (1999). Physical activity in the treatment of the adulthood overweight and obesity: Current evidence and research issues. *Medicine and Science in Sports and Exercise, 31*(suppl.): S547-S552.

Wing, R.R., Venditti, E.M., Jakicic, J.M., Polley, B.A., & Lang, W. (1998). Lifestyle intervention in overweight individuals with a family history of diabetes. *Diabetes Care, 21*: 350-359.

Suggested Readings

For two professional books written by world leaders in the study of obesity, look up the following:

Andersen, R. (2003). *Obesity: Etiology, assessment, treatment, and prevention.* **Champaign, IL: Human Kinetics.**

Bouchard, C. (2000). *Physical activity and obesity.* **Champaign, IL: Human Kinetics.**

Suggested Web Sites

An excellent site from the U.S. government explains the problems of people being overweight and some solutions:

www.cdc.gov/nccdphp/dnpa/obesity

This is the home page for the Department of Health and Human Services information on overweight and obesity.

Three excellent sites offer important information on obesity:

www.nature.com/ijo/index.html

The *International Journal of Obesity* provides an international, multidisciplinary forum for the study of obesity. The journal publishes basic, clinical, and applied studies and also features a quarterly pediatric highlight.

www.naaso.org

For comprehensive information concerning obesity, look at the North American Association for the Study of Obesity Web site.

www.darchives.com/protected/uploaded/ publication/hpcwhpinobesityreportfinal.pdf

Central West Health Planning Information Network. (November 2004). Obesity in adolescents, adults and older adults in Ontario. Hamilton, Ontario. This 171-page report provides information on the prevalence of obesity in Ontario, Canada (numbers could be inferred to other areas in North America).

Two excellent sites from the U.S. government that explain body mass index:

www.cdc.gov/nccdphp/dnpa/bmi/index.htm

BMI—Body Mass Index: Home. Department of Health and Human Services, United States. This site provides excellent information on BMI, including a BMI calculator. It also includes additional links to such topics as nutrition and physical activity.

www.hc-sc.gc.ca/fn-an/alt_formats/hpfb-dgpsa/ pdf/nutrition/weight_book-livres_des_ poids_e.pdf

Office of Nutrition Policy and Promotion. (2003). Canadian guidelines for body weight classifications in adults. Health Canada: It's Your Health. This helpful article on obesity includes links to such topics as calculating your BMI and guides to healthy eating and physical activity.

Moving Your Body

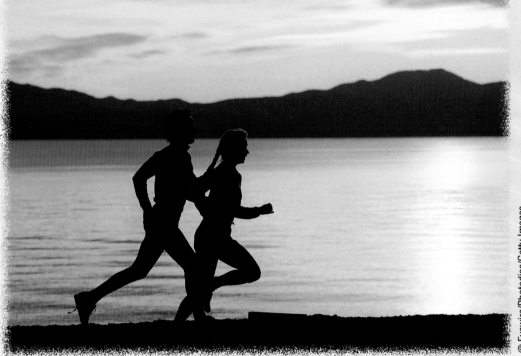

© Eyewire/Photodisc/Getty Images

Cardiorespiratory Assessment and Training

Peter Walters

After reading this chapter, you should be able to do the following:

1. Identify major benefits of cardiorespiratory fitness.
2. Describe three human energy systems.
3. Identify three benefits of cardiorespiratory endurance.
4. Define maximal oxygen consumption and explain physiological adaptations to increased oxygen consumption.
5. Describe several methods to evaluate your cardiorespiratory fitness.
6. Outline exercise prescriptions focused on enhancing cardiovascular endurance.

One of the most remarkable examples of human endurance is recounted by Alfred Lansing in his book *Endurance*. The book is about the failed attempt of English explorer Ernest Shackleton and his men to be the first to cross the continent of Antarctica over land. Unfortunately, they became stuck in some rather desperate conditions during their mission. Their ship was trapped in ice in the Weddell Sea just off the coast of Antarctica. The ice that surrounded their ship eventually tore it to pieces. They were nearly half a continent away from their stored provisions, and most of their supplies were lost as the ship was destroyed by ice. All this occurred at the beginning of a long, cold winter in which darkness ruled both day and night. The author described this season as follows:

> In all the world there is no desolation more complete than the polar nights. This is a return to the Ice Age—no warmth, no life, no movement. Only those who have experienced it can appreciate what it means to be without the sun day after day and week after week. Few men unaccustomed to it can fight off its effects altogether, and it has driven some men mad. (Lansing, 1959, p. 7)

With incredible determination, Ernest Shackleton and his 27 men returned to civilization almost two years later. Throughout the book, the one characteristic that stands out with amazing clarity is that Shackleton refused to quit. No matter the hopelessness of their circumstances, giving up was not an option. This trait was cultivated long before

Defining Terms

Health and fitness professionals use several terms to describe sustained work that builds the fitness of the heart and lungs. Some of the more common are *aerobic endurance*, *cardiorespiratory capacity*, and *cardiovascular fitness*. Most experts use these terms interchangeably to describe the rhythmic movement of larger muscle groups to tax the cardiorespiratory system. For the sake of consistency, the primary term used throughout this chapter is *cardiorespiratory endurance*.

his voyage. Shackleton's official family motto was, "By perseverance we will overcome." The ship that carried him and his men to the South Pole was named *The Endurance*. This dogged determination underlay one of the most amazing survival stories in polar—and human—expedition.

Simply put, Shackleton and his men had staying power. They were indefatigable: untiring, persevering, or incapable of becoming fatigued. That is the primary characteristic of **cardiorespiratory endurance**, which is the focus of this chapter.

Setting the Bar: Primary and Secondary Goals

The fundamental goal of this chapter is to educate and encourage you to move. For most of human history there was little need for movement motivation—survival depended on it. If you didn't move, you wouldn't eat or, perhaps worse, you'd be eaten. Times have changed. Modern conveniences, from premixed peanut butter (you wouldn't want to take the time or trouble to mix peanuts and butter manually) to Segways, which are being touted as human transporters, enable people to live without hardly moving a muscle. On-campus residents attend classes, write papers, and complete exams with little more than a quick stroll from the dorm to an academic building. Off-campus students have the added challenge of walking to their cars and driving to campus. Today, people can get along quite well with minute levels of movement.

I'm sure that our ancestors, who grew or hunted their food, built the homes they lived in, and made the clothes they wore, would consider it quite "odd" that people today walk on treadmills, climb stairs, ride bikes that don't go anywhere, lift weights only to put them back where they started, and perform a host of flexibility movements just to remain mobile. They would no doubt wonder at this sort of "meaningless movement." Yet, it is anything but meaningless to our health and well-being as we will soon learn.

Before we move on, let's be clear that the primary aim of this chapter is about infusing movement into an activity-deficient lifestyle that is zapping our energy and reducing the quality of life we could enjoy. The good news is that you don't have to run marathons or swim the English Channel. Your cardiorespiratory endurance plan can begin with something as simple as walking.

Surprised by the Simplicity

I was a full-time physical education student who also worked at a grocery store and had two volunteer jobs. Although other students and professors in my department were running, cycling, playing intramurals, or working out in the weight room, I thought I had no time for that and didn't participate in any activity that wasn't required of my program. A couple of events changed this. The Christian high school I had attended made no mention of caring for the physical body as part of my responsibility to the Lord. Now, I was learning through classes and readings that, indeed, I needed to be a good steward of my body. I was also learning that activity was a large part of wellness. Although I recognized by that point that exercise was valuable, I didn't really think I could do it; I certainly didn't know how to start. That changed one day when, through the suggestion of friends, God led me to a peaceful trail in the woods where I walked for two hours.

Three widely accepted health standards provide guidance about how much movement to aim for: walking 10,000 steps in a day, getting 30 minutes of physical activity most days of the week, or getting only 10 minutes of exercise several times a day (Centers for Disease Control and Prevention, 2006; Public Health Agency of Canada, 2007; Shape Up America, 2006). These recommendations are discussed in greater detail later in this chapter.

Some secondary objectives of this chapter are to identify the benefits of cardiorespiratory exercise, understand the body's three energy systems, measure your current **cardiorespiratory fitness,** and review several aerobic workouts that can enhance the stamina of your heart and lungs.

Benefiting From Cardiorespiratory Exercise

Most forms of physical activity have scientifically proven benefits. Few, though, can rival the number of rewards from cardiorespiratory exercise. Detailing each of these benefits could easily fill this chapter. Instead, I have focused on three primary benefits.

Fight Heart Disease

It's remarkable, but the body needs very little **aerobic exercise** to substantially lower the risk profile for heart disease. In one study of 2,678 adult men, those who walked only 30 minutes a day cut their risk for having a heart attack by almost 50 percent (McKinnon, 1999).

Cholesterol is often a focus of public discussion because, when elevated above acceptable levels, it is one of the major risk factors for developing heart disease. Most physicians recommend trying to maintain a cholesterol level below 200 mg/dL. Blood cholesterol between 200 and 240 is considered moderately high, while 240 to 270 is high. Any blood cholesterol measurement over 270 is considered very serious.

You probably have heard the term **cholesterol** and have seen TV ads for medications that lower cholesterol. You might also know that what you eat can affect your cholesterol level. However, sufficient cardiorespiratory endurance activity is far more effective, and cheaper, than any medication or "miracle" food.

Several years ago some well-controlled scientific studies brought great attention to the benefit of eating oat bran to lower blood cholesterol. The studies reported that by consistently consuming oat bran as part of the diet, the average person could expect a 1 percent drop in cholesterol (Kerckhoffs et al., 2003; Lovegrove et al., 2000). Compare that, though, to the average effect of cardiovascular exercise, which can lower total blood cholesterol by as much as 24 percent (Hales, 2001). Not only does consistent cardiovascular exercise tend to lower total blood cholesterol, it positively influences the ratio of "good" to "bad" blood cholesterol.

Cholesterol, primarily produced in the liver, is carried throughout the body by lipoproteins. There are two primary types of lipoproteins: low-density lipoproteins (LDL) and high-density lipoproteins (HDL). LDL is often referred to as "bad" cholesterol, because it tends to deposit the cholesterol in the blood stream, where it collects inside blood vessels. This process can ultimately block blood flow enough to cause a heart attack or stroke. Conversely, HDL is called "good" cholesterol, because it recovers, or picks up, cholesterol from the blood vessels and carries it back to the liver, where it is processed and eliminated from the body.

If your LDL is less than 160 and your HDL is greater than 50, the likelihood of your developing heart disease is two to four times less than the average person's. The way to positively affect these ratios is with regular cardiorespiratory exercise. According to Dr. Dianne Hales, the average person can expect a 10 percent drop in LDL and a 6 percent increase in HDL from consistent cardiorespiratory exercise (Hales, 2001).

Lowering blood cholesterol and positively affecting its good-to-bad ratio is just one of the many ways that aerobic exercise lowers the risk for heart disease. Other physical benefits include

- reducing your blood pressure,
- increasing your cardiac output (the amount of blood your heart is able to pump),
- reducing your risk of developing diabetes, and
- reducing your risk of obesity.

These are just some of the other major ways that aerobic exercise helps protect from this killer disease.

Get High on Exercise

Amazingly, some benefits come after only one workout. Researchers have reported elevated mood and reduced anxiety and depression after just one exercise session (Johnson & Morris, 1995). Since the 1970s, studies have consistently shown that regular cardiovascular exercise has a "tranquilizing effect" that decreases levels of anxiety and depression (Stathopoulou et al., 2006). One reason for this is the release of chemical substances by the body during exercise. One of these more popular substances is **endorphins.** Endorphins act as opiates, which decrease pain and produce feelings of well-being. The popular notion of a **runner's high**—a feeling of peace and euphoria reported by long-distance runners—is

suspected to be a result of endorphins. Evidence of this effect can be found in studies that use **naloxone**—a substance that blocks the effects of opiates, thus blocking euphoric feelings. In one study, runners completed two hard 6-mile runs on different days (Cobb, 1989). One day they were administered naloxone, and the other day they were administered a placebo—a pill that looked like naloxone but had no physiological effect. The runners reported no effect after ingesting naloxone; however, after taking the placebo which did not block natural opiates, the runners reported an increase in mood, even to the point of euphoria.

A growing body of research suggests that exercise can be an effective treatment for clinical depression. In one of the initial studies conducted at the University of Wisconsin, 24 patients diagnosed with moderate depression were randomly divided into either an exercise or psychotherapy group. The group that received psychotherapy met with a psychologist once a week, while the exercise group went jogging with a trainer three times a week for 45 to 60 minutes. After 12 weeks, about three-fourths of the patients in each of the groups had recovered from their depression. That by itself doesn't mean much. Depression often lifts within a couple of months, even if a depressed person receives no treatment at all. But the interesting results came later. After one year, half of those in the psychotherapy group returned for additional depression treatment, while none of the subjects in the exercise group returned (Griest et al., 1979).*

More recent, long-term studies suggest similar findings. Harris, Cronkite, and Moos (2006) published the results of a 10-year study examining the relationship between physical activity and exercise among 427 depressed adults. The results clearly indicate that more physical activity is associated with less concurrent depression, even after controlling for gender, age, medical problems, and life events. In fact, physical activity had a significant positive effect on depression to counteract the negative effects of both medical conditions and negative life events. Additional comprehensive reviews also suggest that exercise can be a powerful tool in the fight against depression (Seime & Vickers, 2006; Stathopoulou et al., 2006).

Enhance Immune Function

Recently, a great deal of attention has been paid to the effects of exercise on the immune system

---

*The study did not state whether the exercise group continued to exercise.

(Arey & Beal, 2002; Bruunsgaard & Pedersen, 2000; Gleeson & Nieman, 2004; Pedersen, Rohde, & Ostrowski, 1998). Concern has been raised over the drop in immune cell counts (i.e., lymphocytes, Natural Killer [NK] cells, and T helper and suppressor cells—which all serve to protect our bodies) after continuous endurance exercise and the suggestion that training will regularly suppress immunological responses. This has led to the "open window" theory, which suggests that immunosuppression 3 to 72 hours following exercise may allow viruses and bacteria to take hold. However, other findings support a positive effect of exercise and fitness on immune system function. First, while lymphocytes, a subset of leukocytes, increase during exercise and tend to decrease post-exercise, total leukocytes increase during exercise and continue to increase for at least 2 hours post-exercise. More importantly, resting levels of NK cells are greater in trained individuals compared to untrained individuals. A recent study examined the effects of 1 hour of cycling at 60 percent $\dot{V}O_2$max before and after a

12-week training period involving 30 minutes of cycling at 65 percent to 70 percent $\dot{V}O_2$max, 4 to 5 days per week (Rhind et al., 1996). Resting NK cell counts were 22 percent higher in the trained group and similar acute post-exercise drops of about 56 percent occurred in both the trained and untrained indivuals. Thus, while there may be a drop in immune function immediately following exercise, research supports an overall increase in immune function with increased cardiovascular endurance (Gleeson & Nieman, 2004; Pedersen, Rohde, & Ostrowski, 1998).

It's important to remember that the benefits described above are not exclusively reserved for endurance athletes but can be enjoyed by anyone who regularly participates in moderate aerobic exercise. There is more good news: Aerobic exercise is especially compatible for those who may think they are not athletically gifted. Most forms of aerobic activity (including walking, jogging, and biking) are fairly simple to master and can be performed in most environments. There is no excuse not to reap the rewards of aerobic movement.

 ## Endurance Without Limits

What are the limits to a human's endurance? If you think it's the Ironman Triathon in Hawaii, which involves a 2.4-mile swim, 112-mile bike ride, and 26.2-mile run, guess again. (In metric distances, that's a 3.8-kilometer swim, 179.2-kilometer bike ride, and 41.9-kilometer run.) Women and men have now successfully completed triple Ironman events. In 2002, a Slovenian man swam all 2,360 miles (3,776 km) of the Mississippi River (Aquatic Sports Records, 2002). More recently, the *Chicago Tribune* reported the story of two men who ran 50 marathons in 50 days in 50 U.S. states (Deardorff, 2006).

It's hard to imagine such feats of endurance. Yet, it's even harder to imagine anything or anyone who nevers grows tired. That is exactly what the prophet Isaiah says about God. "Do you not know? Have you not heard? The Lord is the everlasting God, the creator of the ends of the earth. He will not grow tired or weary. . ." (Isaiah 40:28). The Bible is filled with pas-

sages that attest to the immortal (enduring, everlasting) nature of God's plans, faithfulness, and work. Here are some examples:

- "But the plans of the Lord stand forever, the purposes of his heart through all generations" (Psalm 33:11).

- "Blessed is he whose help is the God of Jacob, whose hope is in the Lord his God, the Maker of heaven and earth, the sea, and everything in them-the Lord, who remains faithful forever" (Psalm 146:5–6).

- "I know that everything God does will endure forever; nothing can be added to it and nothing taken from it. . ." (Ecclesiastes 3:14).

When it comes to reading the roster of those with truly "limitless endurance," it's a pretty short list.

Understanding the Three Energy Systems

Here's the challenge: Run as far as you can as fast as you can. At the beginning you start out by sprinting (remember you've got to run as fast as you can). Pretty soon, after about 10 to15 seconds, if you're like most people, your pace will begin to decline from an all-out sprint to what might be considered fast running. Finally, after a couple of minutes of fast running, you will have to slow down to a jog. You will probably be able to jog for quite some time before you're too tired to continue. This example illustrates the three energy systems of the human body:

1. The phosphagen energy system (ATP-PC)
2. The glycolytic energy system
3. The oxidative energy system

Phosphagen Energy System

The body predominantly uses the **phosphagen system,** sometimes called the ATP-PC system, during a sprint. This system uses **adenosine triphosphate (ATP)** stored in skeletal muscle to produce muscular contractions. With regard to work, ATP is the "currency of the body." Without ATP, it's impossible to breathe, blink, or lift a pencil. The structure of ATP consists of adenosine and three phosphates. Energy (from 7 to 12 calories) is produced when the phosphate bonds are broken. ATP chemically becomes adenosine diphosphate (ADP) when one phosphate bond is broken. Fortunately, phosphocreatine (PC) is nearby to rebuild ADP back into ATP. Unfortunately, only enough ATP-PC exists in skeletal muscle to sustain about 10 to15 seconds of maximal muscular contractions.

Glycolytic Energy System

When a runner reduces pace from an all-out sprint to fast running, the body has sufficient time to produce additional energy (ATP) through what is called **glycolysis.** The **glycolytic energy system** takes **glycogen** stored in muscle or **glucose** stored in blood and quickly converts it into ATP so the body can continue working. The good news is that you can continue running at a fairly fast pace; the bad news is that your body produces lactic acid and hydrogen ions. As the hydrogen ions accumulate, muscular force is significantly reduced. Fortunately, if you slow to a jog, another energy system can kick in.

Oxidative Energy System

Going from hard running to a slow jog gives the body time to get rid of **lactate** faster than it is accumulated. Now the body takes stored carbohydrate, fat, and protein and coverts them into ATP; that's why the body can go for such long periods of time using this process to produce energy. This particular energy-producing system is called the **oxidative energy system.**

An important point to remember about these three systems is that oxygen is required only for the production of energy during the last process described. That fact is easy to remember because the process is called **oxidative metabolism.** The phosphagen and glycolytic systems don't require oxygen to complete their metabolic processes. That is the reason that activities that predominately use the first two energy systems are called anaerobic. **Anaerobic** literally means "without oxygen." It is important to remember that the oxygen being used is in reference to metabolic work, not merely respiration. Of course, it's still necessary to breathe oxygen while sprinting and running fast to sustain life, but not to produce the energy required for those activities. Table 5.1 summarizes the primary characteristics of each of the energy systems.

Because this is a fairly extreme example to explain how the energy systems work, two other points need clarification. I challenged you to run as fast and far as you can, but that kind of activity is rare. Most people spend their days sitting, standing, and walking, trying to expend as little energy as possible. They break this pattern occasionally with intermittent periods of exercise and work that call for additional energy resources. This distinction is important because people generally use the energy systems in the opposite sequence I described. The oxidative energy system is used during most daily activities. The body recruits the glycolytic and phosphagen systems when it needs additional energy quickly. This is an important distinction that will be explained in more depth later.

The second item that needs clarification is that the energy systems are not as isolated during most activities as in the example I gave. In reality, all three energy systems are available and contribute to the production of work, but in different proportions. Therefore, exercise physiologists can describe different activities roughly in terms of the percentage of contribution of the aerobic and anaerobic energy systems. Note some of these examples in table 5.2.

Table 5.1   Energy Systems Summary

Characteristics	ATP-PC	Glycolytic	Oxidative
Duration of activity	0 – 10 s	11 – 120 s	More than 2 min
Intensity of activity	High	High	Low to moderate
Rate of ATP production	Immediate	Rapid	Slow
Fuel	Adenosine triphosphate (ATP)	Muscle glycogen and blood glucose	Stored carbohydrate, fat, and protein
Oxygen used?	No	No	Yes

Data from National Strength and Conditioning Association, 2000.

Table 5.2   Approximate Percents of Energy System Contribution

Activity	Anaerobic (ATP-PC and glycolitic)	Aerobic (oxidative)
Tennis	85%	15%
Soccer	50%	50%
Basketball	75%	25%
Volleyball	90%	10%

Adapted from McArdle, Katch, & Katch, 2001.

Evaluating Cardiorespiratory Endurance

The first step in improving your cardiorespiratory endurance is assessing your current condition. Any of the four tests that will be described in this section will give you a good idea of your **cardiorespiratory fitness** level.

Resting Heart Rate Test

As the heart becomes stronger, it doesn't have to work as hard. One reason for this is that as people exercise aerobically, their stroke volume increases. Stroke volume is the amount of blood the heart pumps with each beat. The average adult pumps approximately 2.5 ounces (74 ml) of blood during each beat. As stroke volume increases, the need for the heart to beat as frequently decreases. It's not uncommon for an untrained person to reduce the **resting heart rate** by 8 to 10 beats per minute during the first 10 weeks of aerobic exercise (Nieman, 2003). This adaptation saves the heart about half a million beats each month.

Complete the first application activity at the end of this chapter to get an accurate measure of your resting heart rate.

Maximal Oxygen Consumption Tests

Resting heart rate may provide a general estimate of cardiovascular health, but a better measure of aerobic fitness is **maximal oxygen consumption, or $\dot{V}O_2$max.** In short, that's the maximum amount of oxgen the body is able to use. Maximum oxygen consumption depends on two factors: the delivery of oxygen via the blood and the ability of muscles, more specifically the mitochondria, to extract oxygen from blood and to use it to perform work.

The mathematical equation for calculating $\dot{V}O_2$max is as follows:

$$\dot{V}O_2max = HR \times SV \times (a - \bar{v})O_{2diff}$$

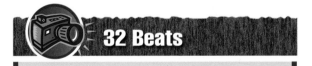

32 Beats

Lance Armstrong, six-time winner of the famous Tour de France bike race (1999-2005), is an extreme example of how much a heart rate can be lowered with regular aerobic exercise. His resting heart rate was an amazingly low 32 beats per minute (Sports Injury Bulletin, 2006).

Cardiorespiratory training results in physiological adaptations to body systems that improve capacity for respiratory oxygen intake, cardiovascular oxygen delivery, and muscular metabolism. Highly trained endurance athletes may have oxygen uptake values higher than 85 ml/kg/min, compared to values in the middle 30s for the untrained adult (Nieman, 2003). The following physiological changes collectively produce the ability to increase oxygen consumption.

- **Increased maximal ventilation:** The maximal capacity for airflow and oxygen diffusion increases due to endurance training. Maximal ventilation (amount of air inspired or expired in a minute) increases as a result of an increased tidal volume (volume inspired and expired during a normal breath) and an increased breathing rate. Highly trained endurance athletes may have ventilations in excess of 220 L·min-1, compared to the untrained adult at 120 L·min-1. Endurance training can easily increase ventilation to about 160 L·min-1.

  Reduced residual lung volume (the amount of air remaining in the lungs after full expiration) is also important. Essentially, this means that more of the lung is being used for gas exchange. Pulmonary diffusion (the amount of gas exchanged in the lungs) increases because greater blood flow to the lungs is available for gas exchange, and greater ventilation means there is more air in the lungs for gas exchange. The lungs become more efficient organs with a much greater capacity to provide oxygen and to eliminate carbon dioxide. It's important to understand that this particular adaptation occurs only during bouts of aerobic training in which maximal or near-maximal demands are made on the respiratory system.

- **Increased stroke volume:** The heart is made of a specialized muscle, called cardiac muscle, that responds to training by getting bigger (hypertrophy) and stronger. As the heart becomes stronger, it becomes more efficient at pumping blood. That is, stroke volume is greater during rest, submaximal, and maximal exercise in fit people than in unfit people. Resting heart rate and submaximal heart rate respond to this increased stroke volume by slowing down. Just as a car requires less fuel to go slower, the body requires less blood and oxygen at rest or during submaximal effort. Because more blood is pumped with each heartbeat, fewer heartbeats are required to provide the required blood and oxygen to the working muscles. Maximal heart rate is unchanged by training and is a function of age.

- **Increased capilarization and blood volume:** Another way the body responds to demands for more oxgen is by increased capilarization, which is sprouting new capillaries (small blood vessels) to carry blood within working tissues. With increased density and dilation of capillaries, more oxgen is available for the heart and working muscles. Additionally, blood volume is increased by small increases in red blood cells and much larger increases in plasma volume, resulting in a lower blood viscosity and, therefore, improved blood flow. In other words, small increases in the number of red blood cells and large increases in plasma volume lower blood viscosity, which improves blood flow.

- **Increased myoglobin and mitochondria:** Endurance training causes structural changes within muscle. One resulting adaptation is that the amount of muscle myoglobin increases. Myoglobin is the oxygen-binding compound in muscle, similar to hemoglobin in the blood, that assists oxygen extraction. In addition, mitochondria, which are the organelles in muscle that house the oxidative energy system, increase in number, size, and efficiency.

All these physiological changes are the body's way of responding to increased demands for oxygen. Collectively they have a dramatic effect on the amount of oxygen your body can use and, probably more important to you, on the amount of work you're able to perform.

Stroke volume (SV) is the amount of blood ejected by the heart in one cardiac contraction (one heartbeat). **Cardiac output** (CO) is the amount of blood pumped by the heart in one minute and is the product of stroke volume and **heart rate** (the number of cardiac contractions or beats in one minute). Arteries supply oxygen to the muscles. After this extraction of oxygen from the arterial blood supply, veins carry the remaining oxygen back to the heart. Therefore, the amount of oxygen used by the muscles is expressed as the arterial-to-venous oxygen difference $(a-\bar{v})O_{2diff}$. Simply put, it is the difference between the amount of oxgen inhaled and the amount exhaled.

It's important to take size into consideration when measuring $\dot{V}O_2$max. A larger person consumes more oxygen because he has more tissues that need oxgen, not because he is more aerobically fit. For this reason, $\dot{V}O_2$max is typically expressed in terms of **milliliters of oxygen per kilogram of body weight per minute** (ml/kg/min). By factoring in weight, it's possible to compare the cardiorespiratory fitness in individuals who are different sizes.

It's not possible to directly measure oxygen consumption without sophisticated laboratory equipment, but field tests exist that can yield indirect estimates of $\dot{V}O_2$max. I describe in the application activities at the end of the chapter three field tests you can use to estimate your $\dot{V}O_2$max: the 3-minute step test, 1.5-mile (1.92-km) run, and the 12-minute walk/run test. Please complete at least one of the tests before you go on to the next section.

Discouraged After Your Aerobic Assessment? Consider This....

How did you fare in your **cardiorespiratory assessment?** If you think the only good news from your test results is that you didn't die from a heart attack, don't be discouraged. The good news is that you have the potential to make dramatic changes to your aerobic fitness level in a relatively short time. If you don't have a genetic disorder or disease, you can reach an excellent level of fitness, according to the standards presented in the assessment section, typically in six to eight months of training. Furthermore, you don't have to run as hard as you can to experience improvement. If you follow the programs outlined later, you'll start off slowly and adapt to higher exercise loads in small manageable steps.

If you are skeptical about your ability to improve, note the following study conducted by Dr. David C. Nieman (2003), a well-known exercise physiologist at Appalachian State University. He measured the average amount of $\dot{V}O_2$max improvement in approximately 1,000 college students who trained for only seven weeks. Each student completed 30 minutes of aerobic exercise five times a week. As you can see from figure 5.1, the average female increased her $\dot{V}O_2$max from 36 ml/kg/min to 41 ml/kg/min. Men increased their $\dot{V}O_2$max from 49 ml/kg/min to 55 ml/kg/min. In summary, the average improvement for both sexes was about 13 percent in less than two months of exercise (Nieman, 2003).

If you completed the cardiorespiratory test with little difficulty, congratulations! You've probably already been doing some type of aerobic activity. Most likely you scored in the "above average" to "excellent" category. If you're not quite in the excellent group, you don't have far to go. With just a little extra push in terms of intensity or time, you'll be there. If you are already where you want to be, you need only a small investment of time for maintenance.

Outlining an Aerobic Exercise Prescription

The acronym FITT works well to help you outline and remember the basics of developing strategies for increasing cardiorespiratory endurance:

- Frequency
- Intensity
- Time
- Type

Understanding the **FITT principle** will help you to design an effective cardio program or, at the very least, to understand the critical components of any exercise prescription.

Frequency

Exercising three times a week for 30 minutes on alternating days is sufficient **frequency** to build aerobic fitness in most people. As your aerobic fitness improves, you may want to increase the number of sessions to between four and six per week. Increased frequency has some advantages. One study showed that six sessions per week were twice as effective as three at building cardiorespiratory fitness (Nieman, 2003).

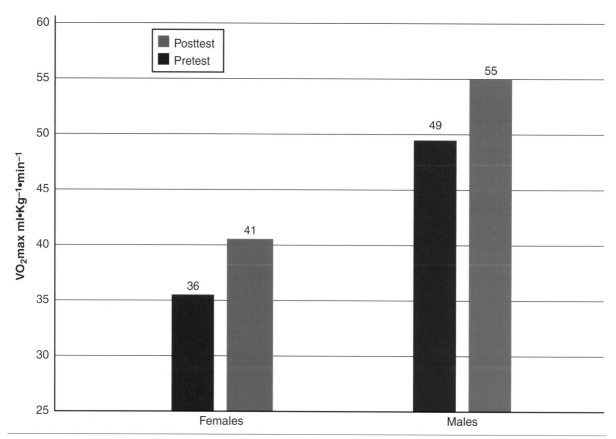

FIGURE 5.1 The average improvement in collegiates' $\dot{V}O_2$max in seven weeks of cardiorespiratory training.
Adapted from Nieman, 2003.

One of the biggest factors to consider when thinking about frequency is intensity, which is discussed next. For now, though, it's important to keep in mind that you'll need more time in between training sessions to allow your body time to recover if you're really pushing the intensity. On the other hand, you can probably train six or even seven days a week with no problem if your training is of relatively low intensity.

Age is another consideration when determining frequency. The younger you are, the more quickly your body recovers. As you age, be sensitive about how your body is feeling. You may need 48 to 72 hours of recovery after a hard cardiovascular workout.

Intensity

Many believe intensity is one of the most important factors in developing cardiorespiratory fitness (McArdle, Katch, & Katch, 2001; Sharkey, 2002). It's easy to make mistakes in one of two ways. If you don't push yourself hard enough, you won't improve. On the other hand, if you push yourself

too hard, you'll be susceptible to exercise-related injuries. So find a challenging, but safe, zone for exercise. There are two ways to determine an appropriate zone for aerobic exercise: target heart rate (HR) and rating of perceived exertion (RPE).

Target Heart Rate Zone

You have probably heard the term *target heart rate* as it relates to aerobic exercise. However, the correct phrase is **target heart rate zone.** A "zone" is important because it's nearly impossible to keep the heart rate at one specific speed, such as 173 beats per minute (bpm). In addition, it's very difficult to be that precise in an exercise prescription without a long history of training information. Therefore, it's necessary to establish a zone that has some variability and can be generalized to a broad group of individuals.

Target heart rate zone consists of a **lower and an upper limit.** For example, if the lower limit is 120 bpm and the upper limit is 153 bpm, an exerciser would work at an intensity level that keeps the heart rate between 120 and 153 bpm. If the heart rate moves above or below those limits, training intensity needs to be adjusted to get back into that zone.

You can calculate your target heart rate zone in different ways; I'll discuss two of them. First, there is a simple method that's easy to calculate and remember, and it's good for beginning exercisers. Those who have been training for a while will appreciate the increased accuracy of the second method.

1. The first, simpler method involves two steps.

   a. Figure your estimated maximum heart rate, or EMHR. You do this by subtracting your age from 220. If you're 18 years old, for example, your estimated maximum heart rate would be 202 bpm. You can tell from this formula that your maximum heart rate decreases with age.

   b. Then determine the lower and upper limit that falls within a range of a percentage of your estimated maximum heart rate. The aim is to work hard enough to maintain or increase cardiorespiratory function without working to the point of injury or dread of exercise because it is so painful. Exercising at less than 40 percent of maximum heart rate won't provide sufficient cardiorespiratory stress to increase or maintain fitness and health in adults (ACSM, 1998). So, the American College of Sports Medicine (Franklin, 2006) established 55 or 65 percent of maximum heart rate as the minimum intensity level for aerobic exercise (ACSM, 1998). In older, sedentary populations, the lesser percentage (40 to 60 percent) is advised. For young adults who are apparently healthy, 65 to 90 percent is recommended. The ASCM recommends not exceeding 90 percent of maximum heart rate as the upper limit.

Here's an example. Sue is 18 years old, so her EMHR is 202 (220 minus age). Her lower limit is 131 beats per minute (202 × 0.65). Her upper limit is 182 beats per minute (202 × 0.90).

2. The second method for calculating training heart rate zone is for those at an intermediate or advanced level of aerobic fitness. The only difference in this calculation and the one for beginning exercisers is that, instead of estimating maximum heart rate, the intermediate or advanced exerciser

New Formula for Estimating Maximum Heart Rate in Older Adults

Few, if any, mathematical calculations are more popular in the fitness and health world than "220 minus age equals estimated maximum heart rate." This calculation has been used in exercise testing and aerobic prescriptions for years. Even so, a group of scientists from Boulder and Denver, Colorado, questioned its validity. After examining heart rate values from 351 studies involving 18,712 subjects, Dr. Hanaka Hirofumi and his collegues discovered that this iconic fitness formula actually underestimated the true maximum heart rate of adults, especially older adults (Tanaka, Monahan, & Seals, 2001). The reason for this error is that studies used to establish the "220 minus age" formula used predominantly young subjects. Individuals 60 years and older were inadequately represented. Therefore, the scientists established a new formula that considered older subjects.

$$208 - (0.7 \times \text{Age})$$

For example, a 32-year-old would have an estimated maximum heart rate of 185.6 beats per minute (208 − [0.7 × 32]).

To further validate their findings, the researchers compared this new equation to actual maximum heart rates for 514 adults. The results of this well-controlled laboratory study reinforced the earlier findings. Therefore, if you're looking for a formula that more accurately determines estimated maximum heart rate in older adults, use this one even though it involves doing a bit more math.

directly measures it in various activities to reduce error.

The margin of error for the estimated maximum heart rate (220 minus age) generally ranges from plus or minus 10 to 12 beats per minute (Franklin et al., 2000). It's important to know that maximum heart rate varies by activity. For example, maximum heart rate during swimming is approximately 7 to 10 beats lower than during a run because the heart doesn't have to overcome as much gravity when the body is in a horizontal position as when it's in a vertical position. So, the bottom line is that determining accurate maximum heart rate through any exercise requires expending maximum effort. The target heart rate zone is more accurate when maximum heart rate is calculated accurately.

After you've calculated your target heart rate zone you will need some way of measuring when you are inside and outside of your zone. The best device for accomplishing this is a **heart rate monitor** (see figure 5.2). Most health and fitness products are gimmicks. However, from time to time a product comes along that can seriously aid anyone who exercises. Such is the case with a heart rate monitor.

A heart rate monitor resembles a traditional wristwatch (see figure 5.2). Wearing the chest strap and watch provides an accurate measurement of heart rate. But how accurate are the monitors? Several brands have the accuracy of a $25,000 ECG unit used in hospitals and research labs. That makes the $60 (U.S.) investment in this monitor quite good.

The alternative to investing in a heart rate monitor is to manually check the pulse during exercise, which is easier said than done. Doing this requires stopping exercise momentarily (which introduces error since the heart is in the process of recovery), finding the pulse, checking it for 10 or 15 seconds, and multiplying the count by 6 or 4, respectively, to estimate the beats per minute. Very few people can do this accurately. I strongly recommend spending a little money to ensure that you're training in the correct zone. Using a monitor is really like having a personal coach giving immediate feedback on your effort.

Rating of Perceived Exertion

A more subjective measure of intensity is perceived exertion. Simply put: How hard do you

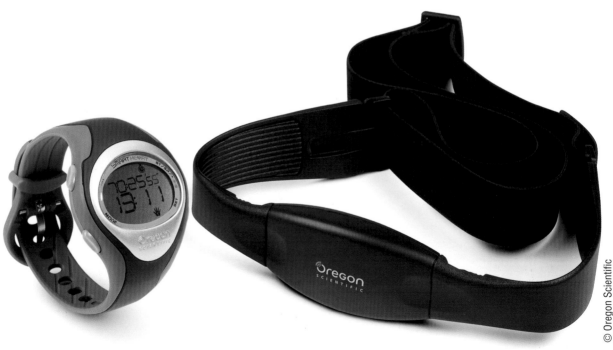

© Oregon Scientific

FIGURE 5.2   A heart rate monitor can be used as your personal aerobic trainer.

feel you are working? The most popular perceived exertion scale was created by Swedish exercise physiologist Gunnar Borg in the late 1950s. Borg studied the level of perceived exertion reported by subjects who worked at various levels of physiological difficulty. What resulted was the Borg Rating of Perceived Exertion scale (RPE; see figure 5.3) (Borg, 1998).

On the Borg scale, numbers run vertically from 6 to 20. Descriptive phrases help users choose the number that best reflects their perception of exercise intensity. Six represents hardly any exertion, while 20 represents the hardest work possible.

Why did Borg use markers of 6 through 20? Borg's early studies showed that in healthy young men, RPE multiplied by 10 was probably equivalent to heart rate. In other words, a heart rating of 60 (6 on the Borg scale) was resting; a rating of 110 (11 on the scale) was "fairly light"; a rating of 150 (15 on the scale) was "hard."

It's important to remember that your perceived exertion and corresponding heart rate may be quite different, because Borg's study included only healthy young men. However, studies do show a fairly linear relationship between exercise heart rate and RPE for a given subject, so individuals who have RPE values for a graded exercise test may be able to use RPE to exercise in their training zones—at least for the exercise mode on which the test was given (Brehm, 1998).

Time

It doesn't take a big investment in time to improve aerobic fitness, especially when beginning an exercise program. One study showed that aerobic fitness improved in low-fit subjects with as little as 10 minutes of cardiorespiratory exercise per day (Howe, 1999). In another study, only 5 minutes of daily, high-intensity exercise caused an increase in cardiorespiratory performance (Franklin et al., 2000). Although very short bouts of exercise yield benefits to someone just starting out, longer sessions are better for those with some experience. The American College of Sport Medicine recommends 20 to 60 minutes of aerobic exercise per session, excluding warm-up and cool-down time (Franklin et al., 2000).

Frequency, intensity, and time are interconnected. As your **aerobic capacity** increases, so will your ability to work longer, more frequently, and with greater intensity. Table 5.3 illustrates this progression.

Type

Cardiorespiratory exercise is continuous physical activity that has the capacity to raise heart rate to a level at which an aerobic benefit can occur.

6	No exertion at all
7	
8	Extremely light
9	Very light
10	
11	Light
12	
13	Somewhat hard
14	
15	Hard (heavy)
16	
17	Very hard
18	
19	Extremely hard
20	Maximal exertion

Borg RPE scale
© Gunnar Borg, 1970, 1985, 1994, 1998

FIGURE 5.3   Rating of Perceived Exertion (RPE).

Reprinted, by permission, from G. Borg, 1998, *Borg's perceived exertion and pain scales.* Champaign, IL: Human Kinetics, 47.

Table 5.3   Progression of Frequency, Intensity, and Time Based on Fitness Level

	Low fitness	Average fitness	Good fitness
Frequency (days/week)	2 – 3	3 – 4	3 – 6
Target heart rate zone (%)	60 – 75	60 – 85	60 – 90
Rating of perceived exertion	12 – 13	13 – 14	14 – 16
Time per workout (min)	10 – 30	20 – 40	30 – 60

Move Beyond Physical Endurance

Despite ability or motivation, there are limits to endurance. Legendary professional football coach Vince Lombardi said, "Fatigue makes cowards of us all" (Draper, 1992, p. 1103). Endurance limits apply not only to cardiorespiratory fitness but also to emotional, relational, academic, and spiritual fitness. There comes a point in almost every aspect of life when it's impossible to endure additional stress.

It seems much easier to accept physical limitations than relational, emotional, or spiritual ceilings. One reason for this is that there are no reliable methods to quantify levels of psychosocial endurance (e.g., trying to identify the point at which faith or hope have been maximized).

Another reason for the lack of clarity surrounding more subjective variables is that when people do seem to reach a breaking point, they rarely acknowledge the event as a true representation of their inner development. Consider, for example, a young man who often explodes in rage. After cooling down, he acknowledges that his anger won't improve the situation and resolves not to explode again. That person is acting as if the specific event is not characteristic of his behavior and that he can extend his tolerance simply by making a commitment to improve.

Denial and lack of reliable psychosocial measures are some of the things that make it easy to deny the fact that limits to patience, hope, and compassion do exist and are as real as **aerobic endurance**. God is in the business of expanding the limits of his children. The writer of Hebrews likens God's purposeful expansion to that of a loving father:

> Endure hardship as discipline; God is treating you as sons. For what son is not disciplined by his father? If you are not disciplined (and everyone undergoes discipline), then you are illegitimate children and not true sons. Moreover, we have all had human fathers who disciplined us and we respected them for it. How much more should we submit to the Father of our spirits and live! Our fathers disciplined us for a little while as they thought best; but God disciplines us for our good, that we may share in his holiness. No discipline seems pleasant at the time, but painful. Later on, however, it produces a harvest of righteousness and peace for those who have been trained by it. (Hebrews 12:7–11)

According to a recent *Newsweek* poll, the second most common reason people give for practicing religion is to become a better person and live a moral life (Adler, 2005). Although most people want personal and moral development, the path to obtaining maturity is not easy. The apostle James coaches, "Consider it pure joy, my brothers, whenever you face trials of many kinds, because you know that the testing of your faith develops perseverance. Perseverance must finish its work so that you may be mature and complete, not lacking anything" (James 1:2–4).

Fortunately (at least for me), God does not lose his patience with his slow-paced children. Paul, in his letter to the Philippians, confidently communicates "that he who began a good work in you will carry it on to completion until the day of Christ Jesus" (Philippians 1:6). Christians can confidently rest in the fact that the Heavenly Father works to expand the limits of our spiritual maturity.

The following section describes some of the more popular forms of aerobic exercise and outlines specific training programs for these types of activites. Don't limit your cardio options to these activities, though. There are literally hundreds of forms of cardiorespiratory exercise.

• **Walking:** This low-impact activity may be the most convenient form of activity in existence.

Walkers can exercise almost any time, in any type of weather conditions (walk indoors during inclement weather), with practically no special exercise equipment.

• **Jogging:** Almost 40 million Americans say they run for exercise (Club Industry, 2006). After a slight decline in the 1990s, jogging is on the rise. From 1998 to 2005, there was an 8 percent increase in the number of individuals in the United States that ran (Club Indusry, 2006).

• **Water workout:** It's not necessary to know how to swim to get an aerobic water workout. Dr. Jane Katz lists dozens of water exercises in her book *Aqua Fit* that get the heart pumping and blood flowing (Katz, 2003). Aqua aerobics can be extremely therapeutic for people with muscular injuries or joint problems.

• **Stair-climbing:** Stair-climbers are popular pieces of aerobic equipment in most fitness gyms. However, it's not necessary to go to the gym to get a good stair-climbing workout. Why not try climbing stairs in a dormitory or office building?

• **Elliptical machines:** Exercise on an elliptical machine is similar to stair-climbing, except that the feet move in an elliptical, or egg-shaped, pattern. This mode of exercise is wonderful for people just beginning a stair-climbing program or who have joint problems that can be exacerbated by compression.

• **In-line skating:** In-line skating can increase aerobic endurance and muscular strength and is less stressful on joints and bones than running or high-impact aerobics. In-line skaters can adjust the intensity of their workouts by skating on different terrain. They can also buy special training wheels and weights to increase resistance and make muscles work harder. One caution: Skaters need to wear protective gear, such as a helmet, knee and elbow pads, and wrist guards.

• **Cross-country skiing:** Data from various studies suggest elite cross-country skiers have the highest $\dot{V}O_2$max of any athletic group (Hales, 2001; see figure 5.4). Physiologist Erlend Hem reportedly measured 8-time Olympic and 9-time World Cross Country Skiing champion Bjorn Daehlie as having a $\dot{V}O2$max of 96 ml/kg/min during the off season (Wikipedia, 2007). Almost every muscle in the body gets a workout. The poles work the arms, shoulders, back, and abdomen, while the kick-and-glide action works most of the leg, hip, and abdominal muscles. Cross-country skiing provides a total-body workout while exposing the hips, knees, and ankles to relatively low levels of compression.

Forget FITT?

Some people find worrying about frequency, intensity, time, and type to be too much of a hassle. They want to just keep things simple. For those people, the 10,000 steps program may be ideal. There is only one requirement: Walk 10,000 steps each day, which is roughly equivalent to 5 miles (8 km).

Purchase a basic pedometer (available for less than $30). Wear it for a week while you continue to follow your normal routine. If you walk fewer than 10,000 steps a day, which most people do (the average person takes between 900 and 3,000 steps per day), set a goal to walk 500 more steps per day for a week. Continue to increase your goal by 500 steps each week until you are consistently walking 10,000 steps a day.

Here are some ways to increase the number of steps you take during the day:

• Walk to places (e.g., work, school, the store) that are close by. If you have to drive, you can still get in some additional steps by parking on the far side of the parking lot.

• Walk up and down flights of stairs instead of taking the elevator.

• Walk with friends to catch up on what's going on in each other's lives.

• Walk while talking to God; you may not come home (see Genesis 5:24).

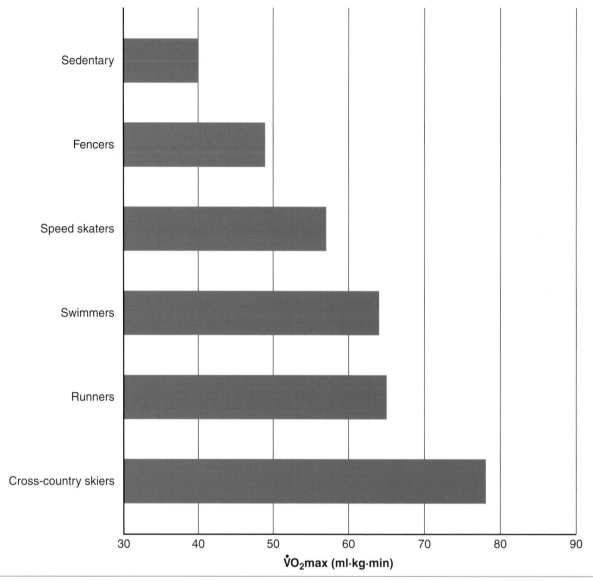

FIGURE 5.4   Cardiorespiratory fitness of various sport populations.

Adapted from Hales, 2001.

Sample Cardiorespiratory Fitness Programs

Although the FITT principle may sound quite basic, there's an art in combining frequency, intensity, time, and type into an effective program. Several sample programs in this section can serve as templates from which you can develop your own aerobic training program.

Walking

If you think walking is for wimps, let me challenge you to go to a track or get on a treadmill and walk 5.5 miles (8.8 km) per hour. My guess is that after 30 minutes you'll be breathing like a locomotive, your tibalis anterior muscles (muscles next to your shins) will be burning, and you will most definitely want to stop! Walking for exercise is quite a bit different than just casually strolling around campus or the neighborhood.

Studies at the University of Colorado that compared fast walking with both running and stepping up and down on a box demonstrated that, when worked with the same intensity, gains in cardiorespiratory fitness were similar for all three activities. What is even more interesting is that the runners missed an average of 11 workout

Guidelines For Putting Your Best Foot Forward

- Walk in comfortable shoes that fit well and have adequate cushioning.
- Walk tall. Maintain good posture.
- Focus your eyes on the horizon, or at least 10 yards (9 meters) in front of your feet.
- Use the heel-to-toe method of walking. The heel of your lead foot should touch the ground before the ball does.

Table 5.4   20-Minute Beginning Walking Program

	Mon., Wed., Fri.	Tue., Thurs., Sat.
Week 1	Easy walk*	Easy walk 5 min
		Moderate walk** 2 min
		Easy walk 5 min
	Time: 20 min	Time: 12 min
Week 2	Easy walk	Easy walk 6 min
		Moderate walk 3 min
		Easy walk 6 min
	Time: 20 min	Time: 15 min
Week 3	Easy walk	Easy walk 6 min
		Moderate walk 4 min
		Easy walk 6 min
	Time: 20 min	Time: 16 min
Week 4	Easy walk	Easy walk 8 min
		Moderate walk 4 min
		Easy walk 8 min
	Time: 20 min	Time: 20 min

***Easy walk** = 60 to 75 percent of estimated maximum heart rate

**Moderate walk = 75 to 85 percent of estimated maximum heart rate

days due to injuries, while the walkers missed only 1.5 days (Chen, 1999).

Walking is convenient, involves no special equipment, can be done alone or with a friend, and has a very low injury rate. Therefore, it's the mode of exercise that most experts recommend for sedentary people. If you had difficulty completing the aerobic assessment due to fatigue, begin with the four-week walking program outlined in table 5.4.

After you complete this program, you may want to make walking the centerpiece of your aerobic training. You could be like Edward Weston who, at the age 28, walked from Portland, Maine, to Chicago in 26 days—a distance of well over 1,000 miles (1,600 km). At age 44 he walked 5,000 miles (8,000 km) in 100 days, averaging 50 miles (80 km) per day. At age 71 he walked from Los Angeles to New York City in an incredible 77 days, averaging a little more than 42 miles (67 kilometers) per day (Wikipedia, 2007). You could save on fuel and walk home for holiday breaks!

If you're really serious, you could try to become an Olympic race walker, but you'd have to walk far and fast. How fast? The average person walks a mile (1.6 km) in 15 to 20 minutes. Michael Takaha, assistant track coach at the University of Houston, says that a good race walker typically walks that distance in about 6 minutes and 30 seconds (Takaha, 1985). One of the best books on improving your walking speed is *Walking Fast* by Therese Iknoian (1998).

If you are not satisfied with walking and want to introduce more variety, you can move to a walk/jog program outlined in the next section.

Should You Use Hand and Ankle Weights?

You may notice people in the gym or on the track with small weights around their wrists or ankles. Do these weights actually improve your workout? Studies show that using these weights provides only small gains in heart rate and number of calories burned (Makalous, 1988); similar gains can be made by exercising a little longer or harder. One other consideration made by some experts, such as Dr. Stephen Nicholas, team physician for the New York Jets, is that running with weights (specifically ankle weights) can dramatically increase your risk of being injured (Barone, 1994).

Jogging or Running

No one agrees on how to define the difference between jogging and running. The general consensus is that jogging is just a slower form of running, and that's sufficient for my purposes.

If you're just beginning but want to do more than just walk, start with the walk/jog program found in table 5.5.

If you want something a little more challenging, you can train for a 5K (3.2-mile) road race. The 12-week program outlined in table 5.6 will ensure that you're prepared to go the distance.

Swimming

Swimming is a popular pastime, but what really matters for aerobic conditioning is getting a good workout, not just getting wet. Your initial goal should be to keep churning through the water for at least 10 minutes using any of the traditional strokes (freestyle, butterfly, breaststroke, or backstroke). After you accomplish that, you're ready for the 20- to 30-minute beginning swimming program outlined in table 5.7.

A lot of people can swim the length of a pool, but few learn how to efficiently breathe, stroke, and kick so they can effortlessly glide through the water. If your technique is poor, you'll end up exhausted in no time. Water is 1,000 times denser

Table 5.5 20- to 30-Minute Walk/Jog Program

	Mon., Wed., Fri.	Tue., Thurs., Sat.
Week 1	Moderate walk*	Moderate walk 6 min
		Jog 1 min
		3 sets
	Time: 20 min	Time: 21 min
Week 2	Moderate walk	Moderate walk 5 min
		Jog 1.5 min
		4 sets
	Time: 24 min	Time: 26 min
Week 3	Moderate walk	Moderate walk 6 min
		Jog 2 min
		3 sets
	Time: 27 min	Time: 24 min
Week 4	Moderate walk	Moderate walk 4 min
		Jog 2 min
		5 sets
	Time: 30 min	Time: 30 min

*Moderate walk = 75 to 85 percent of estimated maximum heart rate

Running Form

Here are some key points on running technique from two top running coaches, Joe Henderson and Hal Higdon (Henderson & Higdon, 2004):

- Run tall. Your back should be erect and your head high.
- Look approximately 10 yards (9 m) ahead of where you are.
- Relax your shoulders and bend your elbows so that your forearms are almost parallel to the ground. When runners get tired, they tend to tighten the upper body, which drains energy and negatively affects fluid running form.
- Don't clench your fists while running. Imagine that you're holding an egg in either hand.

- Be careful not to overstride. When runners overstride, their heads tend to move up and down. This wasted energy distracts from moving efficiently in one direction—horizontally.
- Breathe in through your nose and out through your mouth. Develop a rhythm to your breathing, just as you would do for your stride.
- When you approach a hill, shorten your stride. Lift your knees higher and pump your arms more. If the hill is really steep, lean slightly forward.

Table 5.6 12-Week Plan for Completing First 5K Run

PHASE I 5K RUN PROGRAM			
	Monday	**Wednesday**	**Friday**
Week 1	Moderate run*	Moderate cycle**	Easy run***
	Time: 20 min	Time: 30 min	Time: 25 min
Week 2	Moderate run	Moderate cycle	Easy run
	Time: 24 min	Time: 30 min	Time: 28 min
Week 3	Treadmill run	Moderate cycle	Easy run
	Time: 27 min	Time: 30 min	Time: 30 min
Week 4	Moderate run	Moderate cycle	Easy run
	Time: 30 min	Time: 30 min	Time: 30 min

*__Moderate run__ = 70 to 85 percent of estimated maximum heart rate

**__Moderate cycle__ = 70 to 85 percent of estimated maximum heart rate

***__Easy run__ = 60 to 75 percent of estimated maximum heart rate

PHASE II 5K RUN PROGRAM			
	Monday	**Wednesday**	**Friday**
Week 5	Pace run* 1:15 min:s	Easy run**	Moderate run***
	Recover walk**** 1:15 min:s		2.0 mi (3.2 km)
	10 sets		
	Time: 25 min	Time: 40 min	Timed
Week 6	Pace run 1:30 min:s	Easy run	Moderate run
	Recover Walk 1:30 min:s		2.25 mi (3.5 km)
	8 Sets		
	Time: 24 min	Time: 45 min	Timed
Week 7	Pace run 1:45 min:s	Easy run	Moderate run
	Recover walk 1:45 min:s		2.5 mi (4 km)
	7 Sets		
	Time: 24:30 min:s	Time: 30 min	Timed

(continued)

Table 5.6 *(continued)*

Week 8	Pace run 2 min	Easy run	Moderate run
	Recover walk 2 min		2.75 mi (4.4 km)
	6 Sets		
	Time: 24 min	Time: 50 min	Timed

****Pace Run**= 85% or above estimated maximum heart rate
**Easy Run= 60-75% of estimated maximum heart rate
***Moderate Run= 70-85% of estimated maximum heart rate
****Recover Walk= Slow walking

PHASE III 5K RUN PROGRAM			
	Monday	**Wednesday**	**Friday**
Week 9	Pace run* 1 min	Easy run**	Moderate run***
	Recover walk 30 s		3.0 mi (4.8 km)
	14 sets		
	Time: 21 min	Time: 30 min	Timed
Week 10	Pace run 1:30 min:s	Easy run	Moderate run
	Recover walk 45 s		3.2 mi (5 km)
	10 sets		
	Time: 22:30 min	Time: 50 min	Timed
Week 11	Pace run 2 min	Easy run	Moderate run
	Recover walk 1 min		3.2 mi (5 km)
	6 Sets		
	Time: 18 min	Time: 40 min	Timed
Week 12	Pace run 2 min	Easy run	Race day
	Recover walk 1 min		
	6 Sets		
	Time: 18 min	Time: 10 – 15 min	
RECOVER WALK = SLOW WALKING			

*Pace run = 85 percent or above estimated maximum heart rate
**Easy run = 60 to 75 percent of estimated maximum heart rate
***Moderate run = 75 to 85 percent of estimated maximum heart rate

than air, so if your technique is off a little, your momentum will be impaired. The book *Extraordinary Swimming for Everyone* by Terry Laughlin has excellent instruction for learning proper swimming technique (Laughlin, 2006). Visit the Web site www.totalimmersion.net to find out more about the book and other resources.

Cycling

You can often zip along faster on a bicycle than you can on foot. For this reason, you can use biking to get exercise while running errands, getting to class, commuting to and from work, and just cruising around town. During poor weather, you

Table 5.7 20- to 30-Minute Beginning Swimming Program

	Mon., Thurs.	Tues., Fri.	Wed., Sat.
Week 1	Easy swim*	Moderate swim** 2 min, rest 1 min	Pace swim*** 1 min
		4 sets	Easy swim 2 min
		Easy swim 8 min	5 sets
	Time: 20 min	Time: 20 min	Time: 15 min
Week 2	Easy swim	Moderate swim 2 min, rest 1 min	Pace swim 2 min
		5 Sets	Easy swim 4 min
		Easy swim 5 min	4 Sets
	Time: 22 min	Time: 20 min	Time: 24 min
Week 3	Easy swim	Moderate swim 2 min, rest 45 s	Pace swim 1 min
		5 sets	Easy swim 2 min
		Easy swim 6:15 min:s	5 sets
	Time: 24 min	Time: 20 min	Time: 15 min
Week 4	Easy swim	Moderate swim 2 min, rest 30 s	Pace swim 2 min
		5 Sets	Easy swim 4 min
		Easy swim 7:30 min:s	4 sets
	Time: 26 min	Time: 20 min	Time: 24 min

Note: If you're monitoring your heart rate, know that your maximum heart rate will be 5 to 10 beats slower when you're swimming than when you're running.

*Easy swim = 60 to 75 percent of estimated maximum heart rate

**Moderate swim = 75 to 85 percent of estimated maximum heart rate

***Pace swim = 85 percent or above estimated maximum heart rate

Cycling

Safety is an important concern for outdoor cyclists. Each year in the United States, bicycle crashes kill about 900 people. About 567,000 people go to emergency rooms annually with bicycle-related injuries. Safety helmets can reduce the risk of injury by 85 percent.

Here are a few quick reminders for cycling safety:

- When riding outdoors, be sure to wear a helmet. Look for proof that it conforms to the Consumer Product Safety Commission (CPSC) standard for head protection.

- Make yourself visible. Wear reflective clothing if you can. If you can't, remember that drivers see bright pink, yellow, and orange most easily.

- Always follow the rules of the road—stick to the right, stop at stop signs, heed one-way signs, and so on.

(continued)

(continued)

In most U.S. states bikers are allowed 24 inches of space from the white line on the side of highways. However, automobile driv-ers aren't always aware of this rule, so pick your routes carefully to avoid congested areas.

Table 5.8   20- to 60-Minute Beginning Cycling Program

		Mon., Thurs.	Tues., Fri.	Wed., Sat.
Week 1		Easy cycle*	Pace cycle** 2 min	Moderate cycle***
			Easy cycle 2 min	
			6 sets	
		Time: 30 min	Time: 24 min	Time: 20 min
Week 2		Easy cycle	Pace cycle 4 min	Moderate cycle
			Easy cycle 2 min	
			5 sets	
		Time: 40 min	Time: 30 min	Time: 25 min
Week 3		Easy cycle	Pace cycle 6 min	Moderate cycle
			Easy cycle 2 min	
			3 sets	
		Time: 50 min	Time: 24 min	Time: 30 min
Week 4		Easy cycle	Pace cycle 8 min	Moderate cycle
			Easy cycle 2 min	
			2 sets	
		Time: 60 min	Time: 20 min	Time: 30 min

Note: If you're monitoring your heart rate, know that your maximum heart rate will be 3 to7 beats slower when you're biking than when you're running.

*****Easy cycle** = 60 to 75 percent of estimated maximum heart rate

******Pace cycle** = 85 percent or above estimated maximum heart rate

*******Moderate cycle = 75 to 85 percent of estimated maximum heart rate

can continue cycling using a stationary bike or wind trainer. A 20- to 60-minute beginning cycling program is outlined in table 5.8.

Indoor stationary cycling, also known by the trademarked activity Spinning, was introduced in 1987, and since that time it has become enormously popular. More than 150,000 people in 60 countries participate in indoor cycling classes every day. It has grown in appeal because it is time efficient; doesn't involve high impact on the joints; and people of all ages, skills, and fitness levels can participate (Hales, 2001).

If you enjoy multitasking, you can jump on a stationary bike while checking out your favorite TV programs, studying, or reading.

Can't Stand the Monotony?

Let's be honest: Most forms of aerobic exercise don't require much thought. People beginning an aerobic exercise program complain that aerobic exercise can be just plain boring and the motions are repetitive.

Popular antidotes to the boredom include enlisting a workout partner you can talk to, listening to music, or watching TV if exercising indoors. Another possibility is to meditate. Some Christians are leery of the term *meditation* because of its connotations with religious, New Age, and mystical metaphysical organizations. However, meditation is a spiritual discipline that has been practiced by Christians for thousands of years. David is described in Acts 13:22 as being a man after God's own heart, and David mentioned his practice of meditating on God's word and ways 12 times in the book of Psalms.

Spiritual leader and author J.I. Packer describes meditation this way in his book *Knowing God* (Packer, 1973, pp. 18-19):

Mediation is the activity of calling to mind, thinking over, dwelling on, and applying to oneself the various things one knows about the works and ways and purpose and promises of God.

It is an activity of holy thought, consciously performed in the presence of God, under the eye of God, by the help of God, as a means of communication with God.

Its purpose is to clear one's mental and spiritual vision of God, and to let his truth make its full and proper impact on one's mind and heart.

So why not try soaking in one the fruits of the spirit—kindness—on your next jog? Let the next sidebar be a primer before your next workout.

Kindness

The television cameras showed the air drop of supplies to a country subjected to drought and political oppression. Those who provided that food showed kindness. A few moments later, the cameras showed a young and undernourished boy gently brushing away flies from his dying parents. The boy, too, exhibited kindness.

A scriptural understanding of **kindness** focuses on knowing another's need (especially relatives, guests, and those that in some way depend on you) and helping to fulfill it (Gerhand, 1985). To not be kind, particularly to the poor, shows contempt for God, according to Proverbs 14:31: "But whoever is kind to the needy honors God." Showing kindness also

keeps the devil at bay (Ephesians 4:26–27). Once again, God provides fruit that involves giving to others, and giving this fruit becomes a sign of being one of God's chosen people (Colossians 3:12).

God "exercises kindness" (Jeremiah 9:24), especially through giving Christ Jesus to save humanity from sin. In addition, he is a God who "will meet all your needs according to his glorious riches in Christ Jesus" (Philippians 4:19).

Paul encourages Christians to get rid of things like bitterness and anger and to speak words that are uplifting. A proverb speaks of these kind words as "sweet to the soul and healing to the bones" (Proverbs 16:24). Paul

(continued)

(continued)

also says to be "kind and compassionate to one another, forgiving each other, just as Christ God forgave you" (Ephesians 4:32; see also Colossians 3:8 and 1 Peter 2:1–3).

It's necessary to show kindness to those in need. Furthermore, scripture notes that those who pursue righteousness and kindness will be blessed by finding "life, prosperity and honor" (Proverbs 21:21). Take a moment and pretend to angrily say something to someone, and feel your body become tense. Now pretend to say something kind to someone, and feel the tension release. Kindness helps the well-being of the recipient, and it also gives life and wellness to the giver.

Here are some questions to consider while working out:

1. How have I benefited from the kindness of God?
2. Who do I know who models Christ-like kindness?
3. How can I mature in kindness?
4. What are some of the ways I can begin applying this virtue?

Next Steps

Holding on during stressful circumstances is not only a mark of physical and emotional maturity but also of spiritual maturity (see 2 Peter 1:5–9). The concepts presented in this chapter should help you understand more fully how to increase your physical, emotional, and spiritual endurance.

Key Terms

adenosine triphosphate (ATP)
aerobic capacity
aerobic endurance
aerobic exercise
anaerobic
blood volume
capilarization
cardiac output
cardiorespiratory assessment
cardiorespiratory endurance
cardiorespiratory fitness
cholesterol
easy cycle
easy run
easy swim
easy walk
endorphins
FITT principle
frequency
glucose
glycogen
glycolysis
glycolytic energy system
heart rate

heart rate monitor
kindness
lactate
lower and upper limit
maximal oxygen consumption ($\dot{V}O_2$max)
milliliters of oxygen per kilogram of body weight per minute
mitochondria
moderate cycle
moderate run
moderate swim
moderate walk
myoglobin
naloxone
oxidative energy system
oxidative metabolism
pace cycle
pace run
pace swim
phosphagen system
resting heart rate
runner's high
stroke volume
target heart rate zone

Review Questions

1. Explain how the three energy systems of the body work.

2. Identify the difference between an aerobic and anaerobic exercise.

3. List three major benefits of developing cardiorespiratory endurance.

4. Identify several physiological adaptations that result from aerobic exercise.

5. Discuss the process for evaluating cardiorespiratory fitness.

6. Identify the key components of an aerobic exercise prescription.

Application Activities

1. **Resting heart rate**

Obtaining an accurate resting heart rate is harder than you might think because a lot of preparation is required to get an accurate measurement. The participant should not have eaten or exercised in the previous 3 hours and must lie in a prone position for at least 20 minutes before measuring the resting heart rate. Because of these requirements, most students perform this test after they wake but before getting out of bed in the morning.

If you have a heart rate monitor, simply place the chest strap as recommended by the manufacturer and obtain your heart rate. If you don't have a heart rate monitor, place your forefinger and middle finger on your carotid artery (on your neck) or radial artery (on the inside of your wrist) and count the number of heartbeats in one minute (see figure 5.5a–c). If you are taking this measurement manually, take at least two separate readings. The discrepancy between your readings should be fewer than four beats. Repeat this process until the discrepancy falls within the acceptable range. Take an average of your readings and compare this to the standards for resting heart rate (see table 5.9).

The following are some common mistakes people make while taking resting heart rate:

- Not taking enough time to become fully rested
- Performing the test in a seated instead of a prone position
- Using the thumb instead of the forefinger for palpation

2. **Three-minute step test**

This test requires you to step up and down on a step that measures 16.25 inches high (41.25

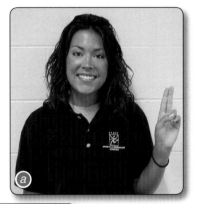
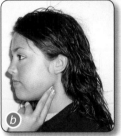
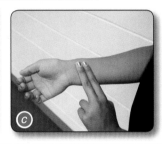

FIGURE 5.5 *(a)* Make sure you use the index or middle finger for taking your pulse; *(b)* measure your pulse at the carotid artery; or *(c)* measure your pulse at the radial artery.

cm) for three minutes (see figure 5.6). Many gymnasium bleachers have a riser height of 16.25 inches. Men step at a rate (cadence) of 24 per minute, while the women step at a rate of 22 per minute. This cadence should be monitored with the help of a metronome. A step cycle has four parts: step up with one leg, step up with the other, step down with the first leg, and finally step down with the last leg. A 24-step-per-minute cadence means to complete the entire step cycle 24 times in a minute. Most participants set the metronome at a cadence of four times the step

Table 5.9 Standards for Resting Heart Rate

Age (Years)	18 – 25		26 – 35		36 – 45		46 – 55		56 – 65		>65	
Gender	M	F	M	F	M	F	M	F	M	F	M	F
Excellent	40 – 54	42 – 57	36 – 53	39 – 57	37 – 55	40 – 58	35 – 56	43 – 58	42 – 56	42 – 59	40 – 55	49 – 59
Above average	55 – 65	58 – 67	54 – 64	58 – 67	56 – 65	59 – 68	57 – 65	59 – 69	57 – 67	60 – 68	56 – 65	60 – 69
Average	66 – 69	68 – 71	65 – 67	68 – 70	66 – 69	69 – 71	66 – 70	70 – 72	68 – 71	69 – 72	66 – 69	70 – 72
Below average	70 – 72	72 – 76	69 – 71	72 – 74	70 – 72	72 – 75	72 – 74	73 – 76	72 – 75	73 – 77	70 – 73	73 – 76
Poor	>73	>77	>72	>75	>73	>76	>75	>77	>76	>78	>74	>77

YMCA, 1989.

rate, in this case 96 beats per minute for men, to coordinate each leg's movement with a beat of the metronome. The women's step rate would be 88 beats per minute.

At the end of the three minutes, immediately stop, and while standing check your heart rate. It is best to use a heart rate monitor to ensure the accuracy of this reading. If a heart rate monitor is not available, manually palpate the pulse at the radial, or wrist, site within 5 seconds of completing the stepping portion of this test and count your pulse for 15 seconds. Multiply your count by 4 to determine your heart rate in beats per minute. Then use the appropriate formula on this page to calculate your $\dot{V}O_2$max. Compare your scores to the standards for maximal oxygen consumption to evaluate your cardiorespiratory fitness level (see table 5.10).

Your $\dot{V}O_2$max is determined from the heart rate (HR) immediately after this test by using the following formulas:

$$\text{For men: } \dot{V}O_2\text{max (ml/kg/min)} = 111.33 - (0.42 \times HR)$$

$$\text{For women: } \dot{V}O_2\text{max (ml/kg/min)} = 65.81 - (0.1847 \times HR)$$

For example, if a man finished the test with a recovery HR of 144 bpm, then

$$\dot{V}O_2\text{max (ml/kg/min)} = 111.33 - (0.42 \times 144)$$

$$\dot{V}O_2\text{max} = 50.85 \text{ ml/kg/min}$$

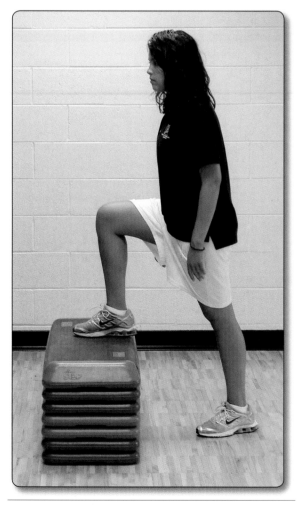

FIGURE 5.6 A step test is one of the fastest ways to estimate cardiorespiratory endurance.

The following are some common mistakes people make on this test:

- Having a box or step set at the wrong height
- Stepping either faster or slower than the required cadence
- Not checking the pulse immediately (within five seconds) after the test
- Not accurately measuring heart rate

3. **1.5-mile run test**

This test requires you to run 1.5 miles (2.4 km) as fast as possible. Setting an appropriate pace for this test is critical. Ensure that the distance for performing this test measures 1.5 miles. A standard 400-meter track would be ideal (6 laps = 1.49 miles, or add 16 more yards to get 1.5 miles). Warm up before you begin this test.

Start a stopwatch when you begin to run. If someone is monitoring this test, ask him or her to give lap times if you're running on a track, because this helps with pacing. Record the total time to complete the test. Use the formula on this page to calculate your $\dot{V}O_2$max. Compare your scores to the standards for maximal oxygen consumption in table 5.10 to evaluate your cardiorespiratory fitness level.

For men and women: $\dot{V}O_2$max (ml/kg/min)
= 3.5 + 483 ÷ time

Time = time to complete 1.5 miles
(2.4 kilometers) in nearest tenth of a minute

For example, if time to complete the distance was 11:12 (11 minutes and 12 seconds), then the time used in the formula would be 11.2 (12 seconds ÷ 60 seconds = 0.2 minute).

$\dot{V}O_2$max (ml/kg/min) = 3.5 + 483 ÷ 11.2
$\dot{V}O_2$max = 46.6 ml/kg/min

The following are some common mistakes participants make on this test:

- Not warming up sufficiently
- Not pacing correctly
- Forgetting how many laps they have completed

4. **12-minute walk/run test**

This test requires you to travel as *far* as you can in 12 minutes by walking, running, or using a combination of walking and running. It is important to warm up before you begin this test.

Start a stopwatch when you begin the test. Run if you are able, because this allows you to cover the greatest amount of distance. When 12 minutes have passed, measure the distance traveled. Note that the distance needs to be expressed in meters. To convert yards into meters, multiply yards by 0.9144. For example, 400 yards × 0.9144 = 365.76 meters. Use the formula that follows to calculate your $\dot{V}O_2$max. Compare your scores to the standards for maximal oxygen consumption in table 5.10 on this page to evaluate your cardiorespiratory fitness level.

Table 5.10 Standards for Maximal Oxygen Consumption ($\dot{V}O_2$max)

Age (Years)	13 – 19		20 – 29		30 – 39		40 – 49		50 – 59		60 +	
Gender	M	F	M	F	M	F	M	F	M	F	M	F
Excellent	≥51.4	≥44.2	≥51.4	≥44.2	≥51.4	≥41	≥48.2	≥39.5	≥45.3	≥35.2	≥42.5	≥35.2
Above average	46.8 – 51.3	38.1 – 44.1	46.8 – 51.3	38.1 – 44.1	46.8 – 51.3	36.7 – 40.9	41.8 – 48.1	33.8 – 39.4	38.5 – 45.2	30.9 – 35.1	35.3 – 42.4	29.4 – 35.1
Average	42.5 – 46.7	35.2 – 38	42.5 – 46.7	35.2 – 38	41 – 46.7	33.8 – 36.6	38.1 – 41.7	30.9 – 33.7	35.2 – 38.4	28.2 – 30.8	31.8 – 35.2	25.8 – 29.3
Below average	39.5 – 42.4	32.3 – 35.1	39.5 – 42.4	32.3 – 35.1	37.4 – 40.9	30.5 – 33.7	35.1 – 38	28.3 – 30.8	32.3 – 35.1	25.5 – 28.1	28.7 – 31.7	23.8 – 25.7
Poor	≤39.5	≤32.3	≤39.5	≤32.3	≤37.4	≤30.5	≤35.1	≤28.3	≤32.3	≤25.5	≤28.7	≤23.8

Data from 6th edition of ACSM's Guidelines for Exercise Testing and Prescription, 2000; Cooper, 1994; Franklin et al., 2000.

For men and women: $\dot{V}O_2$max (ml/kg/min) = $0.0268 \times$ (meters covered in 12 minutes) – 11.3

For example:

If a person completed 1,463 meters in 12 minutes, then

$\dot{V}O_2$max (ml/kg/min) = $0.0268 \times 1{,}463 - 11.3$

$\dot{V}O_2$max = 27.90 ml/kg/min

The following are some common mistakes participants make on this test:

- Not warming up sufficiently
- Not pacing correctly
- Not accurately measuring distance traveled

References

ACSM. (1998). Position statement: The recommended quantity and quality of exercise for developing and maintaining cardiorespiratory and muscular fitness and flexibility in healthy adults. *Medicine and Science in Sports and Exercise, 30*(6): 992.

Adler, J. (2005). Special report: Spirituality. *Newsweek* (September 5): 48.

Aquatic Sports Records. (2002). Ultra distance swimming records. Retrieved August 29, 2006, from www.angelfire.com/electronic/ultramentor/records_aqua.html.

Arey, B.D., & Beal, M.W. (2002). The role of exercise in the prevention and treatment of wasting in acquired immune deficiency syndrome. *Journal of the Association of Nurses in AIDS Care, 13*(1): 29-49.

Barone, J. (1994). Ankle weights: Do they work? *Men's Health, 9*(2): 16.

Borg, G. (1998). *Borg's perceived exertion and pain scales.* Champaign, IL: Human Kinetics.

Brehm, B. (1998). Perceived exertion. *Fitness Management, 14*(7): 35.

Bruunsgaard, H., & Pedersen, B.K. (2000). Effects of exercise on the immune system in the elderly population. *Immunology and Cell Biology, 78*(5): 523-531.

Centers for Disease Control and Prevention. (2006). Physical activity and good nutrition: Essential elements to prevent chronic diseases and obesity. Retrieved December 13, 2006, from www.cdc.gov/nccdphp/publications/aag/dnpa.htm.

Chen, J. (1999). Walk this way. *Women's Sport and Fitness, 2*(6): 2.

Club Industry. (2006). Study reports rise in the number of runners. Retrieved December 14, 2006, from http://fitnessbusinesspro.com/news/rise_runner_numbers.

Cobb, K. (1989). Managing your mile: Are you feeling groovy or burning out? *American Health* (October): 78-84.

Deardorff, J. (2006). 2 extremists teach a physical side to faith. *Chicago Tribune* (August 27): 13.7.

Draper, E. (1992). *Draper's book of quotations for the Christian world.* Wheaton, IL: Tyndale House.

Franklin, B.A. (Ed.) (2006). *ACSM's guidelines for exercise testing and prescription.* Philadelphia: Lippincott Williams & Wilkins.

Franklin, B.A., Whaley, M.H., Howley, E.T., & Balady, G.J. (2000). *ACSM's guidelines for exercise testing and prescription* (6th ed.). Philadelphia: Lippincott Williams & Wilkins.

Gerhand, K. (1985). *Theological dictionary of the New Testament* (vol. 9). Grand Rapids: Eerdmans.

Gleeson, M., & Nieman, D. (2004). Exercise, nutrition and immune function. *Journal of Sports Sciences, 22*(1): 115-125.

Griest, J.H., Eischens, R.R., Klein, M.H., & Faris, J.W. (1979). Antidepressant running. *Psychiatric Annals, 9*(3): 23-33.

Hales, D. (2001). *An invitation to fitness & wellness.* Belmont, CA: Wadsworth.

Harris, A.H.S., Cronkite, R., & Moos, R. (2006). Physical activity, exercise coping, and depression in a 10-year cohort study of depressed patients. *Journal of Affective Disorders, 93*(1): 79-85.

Henderson, J., & Higdon, H. (2004). Running form. Retrieved July 9, 2004, from www.runnersworld.com.

Howe, D.K. (1999). Fitness and exercise. *American Fitness, 17*(2).

Iknoian, T. (1998). *Walking fast.* Champaign, IL: Human Kinetics.

Johnson, P., & Morris, D. (1995). *Physical fitness and the Christian* (2nd ed.). Dubuque, IA: Kendall/Hunt.

Katz, J. (2003). *Aqua fit: Dr. Jane Katz's water workout program with yoga, Pilates, tai chi, and more.* New York: Broadway Books.

Kerckhoffs, D.A., Hornstra, G., & Mensink, R.P. (2003). Cholesterol-lowering effect of beta-glucan from oat bran in mildly hypercholesterolemic subjects may decrease when beta-glucan is incorporated into bread and cookies. *American Journal of Clinical Nutrition, 78*(2): 221-227.

Lansing, A. (1959). *Endurance: Shackleton's incredible voyage.* Wheaton, IL: Tyndale House.

Laughlin, T. (2006). *Extraordinary swimming for everyone.* New York: Total Immersion, Inc.

Lovegrove, J., Closessy, A., Milon, H., & Williams, C. (2000). Modest doses of B-glucan do not reduce concentrations of potentially atherogenic lipoproteins. *American Journal of Clinical Nutrition, 72*(1): 29-55.

Makalous, S. (1988). Energy expenditure during walking with hand weights. *Physician and Sportsmedicine, 16:* 139-143.

McArdle, W D., Katch, F.I., & Katch, V. (2001). *Exercise physiology* (5th ed.). Baltimore: Lippincott, Williams & Wilkins.

McKinnon, M. (1999). Walk your way to total health. *American Health, 18*(8): 74.

National Strength and Conditioning Association. (2000). *Essentials of strength training and conditioning* (2nd ed.). Champaign, IL: Human Kinetics.

Nieman, D. (2003). *Exercise testing and prescription: A health-related approach.* Boston: McGraw-Hill.

Packer, J.I. (1973). *Knowing God.* Downers Grove, IL: InterVarsity Press.

Pedersen, B.K., Rohde, T., & Ostrowski, K. (1998). Recovery of the immune system after exercise. *Acta Physiologica Scandinavica, 162*(3): 325-332.

Public Health Agency of Canada. (2007). Get active your way every day—for life. Retrieved June 8, 2007, from www.phac-aspc.gc.ca/pau-uap/paguide/start.html.

Rhind, S., Shek, P., Shinkai, S., & Shepard, R. (1996). Effects of moderate endurance exercise and training on in vitro lymphocyte proliferation, interleukin-2 (IL-2) production, and IL-2 receptor expression. *European Journal of Applied Physiology, 74:* 348-360.

Seime, R.J., & Vickers, K.S. (2006). The challenges of treating depression with exercise: From evidence to practice. *Clinical Psychology: Science and Practice, 13*(2): 194-197.

Shape Up America. (2006). 10,000 steps program. Retrieved August 30, 2006, from www.shapeup.org/shape/steps.php.

Sharkey, B. (2002). *Fitness and health* (5th ed.). Champaign, IL: Human Kinetics.

Sports Injury Bulletin. (2006). Lance Armstrong. *Sports Injury Bulletin.* Retrieved December 14, 2006, from www.sportsinjurybulletin.com/archive/lance-armstrong.html.

Stathopoulou, G., Powers, M.B., Berry, A.C., Smits, J.A.J., & Otto, M.W. (2006). Exercise interventions for mental health: A quantitative and qualitative review. *Clinical Psychology: Science and Practice, 13*(2): 179-193.

Takaha, M. (1985). *Race walking.* Oral presentation, Houston, TX.

Tanaka, H., Monahan, K., & Seals, D. (2001). Age-predicted maximal heart rate revisited. *Journal of the American College of Cardiology, 37*(1).

Wikipedia. (2007). Edward Payson Weston. Retrieved May 28, 2007, from http://en.wikipedia.org/wiki/Edward_Payson_Weston.

Wikipedia. (2007). Max Vo2. Retrieved May 28, 2007, from http://en.wikipedia.org/wiki/V02_max.

YMCA. (1989). *Y's way to physical fitness* (3rd ed.). Champaign, IL: Human Kinetics.

Suggested Readings

Bishop, J.G. (2005). *Fitness through aerobics* **(6th ed.). San Francisco: Pearson/Benjamin Cummings.**

Methodologies for performing all types of aerobic dance exercises are outlined. It illustrates step-by-step exercises, highlights various exercise methodologies, and teaches injury prevention.

Cooper, K.H. (1991). *The aerobics program for total well-being: Exercise, diet, emotional balance.* **New York: Bantam.**

This book from the originator of the term "aerobics" discusses how cardiovascular fitness fits into a holistic health.

Foran, B. (2001). *High-performance sports conditioning.* **Champaign, IL: Human Kinetics.**

Everyone from "weekend warrior" to competitive athletes can benefit from this guide to aerobic training for athletes.

Lee, B. (2003). *Jump rope training.* **Champaign, IL: Human Kinetics.**

Think jumping rope is for grade-school children? Think again. This book shows you how to get an incredible cardiovascular workout in minutes. One of the best things about learning to jump rope for exercise is that you can do it almost anywhere.

Stokes, R., & Trapp, D. E. (2003). *Aerobic fitness everyone!* **(3rd ed.). Winston-Salem, NC: Hunter Textbooks.**

Designed as a textbook for aerobic conditioning and dance. The goal of this book is to teach students to maximize their cardiovascular function.

Suggested Web Sites

www.phac-aspc.gc.ca/new_e.html

Canadian guidelines for physical activity and nutrition. A well-designed site with excellent health information.

www.totalimmersion.net

Instructional swimming material. One of the best resources for learning how to swim efficiently and for long enough to get a cardiovascular workout.

www.shapeup.org/shape/steps.php

Shape Up America: 10,000 steps program. A wealth of walking information targeted toward individuals who are just getting started on a fitness program.

www.fitness.gov/

President's Council on Physical Fitness and Sports. Although the target audience is primarily grade school–age children, a host of health-related material is available.

www.halhigdon.com

One of the best sites for beginning to intermediate runners who are running anything from a 5K to marathon road races.

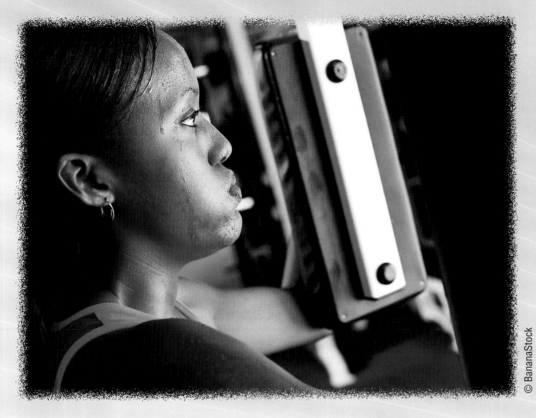

© BananaStock

Muscular Strength Assessment and Training

Peter Walters

After reading this chapter, you should be able to do the following:

1. Outline the benefits of strength training.
2. Learn how to evaluate muscular strength and endurance.
3. Understand basic muscle anatomy.
4. Identify four primary types of resistance training.
5. Outline a beginning strength-training program.
6. Learn seven guidelines for safe weightlifting.

The Greek civilization flourished politically, scientifically, intellectually, and architecturally during the sixth, fifth, and fourth centuries BC. Democracy was invented, astronomy was developed, Plato philosophized, and Sophocles wrote his great tragedies. People thanked the gods for this, and they held religious festivals in their honor. Athletic competitions, which began as peripheral parts of these celebrations, soon became the main attractions. None was more famous than the Olympic Games (Harris, 1993).

Probably the greatest champion of the ancient Olympics was the wrestler Milo of Croton (Harris, 1966). Born near the end of the sixth century BC, Milo competed until he was more than 40 years old, and was the only man ever to win six consecutive Olympic victories. Legend has it that Milo could break a ribbon tied across his brow just by expanding the veins in his forehead. After his victories, Milo reportedly cooked a small bull,

ate all of it, and washed it down with nine quarts of wine (Harris, 1966). Unlike Hercules, Milo's mythical hero, Milo achieved his great strength through training.

Setting the Bar

The goal of this chapter is not to teach you how to obtain the strength and muscular size of Paul Anderson, reputed to be the world's strongest man (see sidebar on this page). It is to help you obtain lifelong health benefits, such as reducing your risk of injury, strengthening your muscles and skeleton, increasing your metabolic rate, pleasantly altering your body shape, and having the strength to act with **goodness** toward God, others, and yourself (see sidebar on page 107). I have written this chapter for people who are new to strength training, so if you have been intimidated by athletes

World's Strongest Man

Paul Anderson was born in Taccoa, Georgia, on October 17, 1932. He would ultimately become one of the most dominant strongmen in the world. At 5 feet 9 inches (175 centimeters) and 360 pounds (163 kg), Anderson was the first man to lift 450 pounds (204 kg) from the floor to overhead. Olympic, World, and two-time U.S. national champion, Anderson held 18 American and 9 world records. In 1957, Anderson earned the title of world's strongest man from Guinness World Records because he lifted 6,270 pounds (2,844 kilograms) off the ground (Guinness World Records, 1957).

After achieving stardom, Anderson traveled around the world giving approximately

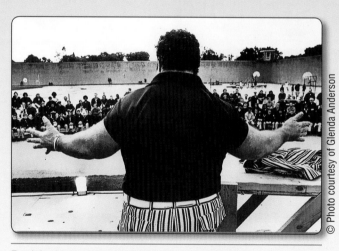

© Photo courtesy of Glenda Anderson

Paul Anderson speaking to a group of prison inmates.

500 strength exhibitions each year. During the demonstrations, Anderson would lift a platform holding 8 to 10 adult men and drive a 20-penny nail through a 2-inch (5 cm) board with his bare hands. Such feats are inconceivable to most people. To Anderson, who on some occasions repeated these performances three times in one day, they seemed like child's play. Yet this behemoth of a man concluded almost every incredible display of strength by simply saying, "They call me the world's strongest man, but I'm telling you that the world's strongest man could not live one day without Jesus Christ" (Jenkins, 1975). Whose strength do you rely on?

Goodness

The end result of developing strength is not about bulging biceps, bench pressing double your body weight, or even preventing neuromuscular injuries. In the final analysis, we want strength to bring about goodness – the goodness of God. At times, goodness must be supported by strength.

In his day, Jesus recognized the existence of evil forces whose primary aim was to steal, kill, and destroy any goodness in the lives of the people (John 10:10). Not only did he recognize evil, he moved powerfully against it. One of the most common miracles that Jesus performed was driving out evil spirits. When a group of religious zealots, called the Pharisees, saw Jesus casting out demons, they said he did this by the power of the "prince of demons" (Beelzebub). Notice Jesus's reply in Matthew 12:24–29:

> Every kingdom divided against itself will be ruined, and every city or household divided against itself will not stand. If Satan drives out Satan, he is divided against himself. How then can his kingdom stand?...But if I drive out demons by the Spirit of God, then the kingdom of God has come upon you. Or again, how can anyone enter a strong man's house and carry off his possessions unless he first ties up the strong man?

Not only did Jesus refute their claims on the basis of simple logic, he specifically mentioned superior strength as a necessary ingredient for this type of goodness. Moving into Satan's territory is just as fierce as claiming gang turf in any urban area of a major city. It's not work for the weak.

The prophet Micah outlines a less confrontational form of goodness in Micah 6:8: "He has showed you, O man, what is good. And what does the Lord require of you? To act justly and to love mercy and to walk humbly with your God."

This goodness sounds softer and more genteel than casting out demons. But if you think justice, mercy, and humility come from being weak, you've probably never tried to help oppressed people receive justice or to walk in humility in a culture that promotes self-promotion. This type of goodness is not only difficult – it is impossible. The apostle Paul recognized this when he wrote, "I have the desire to do what is good, but I cannot carry it out" (Romans 7:18). We should be thankful that we have a power (the Holy Spirit) that transcends our human strength and bears the fruit of goodness. It is only through God's power that we can bring about goodness in this world.

Goodness: Describe at least one act of justice, mercy, or humility that you would like to carry out in the next four weeks. Admit your lack of strength, and ask God for his strength to bring about this specific action.

_____

_____

_____

_____

_____

_____

_____

_____

grunting and screaming or by the complexity of equipment in most weight rooms, this chapter is for you. At the end of this chapter you'll find an effective, easy-to-follow, step-by-step program for college women and men to dramatically alter their level of strength.

Benefits of Strength Training

Although you may not have Olympic aspirations, you may have considered "pumping iron" to make your body stronger and firmer. What you may not know is that lifting weights can also help speed up your metabolic rate, develop strong bones, and increase your ability to work.

Shapes Your Body

A common misconception (and sometimes fear) among women is that if they lift weights they may end up with muscles like a man's. Actually, women have nothing to fear. Women do have hypertrophic capacities (see figure 6.1). **Hypertrophy** means muscle enlargement and is the opposite of **atrophy**, or muscle shrinkage. However, women's capacity to enlarge their muscles is much more limited than men's. The main reason is hormonal; men have 20 to 30 times more testosterone than women do, as figure 6.2 illustrates (McGlynn & Moran, 1997). High levels of testosterone help create a positive environment for building muscle.

Anatomical differences also limit women's hypertrophic capacity. Women on average have about half (40 to 60 percent) of the upper-body strength and three quarters of the lower-body strength of males because, although they have the same number of muscles as men, women have fewer individual muscle fibers (Incledon, 2005).

Women who lift weights are much more likely to achieve results like those seen in figures 6.3 and 6.4. These before-and-after photographs depict females who participated in an experimental 16-week resistance-training course. **Resistance training** specifically refers to lifting weights of various size in order to develop increased muscular tone and strength.

These pictures, rather than figure 6.1, illustrate the more typical body composition changes women can achieve through strength training. The average female in this 16-week class lost 11.7 pounds (5.3 kg) of fat while gaining 3.7 pounds (1.7 kg) of muscle. (Body composition changes were measured with a Bodpod, which measures changes in body composition via air displacement. This method of testing body composition is comparable to hydrostatic measures.). This experimental class was required to adhere to a strict regimen of not only resistance training but also of diet. Therefore, these changes are not representative

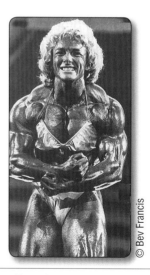

FIGURE 6.1　Bev Francis, champion female bodybuilder.

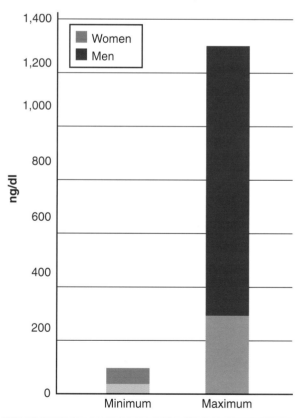

FIGURE 6.2　Men have 20 to 30 times more testosterone than women have.

Data from McGlynn and Moran, 1997.

of people who lift weights only. These pictures are not included to identify precise changes in body composition associated with strength training, but are used to provide evidence that women who train with weights will not develop large, bulky muscles.

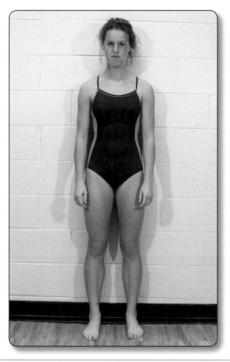 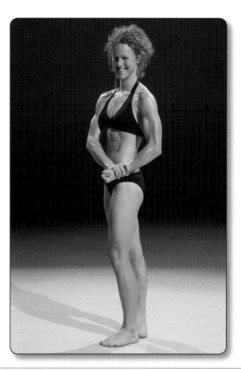

FIGURE 6.3   Corrie Walters lost 10 pounds (4.5 kg) of fat and gained 4.2 pounds (1.9 kg) of muscle.

Photos courtesy of Zachary Wenger

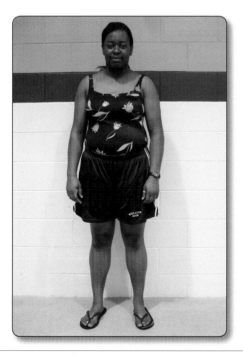 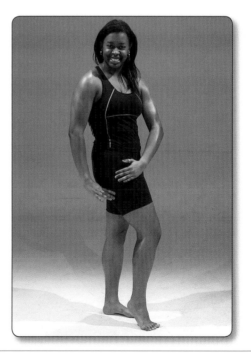

FIGURE 6.4   Elizabeth Woodson lost 22 pounds of fat (10 kg) and gained 3.8 pounds (1.7 kg) of muscle.

Photos courtesy of Zachary Wenger

Helps Boost Fat-Burning Metabolism

Weight training turns the body into a fat-burning machine. Simply put, **body composition** is the body's ratio of fat to nonfat. Everything that is not fat is lumped into the category of **lean body mass (LBM).** Muscle is the largest and heaviest component of LBM, but bones, organs, blood vessels, connective tissue, and other things are part of it as well. Since changes in body weight are nearly always changes in either fat or muscle, I have focused on those.

Different exercise methods bring about different results. In one study (Westcott, 1994), 72 men and women agreed to exercise for 30 minutes a day, three days a week, for 12 weeks. Twenty-two of the participants spent the entire 30 minutes in endurance exercise. The other 50 participants divided their workouts into 15 minutes of aerobic exercise and 15 minutes of strength training. Table 6.1 shows the changes in body composition for each group. The group that did strength training lost considerably more fat and gained more muscle than the group that did only aerobic exercise.

In this study, Westcott reported that the resistance-training group had greater fat loss because of how lean body mass affects resting metabolic rate. **Resting metabolic rate (RMR),** the rate at which the body burns calories when completely inactive, is profoundly affected by the amount of

lean body mass a person has. Each pound (0.45 kg) of muscle burns 30 to 40 calories per day at rest (Westcott, 1994; Darden, 1995), making it the most metabolically active substance in the body. (By contrast, a pound of fat burns one to two calories per day.) It follows that a person who gains 5 pounds of muscle (2.3 kg) will burn 150 to 200 more calories per day *doing nothing*.

The average adult between the ages of 30 and 65 loses half a pound (0.2 kg) of muscle per year (Westcott, 1994). This means that if caloric intake is unchanged, adults burn approximately 6,387.5 fewer calories (0.5 lb. of muscle burns 17.5 calories per day, since 1 lb of muscle burns approximately 35, times 365 days = 6387.5) per year. No wonder

Table 6.1 Changes in Body Composition as a Result of Strength and Endurance Training

Exercise	Weight change	Fat	Muscle
Strength + endurance	-8.0 lb (17.6 kg)	-10.0 lb (22 kg)	+2.0 lb (4.4 kg)
Endurance only	-4.0 lb (8.8 kg)	-4.0 lb (8.8 kg)	+0 lb

Effect of 5,004 Sit-Ups on Abdominal Fat

Dr. Frank Katch and other investigators set out to determine the effect of 5,004 sit-ups on abdominal fat (Katch et al., 1984). After measuring total body fat hydrostatically (underwater) and taking fat biopsies of the abdomen, subscapular, and gluteal regions, 13 men began a progressive sit-up routine for 27 days. As a group, the men performed a total of 5,004 sit-ups. Although cell diameter at all three biopsy sites decreased significantly, the study measured no significant differences in the rate of fat change in the abdominal area compared to the other areas measured (e.g., the gluteal tend subscapular).

This study was one more well-designed and controlled investigation that refutes the myth of spot reduction. The theory of spot reduction

suggests that, by exercising muscles around the region of the body that has too much fat, a person can reduce fat in that spot. For example, a person who wants to burn fat on the thighs would do many exercises that involve the quadriceps and hamstring muscles.

One study that tested this theory in a clever manner involved competitive tennis players. Tennis players exercise their dominant arms much more than their nondominant ones, so if spot reduction were possible, it would be evident among this group. When researchers measured the composition of muscle and fat in both arms, they found that the amount of muscle was significantly different, but there were no significant differences in the amount of fat (Gwinup, Chelvam, & Steinberg, 1971).

most adults experience creeping obesity, a gain of one or two pounds, or a kilogram, of fat per year as they get older.

Figures 6.5 and 6.6 graphically illustrate changes that occurred in two men who participated in the 16-week resistance-training experiment cited earlier. The average man in this study, whose aim was to lose fat while building muscle, lost a little more than 1 pound (0.45 kg) of fat per week, or 18.3 pounds (8.3 kg) overall.

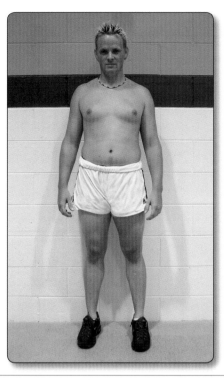
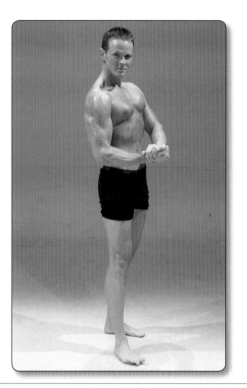

FIGURE 6.5 Brandon Lochstampfor lost 16.8 pounds (7.6 kg) of fat.
Photos courtesy of Zachary Wenger

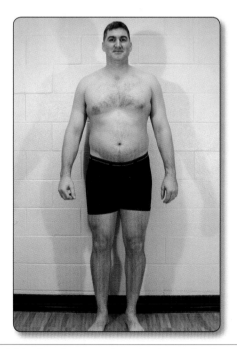
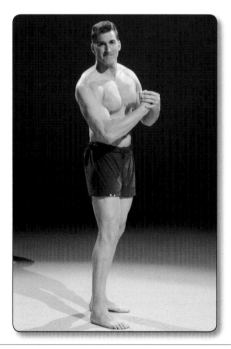

FIGURE 6.6 Bob Norris, who started at a body weight of 264.7 pounds (120 kg), lost 39.3 pounds (17.8 kg) of fat.
Photos courtesy of Zachary Wenger

Builds Strong Bones

Weight training delays and prevents the loss of bone tissue. Most people know that systematic resistance training strengthens muscles, but many people do not realize that it strengthens bones as well. Bones consist of weblike structures of collagen, calcium, and other minerals; the spaces in between the web are filled with marrow and blood vessels. **Osteoporosis** (derived from the Greek words for *bone* and *porous*) is the breakdown of the bone mineral web, making it more vulnerable to compression and shear fractures. This process tends to happen with aging: 55 percent of people over age 50 have low bone density (National Osteoporosis Foundation, 2003). Figure 6.7*a* is a magnified photograph of a healthy bone, and figure 6.7*b* is an unhealthy bone (National Osteoporosis Society, 2003).

Although scientists don't completely understand the causes of osteoporosis, the general progression is well documented. Bones are constantly being broken down (**osteoclast**) and rebuilt (**osteoblast**). In young people, the latter process more than compensates for the former; but sometime between ages 20 and 30, bone density peaks, and then bones begin breaking down faster than they are rebuilt. Because estrogen inhibits this breakdown, and estrogen levels decrease after menopause, the decline is especially dramatic in women.

Researchers have known for a long time that calcium supplements help prevent osteoporosis, but recent research indicates that resistance training is another critical component to consider. In one study, 39 women were divided into two groups. Both groups had adequate calcium intake, but the first group did strength training twice a week while the second group did not. After a year, tests showed that, on average, bone mineral density in the second group decreased by 2 percent, while it increased in the first group by 1 percent (Dornemann, 1997).

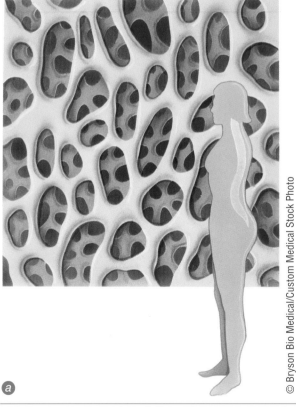

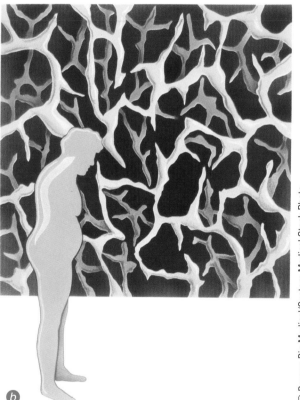

© Bryson Bio Medical/Custom Medical Stock Photo

FIGURE 6.7   Bone mineral density begins deteriorating in most people after age 25. *(a)* Healthy bone mineral density; *(b)* deteriorating bone mineral density.

Enables Endurance

Weight training enables harder and longer work. The ability to do physical work is called **functional capacity**. The average person's functional capacity peaks between the ages of 20 and 25, is maintained until about age 30, and then slowly begins to decline. Of the many factors that influence functional capacity, muscular strength is one of the most important. It's impossible to move without contracting a muscle.

An increase in muscular strength—that is, the ability to exert more force—is perhaps the biggest result of weight training and the first one you will notice when you begin a training program. Gains happen fastest at the beginning; several studies report a 30 to 40 percent increase in strength after only three months (Westcott, 1994). Weight training benefits people of all ages, too. Participants in a study of people over age 90, on average, more than doubled their strength after three months of weight training (Fiatarone, 2002).

People with sedentary desk jobs may think it's not important for them to have muscular strength, but they're wrong. One study showed that participants lost, on average, 30 percent of their neck strength simply by sitting at a desk for eight hours (Westcott, 1994). Subtle changes like these decrease energy and drain levels of productivity.

To summarize: Weight training will increase your muscular strength, metabolic rate, bone mineral density, and ability to work and play. Do you need any more incentives?

Assessing Muscular Strength

To know how to get where you're going, you first need to know where you are. Any strength-training program should begin with a measurement of your current strength level. At the beginning of his program, Milo could carry a newborn calf that weighed between 60 and 90 pounds (27 and 41 kg) the length of the Olympic stadium, which was a little more than 100 meters. Fortunately, things have changed somewhat since Milo's day, and you can assess your ability without bearing barnyard beasts on your back. The application activities at the end of this chapter include tests that measure both muscular strength and muscular endurance.

Muscular strength is the ability of a muscle or muscle group to generate maximal force, and it is usually tested by trying to lift as much weight as possible one time. **Muscular endurance** is the ability of a muscle or muscle group to perform repeated submaximal contractions or to maintain an isometric contraction. Muscular endurance is usually tested by lifting a submaximal load as many times as possible.

In the application activities at the end of this chapter, five specific strength tests are described. They are the grip test, the one-minute push-up test, the one-minute sit-up test, the bench press **one-repetition maximum (1RM)** test, and the leg press one-repetition maximum (1RM) test. Although both muscular strength and endurance tests are included, many strength professionals have noted strong relationships between these two components (Stone et al., 2006). Theoretically, people with a high degree of muscular strength should also be able to perform well on muscular endurance tests. If you make comparisons between muscular strength and muscular endurance, make sure that you test the same muscle groups during both examinations. For example, the one-repetition maximum (1RM) bench press and the one-minute push-up test would be a fair comparison, because both exercises use virtually the same muscles.

Strength: Encouragement and Possibilities

If you're disappointed with your existing strength, consider that one study (ACSM, 1998) found that 40 percent of boys and 70 percent of girls aged 6 to 12 can't do more than one pull-up. In fact, the average man can do only one, and the average woman can't do any. Well over half of all older women can't lift 20 pounds (9 kg) over their heads with one arm (ACSM, 1998). No matter how old or weak you are, you can get much stronger if you commit to a consistent strength-training schedule.

So how strong can you become? Here are some records from the *Guinness World Records 2004* (Guinness Book of World Records, 2004):

- *Most push-ups in one minute*: 133, by Jack Zatorski, USA, 2003

- *Most push-ups in one hour*: 3,416, by Roy Berger, Canada, 1998

- *Most one-arm push-ups in five hours*: 8,794, by Paddy Doyle, UK, 1990

Grip Strength

Force of grip has long been associated with strength (Baldo, 1996). Strongmen of old did not have Olympic barbells, dumbbells, or sophisticated equipment with which to measure and compare their strength. So they used what was readily available to them—coins, horseshoes, and rope.

Peter the Great, the first czar of Russia, was said to be able to break silver coins with the strength of his hands and fingers. Charles Vansittart, billed as "the man with the iron grip," could bend an Old English penny by holding it in one hand with finger and thumb and pressing it against the ball of his other thumb. John Marx, the Luxembourg strongman, was able not only to bend but also to completely break iron horseshoes in half. In the Middle Ages, Richard Joy from Kent, England, was reportedly able to break a rope that had a breaking strain of over 35,000 pounds (1,588 kg) with his bare hands (Gentle, 2000).

So how strong is your grip? Ironmind Enterprises (www.ironmind.com) has reignited interest in grip strength. Inexpensive plastic hand grippers targeted at enhancing grip have been available for years. Ironmind took this old concept to a whole new level. The company manufactures seven types of grippers with different resistances. The gripper that's easiest to close (to touch the ends together; see figure 6.8) requires 60 pounds (27 kg) of grip strength. The most challenging gripper requires 365 pounds (166 kg) of grip strength to close. Only five people on the planet have been able to accomplish that feat of strength at the time of this writing (Strossen, 2007).

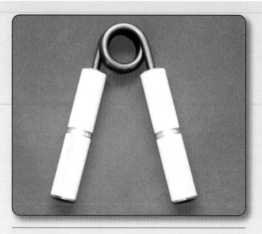

FIGURE 6.8   These all-metal grippers require a strong grip to close.

What would it feel like to shake hands with someone who can exert 365 pounds of pressure on your hand? It would be frightening if he wanted to cause harm. But if you were dangling from the rooftop of a high building or drowning in open water, you'd welcome a very strong grip in a loving friend. When Jesus' disciples were about to become very familiar with a world running in opposition to Christian thinking, he reminded them that they were safe in his grip. Jesus emphatically declared that "no one can snatch [sever or break] them [his followers] out of my hand" (John 10:28). He reinforced their secure position by adding that not only are they in his grip, but they also are in the grip of God the Father, who is strongest of all. "My Father, who has given them [his disciples] to me, is greater than all, no one can snatch them out of my Father's hand" (John 10:29). Rest assured: You're in good hands with God.

- *Most push-ups in one year:* 1,500,230, by Paddy Doyle, UK, 1988–1989

- *Most consecutive one-finger push-ups:* 124, by Paul Lynch, UK, 1992

You probably do not have the time or desire to better these records. But unless you have a debilitating disease, you should be able to meet the following standards, considered benchmarks of excellent physical strength, if you work at it.

The U.S. Army Challenge for Body-Weight Exercises

- *Men:* 71 push-ups and 78 sit-ups (a two-minute time limit is allowed for each exercise)

- *Women:* 42 push-ups and 78 sit-ups (a two-minute time limit is allowed for each exercise)

Weightlifting Exercises (One Repetition)

- *Men:* Bench press 1.5 times your body weight
- *Women:* Bench press your body weight
- *Men:* Parallel squat twice your body weight
- *Women:* Parallel squat 1.5 times your body weight

Basic Muscle Anatomy

Muscle comes in three types: cardiac, smooth, and skeletal. **Cardiac muscle**, found only in the heart, pumps blood through the circulatory system. **Smooth muscle** is found in the blood vessels and internal organs, including the digestive and reproductive systems, and performs a variety of functions. These two muscle types are involuntary, controlled automatically by the central nervous system. Only **skeletal muscle**, so named because it is attached to the bones, is under voluntarily control. Skeletal muscle is what people usually think of when they hear the word *muscle,* and that's the focus of this chapter.

Voluntary Neuromuscular Contraction

All voluntary muscle contractions originate in one place: the brain. When a person decides to move, the brain sends a message to the muscles through the spinal cord and nerve fibers, called **motor neurons**.

Like the roots or branches of a tree, these motor neurons split into tiny threads that activate each muscle fiber. Together, the motor neuron and the fibers it innervates are called a **motor unit.** Small motor units allow for precise, delicate movements (such as swiveling the eyeballs). Large motor units, like the ones in the thighs, enable heavy-duty tasks like running and jumping. Every fiber contracts either 100 percent or not at all, and the number and size of the fibers recruited by motor neurons determine the strength of the total contraction. For example, when biceps exert half the force they are capable of, it is because only half of the fibers are fully contracted, not because all of the fibers are half contracted. The nervous system recruits more motor units for stronger contractions.

Surrounding the entire muscle is a sheath of connective tissue called the **epimysium** (see figure 6.9). Within that are bundles of muscle fibers, called **fascicles** (a single bundle is called a fasciculus), each held together by an extension from the epimysium called the **perimysium.** Within the fascicle, the individual muscle fibers are separated by yet another layer of connective tissue, the **endomysium.** The muscle fibers themselves consist of thousands of **myofibrils**, the protein filaments that interact and slide by one another during muscle contraction.

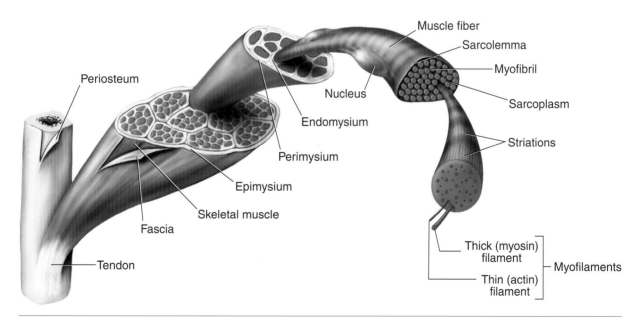

FIGURE 6.9   The structure of skeletal muscle.

Each myofibril comprises even smaller protein strands called **myofilaments.** The two types of myofilaments are **myosin** and **actin**, and they're arranged in units called **sarcomeres.** Sarcomeres are lined up end to end to form the myofibril (see figure 6.10). During a muscle contraction, the myosin reaches out with its hairlike arms, attaches to special sites along the actin, and pulls the two filaments past each other. It releases, reattaches, and continues pulling until the full contraction is achieved.

Although it is interesting to know the mechanisms for muscular contraction, it is critical to know the major muscles of the body. Everyone, male or female, has 614 muscles, but for the purposes of strength training you need to be familiar with only about two dozen of them. Figure 6.11 highlights the primary muscles you should be familiar with (National Strength and Conditioning Association, 1994).

Figures 6.13 and 6.14 on page 119 show two exercises that specifically target the erector spinae muscles. You can adjust the resistance in the incline back extension exercise by changing your arm placement. Placing your arms beside the hips is a good place to start, because that reduces the amount of resistance you are working against.

When your lower back gets stronger, try crossing your arms in front of your chest while performing this movement (see figure 6.13 on page 119). Doing so raises your center of gravity, increasing the resistance. If that doesn't make this movement hard enough, extend your arms above your head as if you were going to surrender to an enemy.

Training Concepts

Carrying a 90-pound (41 kg) calf is not an amazing feat. But Milo carried his calf day after day. As the calf grew larger, Milo grew stronger. According to legend, Milo could still carry the calf when it weighed more than 1,000 pounds (454 kg) (Harris, 1993). Milo had discovered the fundamental insight of strength training, now known as the **overload principle**: The way to get stronger is to subject muscles to gradually increasing resistance.

Sets, **repetitions**, **rest intervals**, and many other elements—not to mention the hundreds of possible exercises—make strength training seem very complicated. An understanding of a few terms and principles, however, can clear things up quickly. The following section on types of strength training covers those terms and principles.

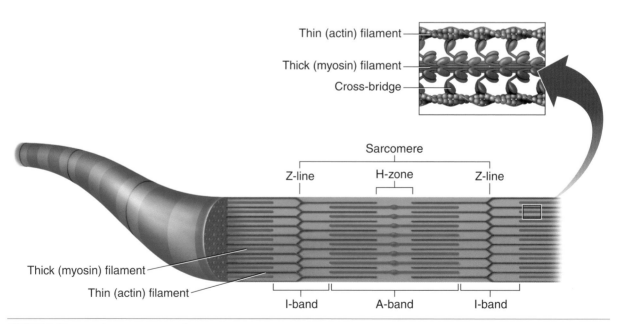

FIGURE 6.10 The functional unit of skeletal muscle is the sarcomere.

Reprinted, by permission, from R. Behnke, 2006, *Kinetic anatomy*, 2nd ed. (Champaign, IL: Human Kinetics), 14.

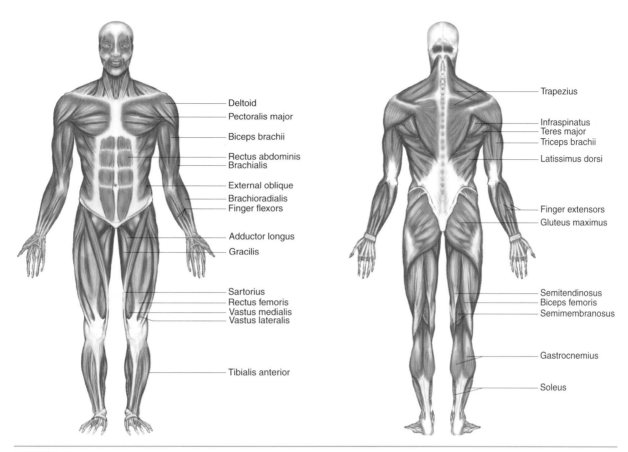

FIGURE 6.11 Major muscles targeted during strength training.

Reprinted, by permission, from National Strength and Conditioning Association, 2000, *NSCA's essentials of strength training and conditioning,* 2nd ed. (Champaign, IL: Human Kinetics), 29.

The Weakest Link

Lower-back pain is the second most common health problem in the United States, ranking just below the common cold (Wipf & Deyo, 1995). Eight out of ten people will have lower-back pain at some point (Eidelson, 2006). Back pain is responsible for more days in the hospital than any other medical condition except childbirth (Reynolds et al., 1990). At any given time, 31 million Americans have lower-back pain; 80 million Americans have recurring back distress (Sharkey, 2002). All this pain and suffering costs individuals, companies, and the entire health care system a significant amount of money. The average cost for an American with lower-back pain is $6,000 per occurrence. Liberty Mutual Insurance Company, the largest payer of workers' compensation claims, pays out $1 million each day to cover claims from people with lower-back maladies. The total estimated cost of lower-back pain is $16 billion per year (Hochschuler, 1991). These statistics have been used to argue that the lower back is the weakest link in the human muscular chain. Although that is debatable, there is no argument that lower-back pain is a serious health care concern.

Although the role of strength training in preventing and treating back injuries is still being investigated, growing evidence suggests that the strength of the lower back plays an important role. One long-term study examined the effect of lower-back strengthening on 50

(continued)

postmenopausal women. Those who engaged in resistance exercises not only had greater bone mineral but also experienced far fewer back injuries. In fact, the control group, which didn't perform any resistance exercises for the lower back, had 2.7 times more lumbar factures than the strength-training group during an eight-year period (Sinaki et al., 2002). This is only one of the many studies suggesting a positive relationship between lower-back strength and reduced lower-back pain and injury (Seung-Houn, Sung-Hwan, & Ji-Han Seo, 2004; Wheeler, 1995). One of the primary muscle groups responsible for lower back strength is the erector spinae (see figure 6.12).

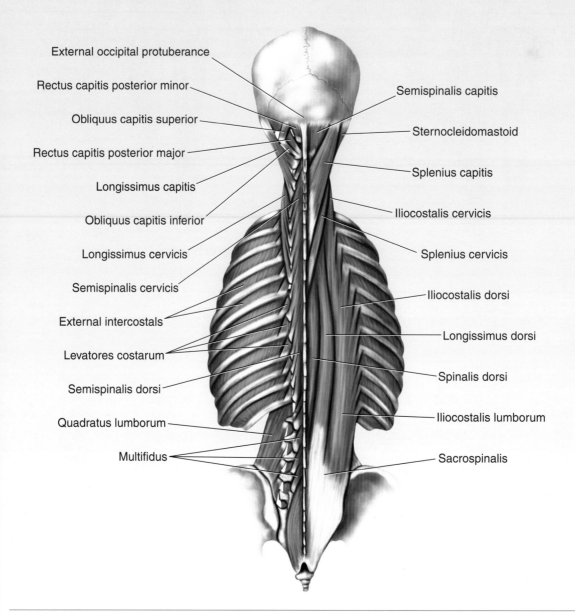

External occipital protuberance
Rectus capitis posterior minor
Obliquus capitis superior
Rectus capitis posterior major
Longissimus capitis
Obliquus capitis inferior
Longissimus cervicis
Semispinalis cervicis
External intercostals
Levatores costarum
Semispinalis dorsi
Quadratus lumborum
Multifidus

Semispinalis capitis
Sternocleidomastoid
Splenius capitis
Iliocostalis cervicis
Splenius cervicis
Iliocostalis dorsi
Longissimus dorsi
Spinalis dorsi
Iliocostalis lumborum
Sacrospinalis

FIGURE 6.12 The erector muscles run parallel to the spine and are essential to a strong lower back.

Reprinted, by permission, from R. Behnke, 2006, *Kinetic anatomy,* 2nd ed. (Champaign, IL: Human Kinetics), 134.

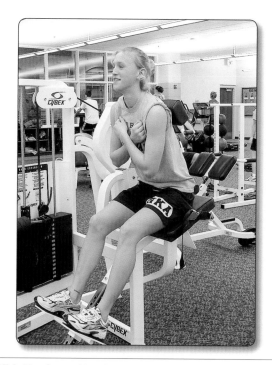 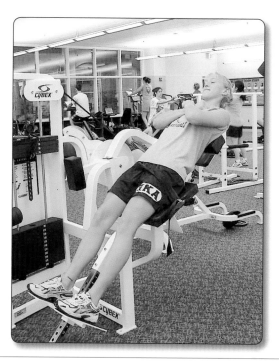

FIGURE 6.13   Seated back extension. Lean back so your upper back is in a straight line with your legs.

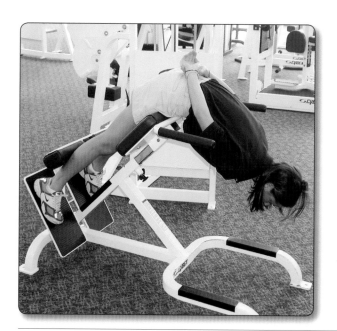 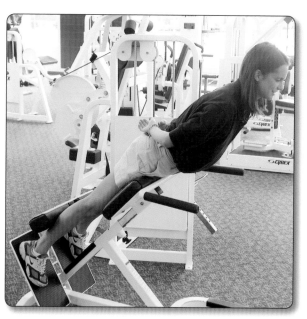

FIGURE 6.14   Incline back extension. Rise up so your upper back is in a straight line with your legs.

Types of Strength Training

Today, most people think of dumbbells, barbells, and weight machines when they hear the words *strength training*. Those words simply name types of equipment used to create four fundamental methods of resistance:

1. Isometric
2. Isokinetic
3. Isotonic
4. Variable resistance

• **Isometric** means "equal length." In isometric exercise, muscles contract without the body's moving. Standing in a doorway and pushing against the frame with the arms is an example of isometric exercise. In the 1920s, Charles Atlas popularized this method of strength training, which he called dynamic tension. Atlas promised that even the "98-pound weakling" who followed his mail-order program would never again "have sand kicked in his face" (Atlas, 2003). Few people today train with isometric exercise, though, because it develops strength within a very small range of motion (at most, 20 degrees in each direction from the point of contraction) (National Strength and Conditioning Association, 1994).

• **Isokinetic** means "equal motion." The rate of movement is controlled in isokinetic exercise. Machines are specially designed so that no matter how hard an exerciser pushes or pulls the set speed remains constant. This type of resistance training is most often used by athletic trainers and physical therapists measuring or rehabilitating patients from injury.

• **Isotonic** means "equal tension," where force remains constant. Free weights and many machines are in this category. A 50-pound (23 kg) dumbbell, for instance, weighs 50 pounds throughout a lift. Even though the weight stays the same, research shows that the force exerted by the muscles varies because of mechanical advantage and other factors (Fleck & Kraemer, 1997).

• Machines with levers, cams, and pulleys, or barbells with bands and chains attached facilitate **variable resistance** exercise. Variable resistance exercises change the resistance to compensate for changes in mechanical advantage. For example, during an arm curl the biceps work the hardest when the angle of the elbow is between 80 and 100 degrees, so an exerciser should be able to handle more resistance at the beginning (between 180 and 100 degrees) and at the end (between 80 and 5 degrees) of the movement.

Few weight trainers talk about those four methods of resistance. They simply refer to using either free weights or machines. Resistance machines are designed for safety, simplicity, speed, and specificity. It's almost impossible to use incorrect form when training on a resistance machine. The body may not be at the perfect height or angle out of ignorance of specific adjustments or failure to take the time to make personalized changes to individual machines, but resistance machines guide the user through predetermined planes of movement. In some ways, using the machine is like having a spotter who will not allow the arms, torso, or legs to move in a manner other than the correct one. These controlled movement patterns are especially helpful for beginners learning new movements.

Speed is another benefit of using machines. They provide faster workouts because it doesn't take much time to change resistance. Sometimes all it takes is moving a metal pin. When using free weights, it's necessary to load plates and secure **barbell collars;** with machines, moving a pin up and down a stack of weights provides the right amount of resistance.

As they gain experience with weightlifting, most people begin incorporating free-weight exercises into their lifting programs. This change increases muscle stimulation, primarily by involving supportive muscles which guide movement. In other words, muscle, not a machine, controls movement when using free weights.

In addition to increasing muscle stimulation, free weights let an exerciser vary exercises more. The hand spacing, angles of movement, and range of motion can almost always be altered more when using free weights than when using a machine. One

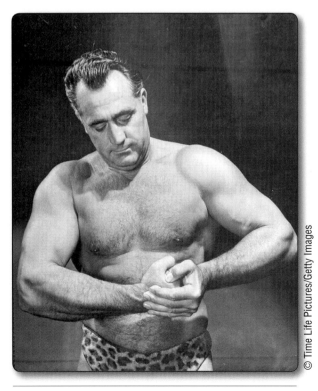

Charles Atlas popularized isometric training.

final benefit is that many exercises performed with free weights replicate real-life activity much more closely than machine exercises do. This helps increase strength needed in daily activities.

A Three-Phase Strength-Training Program

The program in this section is perfect for people who've never done strength training or who have been lifting weights for fewer than six months. Although it is meant for beginners, it contains advanced training principles that more experienced lifters can benefit from. On average, beginners who complete all three phases of this program increase their overall strength by approximately 30 percent. (See appendix C to find a version of the workout program that is easy to tear out.) Of course, your results will be less significant if you have already been lifting weights. As you preview the workout program in the next few pages, you'll most likely have some questions, so I've answered some of the most common ones here:

1. What am I supposed to do on the first day of any phase?

The first day will be your longest workout, because, after you do a brief warm-up, you'll need to become familiar with the exercises, establish the proper fit of each machine, and determine the right weight and repetitions for each exercise. First, find the right piece of exercise equipment. You'll find photographs of the beginning and end of each exercise in the program to help you with this task. Your workout facility may not have the exact piece of equipment in the pictures, but most weight rooms have similar equipment, so you should be able to find an appropriate substitute.

After you find the right equipment you may need to make some minor fitting adjustments, such as moving the seat up or down. Most machines have diagrams to help you with this procedure. If yours do not, ask a personal trainer or fitness professional to help you. Record your individual fitting adjustments in the notes section of day 1.

Every phase I: day 1 workout card has several specific items across the top: sets/effort, repetitions, **repetition speed**, and rest intervals (see figure 6.15).

Sets/effort refers to the number of sets per exercise and the amount of effort you'll exert, ranging from 0 to 100 percent. You'll do only one set of each exercise in each phase and exert 85 to 100 percent of your maximum effort. During each set in phase I, you will do 12 to 15 repetitions at a speed of four seconds (2/0/2) per repetition. Repetition speed refers to the number of seconds it takes to raise and lower the weight. The speed will remain the same in each phase. Take 2 seconds to raise the weight and 2 seconds to lower it, and don't stop in between. (I talk more about repetition speed later in the chapter.) Finally, you will rest for 60 to 90 seconds between each set. The program doesn't specify the amount of resistance you will need for each exercise. You'll have to determine that through trial and error.

2. How do I determine how much weight to start with?

Scientists and coaches have come up with various formulas for determining how much you should begin lifting, but none has a high degree of reliability. Therefore, you'll need to experiment to determine the weight that is right for you. First, perform the exercise without any resistance to help your brain and motor memory become familiar with the movement. Next, perform the movement with a small amount of resistance as a warm up to further ingrain the motor program into memory. Finally, continue adding resistance until you find the amount of weight you can lift for the indicated number of repetitions (12 to 15 reps in phase I) while exerting approximately 85 percent of your total effort. You shouldn't begin with a 100 percent effort, because you will be adding weight and repetitions very soon; you want to give yourself a little room for growth. Second, too much weight might cause you to sacrifice form. Third, beginning with around 85 percent effort "leave a little extra fuel in the tank" at the beginning of your program so you'll quickly be able to add more resistance.

Phase I: day 1	Sets/effort	Repetitions	Repetition speed	Rest between sets
	1/85-100%	12-15	2/0/2	60-90 s

FIGURE 6.15   Each of these items is listed on every workout program.

3. **Why just one hard set?**

Die-hard lifters might laugh at the idea of doing only one set, but several well-designed studies suggest that one set is virtually as effective as three for beginners (Rhea et al., 2002). Researchers at the University of Florida divided a total of 42 male and female beginning lifters into two groups. The first group performed one set of 8 to 12 repetitions on nine different machines; the second group performed three sets. After 13 weeks, there were no significant differences between the two groups in strength, endurance, or body composition (Hass, 2000).

As you become more experienced, you will probably want to add additional sets to your exercises. However, if you've been training for fewer than six months, you can cut your workout time by two thirds (traditional strength-training programs suggest doing three sets of each exercise) and get the same benefit.

4. **What do I write on the workout card?**

On the first workout of each phase you will need to record three items for each exercise: the resistance used, number of repetitions completed, and any notes pertaining to a particular exercise you may want to remember, such as the seat position or where the machine is located. After completing the first workout, transfer the weight and repetitions used for each exercise to the opposite side of the card in the week 1, day 1 column. An example is shown in figure 6.16.

After transferring the weight and repetitions to your workout card, the only things you'll need to record on your workout cards are the weight and repetitions used for each exercise, which you'll increase over time.

5. **How quickly should I progress?**

Don't try to progress as quickly as possible. That's right: *Don't try to progress as quickly as possible.* You will probably discover that it's easy to make rapid gains during week 1, but that's not the goal. The goal is to increase the resistance gradually, not for 1 week but for 12 weeks. To make steady improvement, carefully follow these guidelines:

1. Do not add more than one repetition to any exercise from one workout to the next. If the resistance feels too easy, slow

Phase I: day 1	Sets/effort	Repetitions		Repetition speed	Rest between sets
	1/85-100%	12-15		2/0/2	60-90 s
Seated leg extension	Wt	Notes			
	50				
	Reps				
	12				

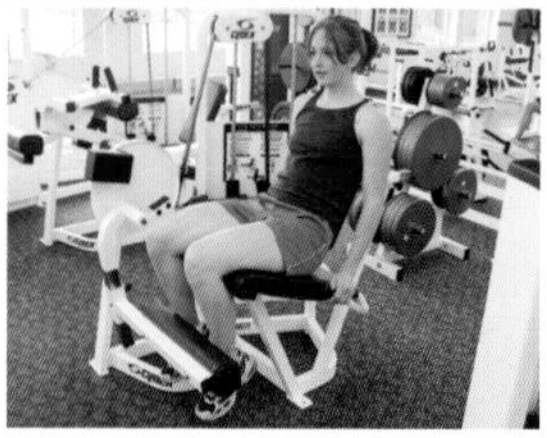

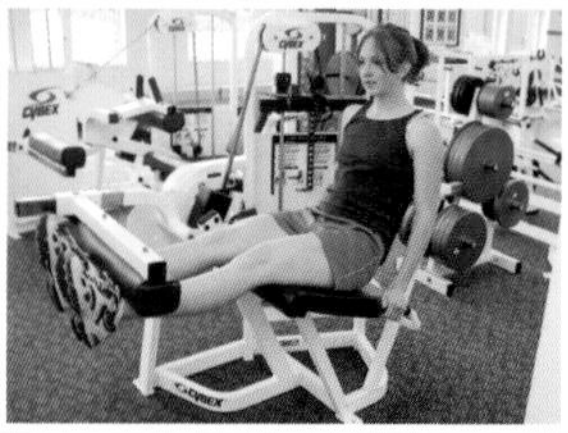

Phase I **strength-training program**

Weeks 1-2	WEEK 1			WEEK 2		
	Day 1	Day 2	Day 3	Day 1	Day 2	Day 3
Seated leg extension	Wt	Wt	Wt	Wt	Wt	Wt
	50					
	Reps	Reps	Reps	Reps	Reps	Reps
	12					

FIGURE 6.16   After the first workout, transfer weight and repetitions to the weekly workout section.

down the repetition speed to make the exercise more difficult without increasing resistance.

2. When you have reached the highest number of repetitions for the phase (15 repetitions are the most you should do in phase I), add resistance. The rule for adding resistance is to add 5 pounds (2.2 kg) for upper-body exercises and 10 pounds (4.5 kg) for lower-body exercises. Upper-body exercises are movements that train muscles from the waist up. Muscles from the waist down are classified as lower-body exercises.

3. When you add weight, reduce the number of repetitions to the lowest number for that phase. See figure 6.17 for an example of this progression for a phase I exercise in which the target repetitions are 12 to 15.

6. Can I substitute an exercise I like better than the ones listed?

You can, but keep one thing in mind. Novice lifters often make the mistake of focusing on certain body parts and ignoring others. Men usually want bigger and more defined chest, arms, and abs; and women usually want to tone the abdomen, hips, and thighs. The resulting muscular imbalances can increase your chance of muscular injury (and they make you look funny). For instance, athletes who spend a lot of time on their quadriceps but ignore their hamstrings are more susceptible to leg injuries. You need to include six major muscle groups in every strength-training program: legs, back, abdominals, chest, shoulders, and arms. Memorize the mnemonic phrase "little **b**oys always **c**atch **s**limy **a**nimals" to help you remember all six major muscle groups. Remember: You can substitute exercises, but when you do, make sure you are doing not only exercises that you prefer but also movements that train all major muscle groups. Exercises for all the major muscle groups are included in each phase, so substitute those that work the same muscle or muscle group if you choose to switch exercises.

7. Do I need to complete the exercises in this order?

Yes, if you can. Exercises are listed in order according to the big-to-small principle. Exercises for body parts with the greatest muscle mass come before those with the least—again, "little boys always catch slimy animals." Improvement will happen a little bit faster if you follow this sequence. More advanced lifters can rearrange the order in which the muscles are trained to add variety to their workouts.

8. Why so many different workouts?

After three to four weeks repeating the same exercises, most exercisers reach a plateau, and progress slows dramatically. The world's top athletes frequently change their exercise programs. The Westside Barbell Club, just outside of Columbus, Ohio, provides a great example. In 2004, they had more than 40 people who could bench press in excess of 500 pounds (227 kg) (Simmons, 2005). Most gyms would boast if they had one person accomplish such a feat. What is the Westside Barbell Club's secret? Members change their training regimens every two weeks! The continual change forces increased muscle stimulation. That strategy supports the rationale for each phase being only two weeks long.

Phase I strength-training program   Name

Weeks 1-2	WEEK 1			WEEK 2		
	Day 1	Day 2	Day 3	Day 1	Day 2	Day 3
Seated leg extension	Wt	Wt	Wt	Wt	Wt	Wt
	50	50	50	50	60	60
	Reps	Reps	Reps	Reps	Reps	Reps
	12	13	14	15	12	13

FIGURE 6.17 The seated leg extension is a lower-body exercise, so 10 pounds (4.5 kg) are added after 15 repetitions are completed.

9. What do I do after I complete all three workout phases?

After you finish the last phase go back to the beginning and repeat each phase again. Note the amount of resistance you used during your first phase. You will be amazed at how easy that beginning weight feels now that you're stronger. Don't go back to the weight you started using, though. Instead, start the new phase I just as you did at the beginning (12-15 reps, 85% effort), except calibrated to your newly developed strength. After you go through the entire program twice (12 weeks), you will need to move on to an intermediate training program. One of the best books for intermediate workout ideas is *Serious Strength Training* (Bompa, Di Pasquale, & Cornacchia, 2002).

10. Do I need to warm up before each exercise session?

Yes. It is important to do a general warm-up, such as riding a bike, running, or doing some calisthenics for 5 to 10 minutes, before you do any lifting. The warm-up increases blood flow throughout your body and prepares your muscles to perform work. After the general warm-up you can do a specific warm-up for added protection. A specific warm-up prepares a particular muscle region for targeted work. The targeted warm-up can be a light set before your first set at 85 to 100 percent effort. Use approximately 50 percent of the weight for this warm-up set that you intend to use for your hard set, and complete 6 to 10 repetitions. Doing a general and a specific warm-up not only protects you from injury but also prepares your muscles to work harder.

You will no doubt notice that all the exercises in phase I use machines (see figure 6.18). I told you the reasons for that earlier. Also note the order in

Should Women Train Differently Than Men?

Women, on average, have two-thirds the strength of men (Lauback, 1976) largely because of the hormonal differences cited on page 106. The influence of hormones becomes obvious as children experience puberty. Before puberty, there are essentially no differences in height, weight, body size, lean body mass, and adipose tissue between boys and girls. During puberty, the production of estrogen in girls increases their percentage of body fat, whereas testosterone production in boys increases bone formation and muscle mass. The net effect of these changes in terms of muscle mass is that men develop more muscle tissue and have taller and wider skeletal frames that support additional muscle.

These differences suggest to some that men and women should perform resistance training differently. Others believe there is no sensible reason why women's resistance-training programs need to be different than men's.

Thomas Baechle and Roger Earle, who have written "*the* manual" for most strength-training professionals, state the following (National Strength and Conditioning Association, 2000, p. 180):

It is a misperception that resistance-training programs for women should be different from those for men or that women lose flexibility or develop "bulky" muscles if they train with weights. The only real difference between training programs for men and women is generally the amount of resistance used for a given exercise.

Although there may not be physiological differences in men's and women's muscle tissue, there are other factors to consider.

The first is that women generally have different goals for strength training than men have. While many men seek muscular strength and size, women desire firmness and muscular definition. These goals should be reflected in strength prescriptions. A second difference is susceptibility to injury. Some studies suggest that females are more susceptible to knee injuries than males are (Arendt & Dick, 1995; Baker, 1998). In one NCAA report, female basketball players were six times more likely to incur an anterior cruciate ligament tear than the male players were (National Collegiate Athletic Association, 1994). Review the literature on this controversial issue and develop an informed opinion.

Phase I: day 1	Sets/effort 1/85-100%		Repetitions 12-15	Repetition speed 2/0/2	Rest between sets 60-90 s
Seated leg extension	Wt		Notes		
	Reps				
Lat pull-down	Wt		Notes		
	Reps				
Seated back extension	Wt		Notes		
	Reps				
Abdominal crunch	Wt		Notes		
	Reps				
Chest press	Wt		Notes		
	Reps				
Lateral raise	Wt		Notes		
	Reps				
Arm extension	Wt		Notes		
	Reps				
Arm curl	Wt		Notes		
	Reps				

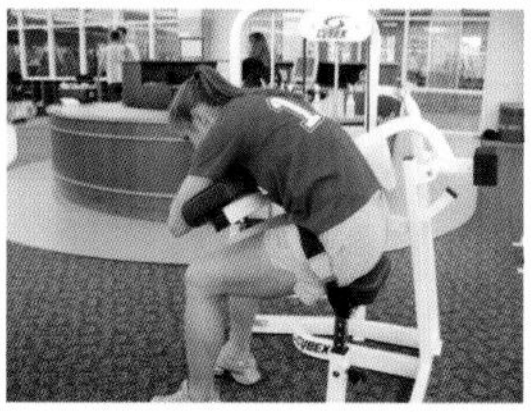

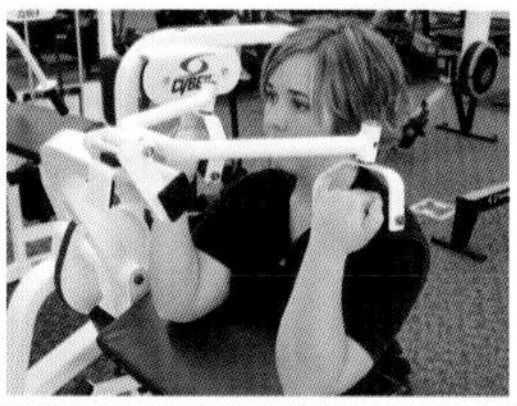

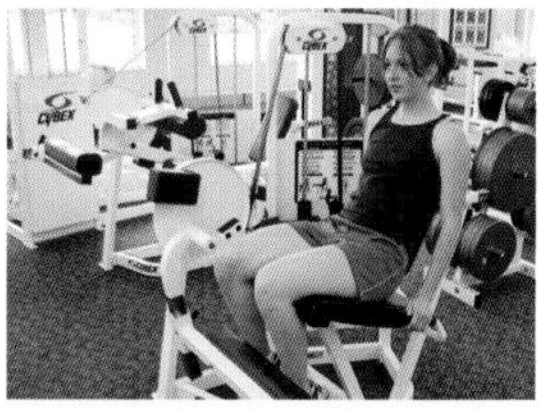

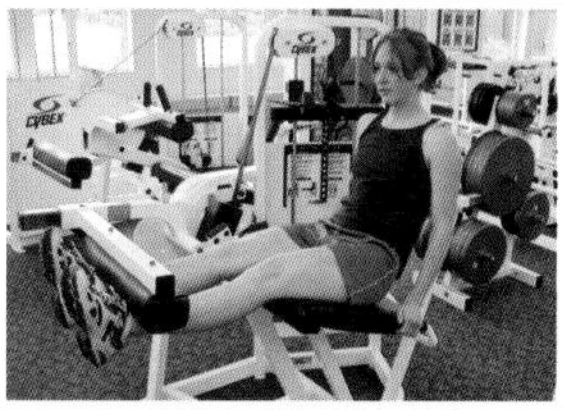

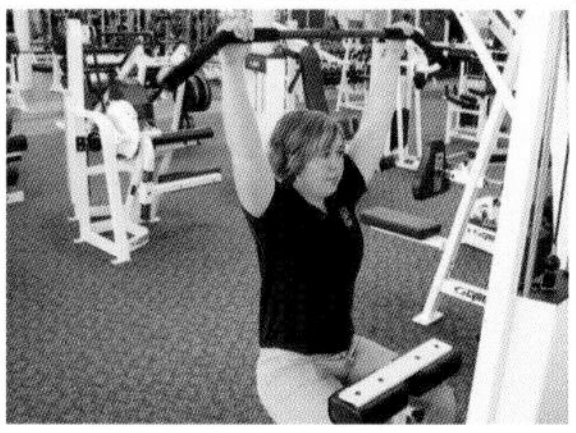

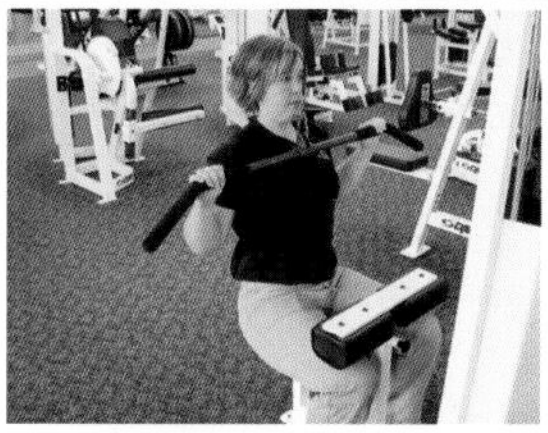

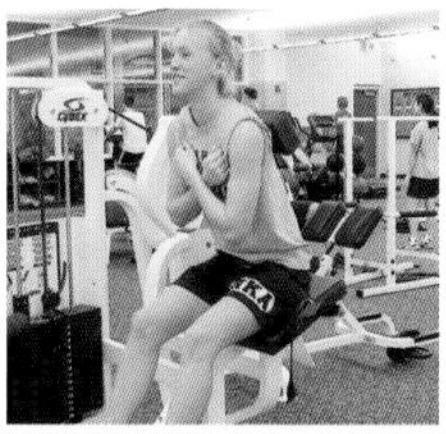

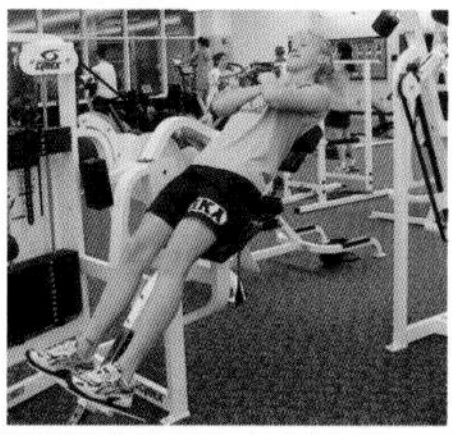

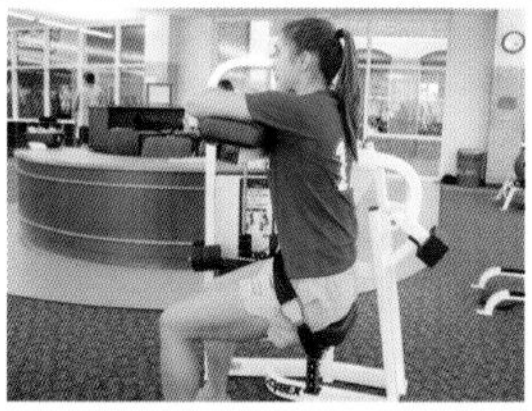

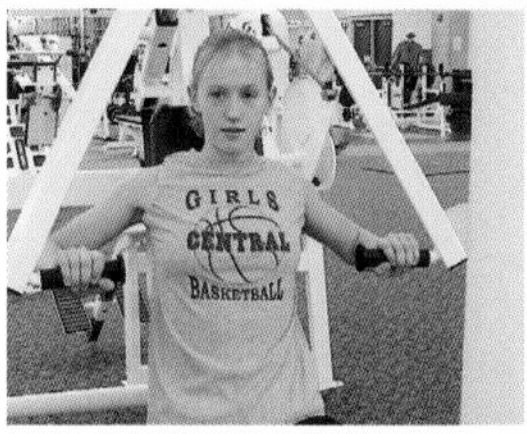

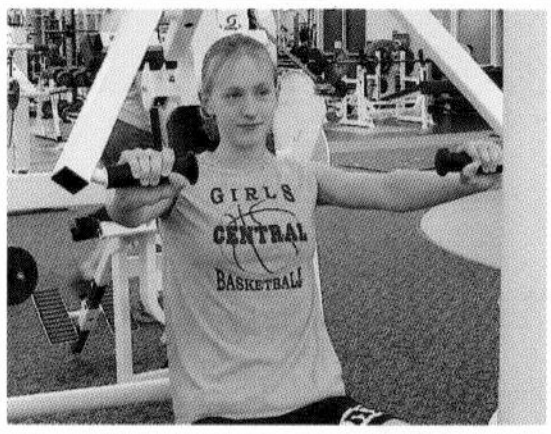

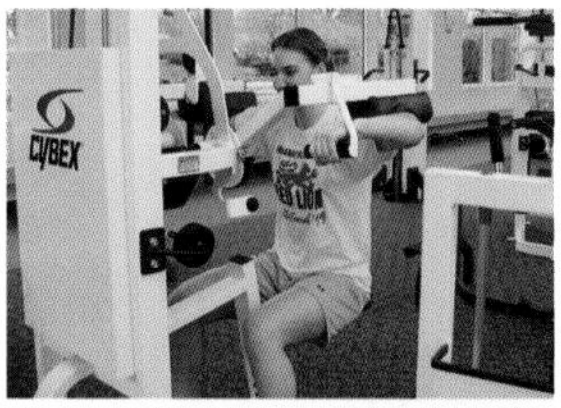

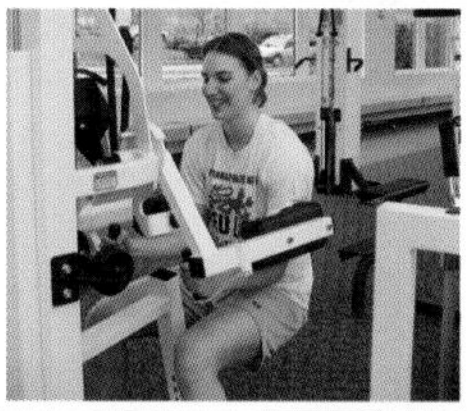

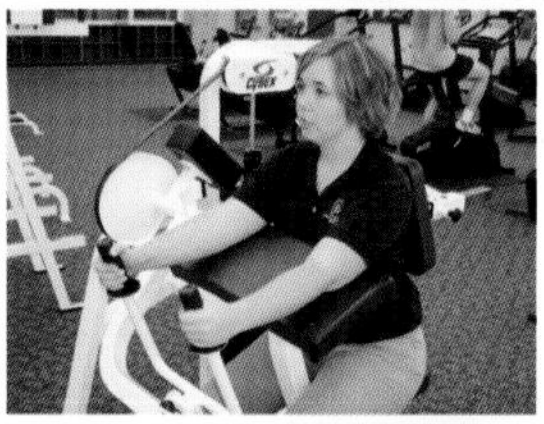

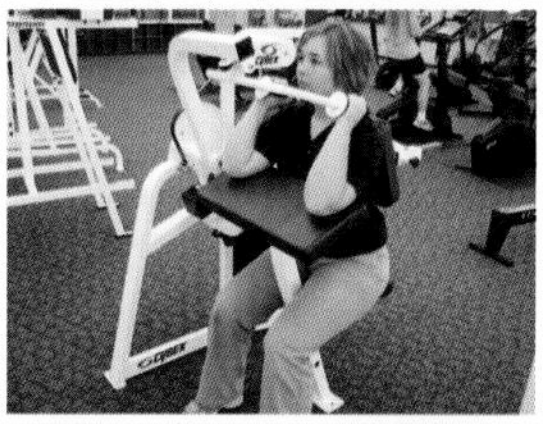

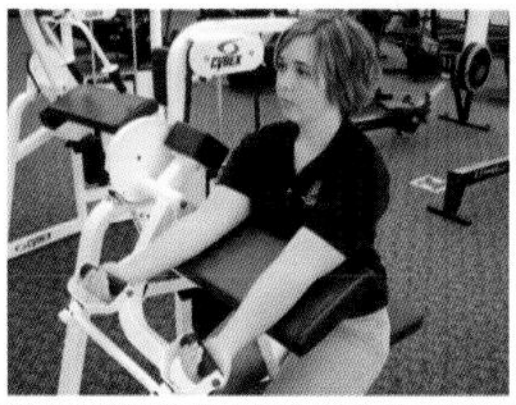

FIGURE 6.18   This is the first of three progressive workout programs.   *(continued)*

Phase I strength-training program

Weeks 1-2	WEEK 1			WEEK 2		
	Day 1	Day 2	Day 3	Day 1	Day 2	Day 3
Seated leg extension	Wt	Wt	Wt	Wt	Wt	Wt
	Reps	Reps	Reps	Reps	Reps	Reps
Lat pull-down	Wt	Wt	Wt	Wt	Wt	Wt
	Reps	Reps	Reps	Reps	Reps	Reps
Seated back extension	Wt	Wt	Wt	Wt	Wt	Wt
	Reps	Reps	Reps	Reps	Reps	Reps
Abdominal crunch	Wt	Wt	Wt	Wt	Wt	Wt
	Reps	Reps	Reps	Reps	Reps	Reps
Chest press	Wt	Wt	Wt	Wt	Wt	Wt
	Reps	Reps	Reps	Reps	Reps	Reps
Lateral raise	Wt	Wt	Wt	Wt	Wt	Wt
	Reps	Reps	Reps	Reps	Reps	Reps
Arm extension	Wt	Wt	Wt	Wt	Wt	Wt
	Reps	Reps	Reps	Reps	Reps	Reps
Arm curl	Wt	Wt	Wt	Wt	Wt	Wt
	Reps	Reps	Reps	Reps	Reps	Reps

FIGURE 6.18 *(continued)*

which the exercises, from top to bottom, include all major muscle groups and are sequenced from the largest muscle groups to the smallest.

Phase II combines both free weight and machine exercises (see figure 6.19). You will still do only one set with 85 to 100 percent effort. Repetition speed and the rest between sets also remain consistent.

Yet notice there is a change in the repetition range. Instead of doing 12 to 15 repetitions, you will now do 9 to 12 reps. Reducing the number of repetitions allows you to increase resistance. Take your time on the first day of this workout to determine the appropriate amount of resistance. After completing day 1, transfer the weight and repetitions

Phase II: day 1	Sets/effort	Repetitions	Repetition speed	Rest between sets
	1/85-100%	9-12	2/0/2	60-90 s
45-degree leg press	Wt Reps	Notes	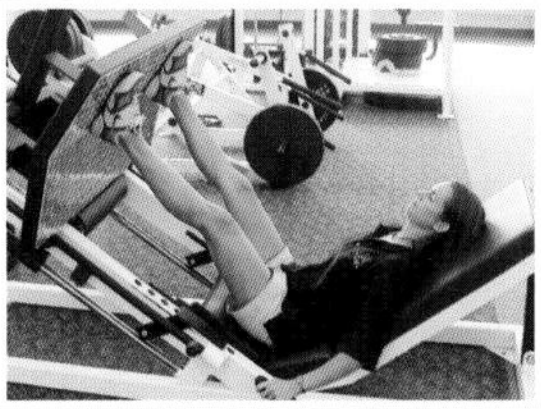	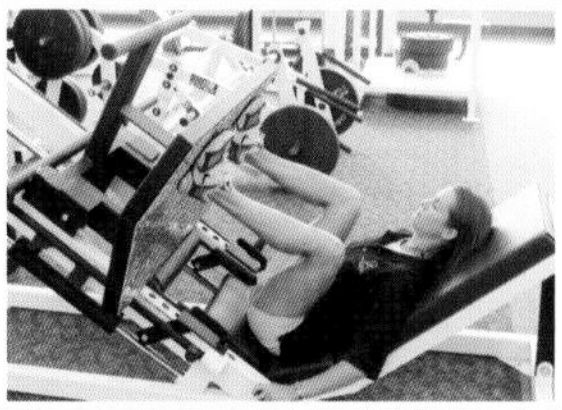
Leg curl	Wt Reps	Notes	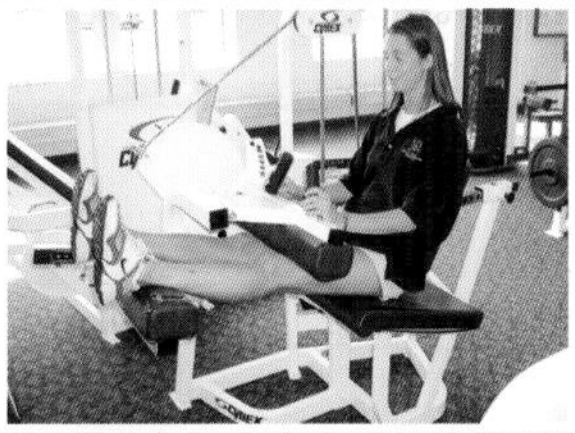	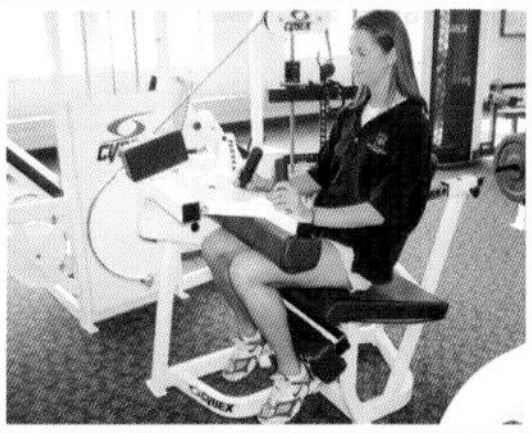
Low row	Wt Reps	Notes	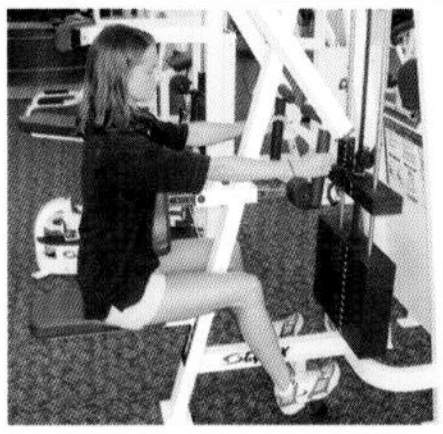	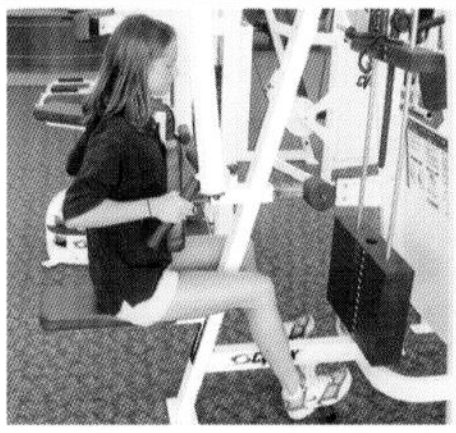
Incline back extension	Wt Reps	Notes	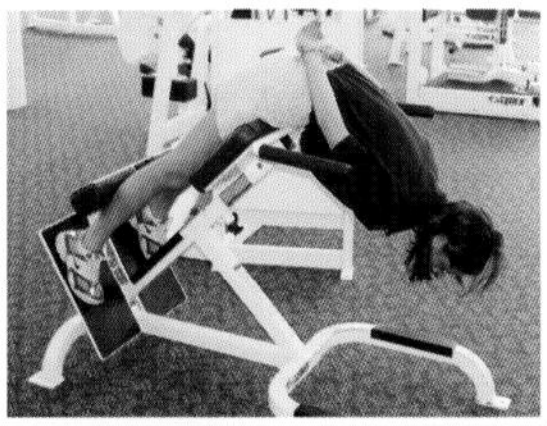	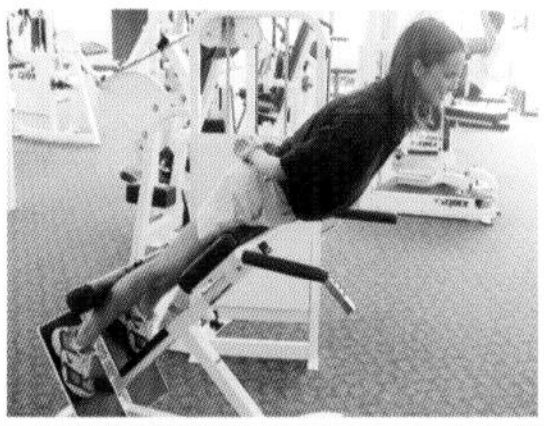
Torso rotation	Wt Reps	Notes	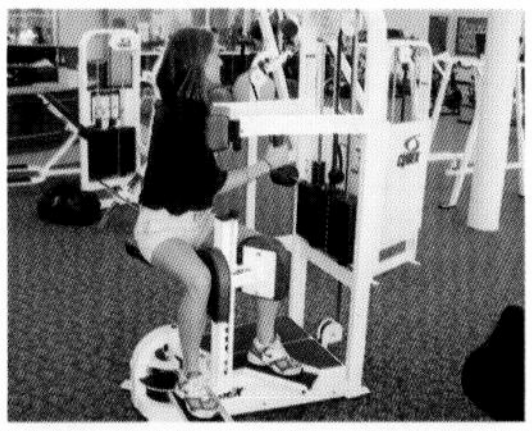	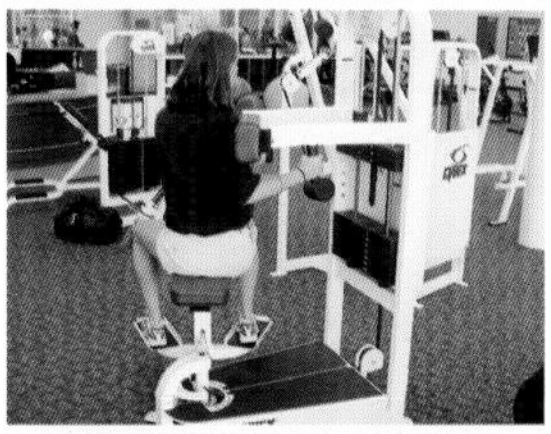
Reverse crunch	Wt Reps	Notes	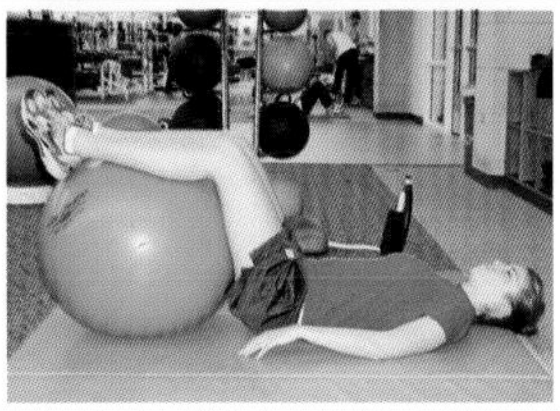	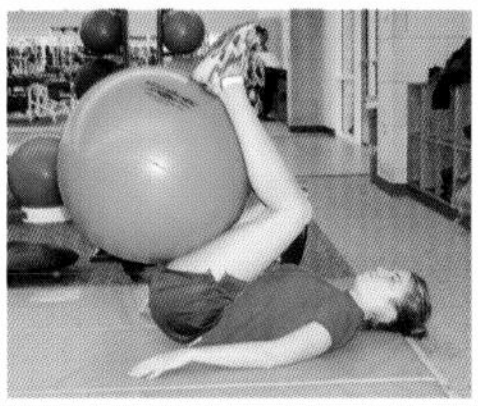

FIGURE 6.19 Phase II combines free-weight and machine exercises.

(continued)

Phase II: day 1	Sets/effort	Repetitions	Repetition speed	Rest between sets
	1/85-100%	9-12	2/0/2	60-90 s
Chest fly	Wt	Notes	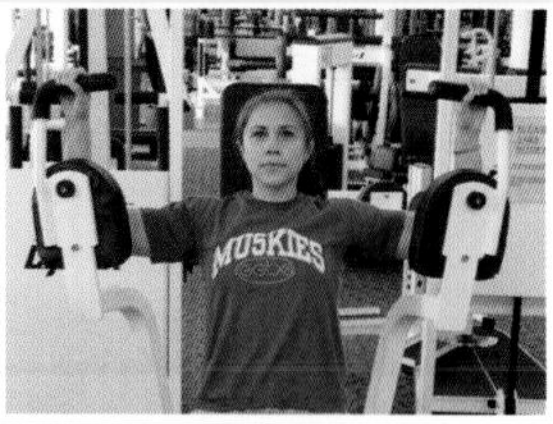	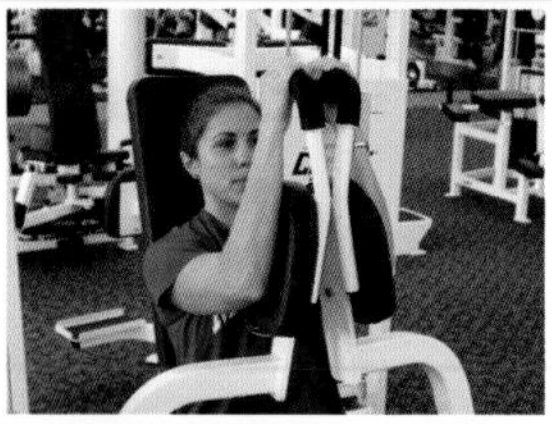
	Reps			
Bent-over rear cable raise	Wt	Notes	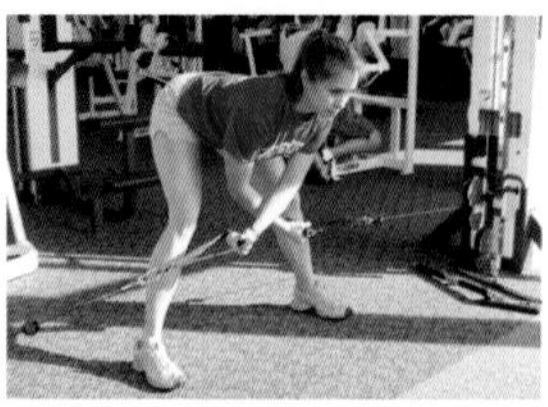	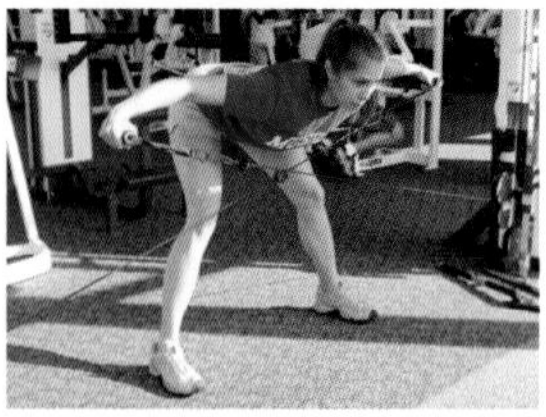
	Reps			
Standing dumbbell curl	Wt	Notes	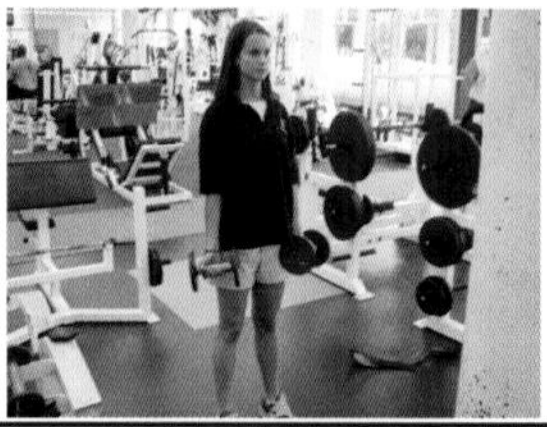	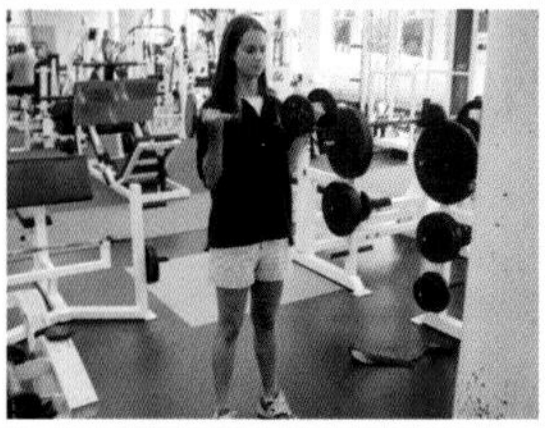
	Reps			
Triceps push-down	Wt	Notes	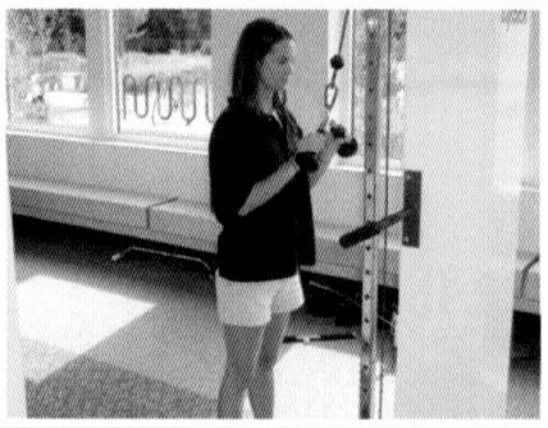	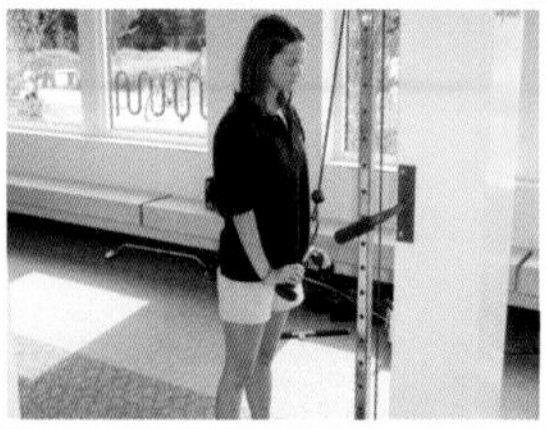
	Reps			

Phase II strength-training program

Weeks 3-4	WEEK 3			WEEK 4		
	Day 1	Day 2	Day 3	Day 1	Day 2	Day 3
45-degree leg press	Wt	Wt	Wt	Wt	Wt	Wt
	Reps	Reps	Reps	Reps	Reps	Reps
Leg curl	Wt	Wt	Wt	Wt	Wt	Wt
	Reps	Reps	Reps	Reps	Reps	Reps

(continued)

FIGURE 6.19 *(continued)*

Weeks 3-4	WEEK 3			WEEK 4		
	Day 1	Day 2	Day 3	Day 1	Day 2	Day 3
Low row	Wt	Wt	Wt	Wt	Wt	Wt
	Reps	Reps	Reps	Reps	Reps	Reps
Incline back extension	Wt	Wt	Wt	Wt	Wt	Wt
	Reps	Reps	Reps	Reps	Reps	Reps
Torso rotation	Wt	Wt	Wt	Wt	Wt	Wt
	Reps	Reps	Reps	Reps	Reps	Reps
Reverse crunch	Wt	Wt	Wt	Wt	Wt	Wt
	Reps	Reps	Reps	Reps	Reps	Reps
Chest fly	Wt	Wt	Wt	Wt	Wt	Wt
	Reps	Reps	Reps	Reps	Reps	Reps
Bent-over rear cable raise	Wt	Wt	Wt	Wt	Wt	Wt
	Reps	Reps	Reps	Reps	Reps	Reps
Standing dumbbell curl	Wt	Wt	Wt	Wt	Wt	Wt
	Reps	Reps	Reps	Reps	Reps	Reps
Triceps push-down	Wt	Wt	Wt	Wt	Wt	Wt
	Reps	Reps	Reps	Reps	Reps	Reps

FIGURE 6.19   *(continued)*

over to the weekly workout and use the same progression scheme for increasing repetitions and resistance as you did in phase I.

Most of the exercises in phase III are free-weight exercises (see figure 6.20). Only the exercises and the number of repetitions change in this workout. Only perform six to nine repetitions for each exercise during this phase. As you did in the previous phases, determine your starting weight on day 1, and follow the same system of progression.

Phase III: day 1	Sets/effort	Repetitions	Repetition speed	Rest between sets
	1/85-100%	6-9	2/0/2	60-90 s
Box squat	Wt / Reps	Notes	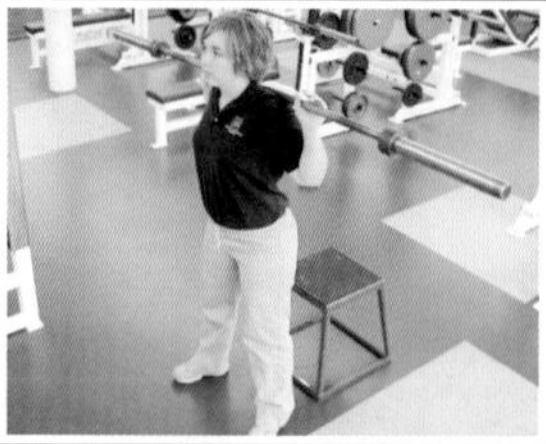	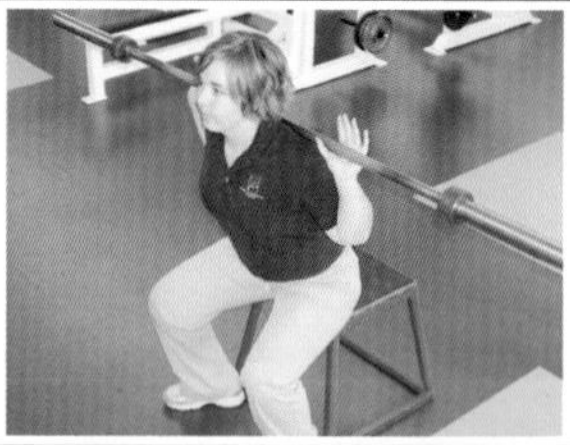
Leg adduction	Wt / Reps	Notes	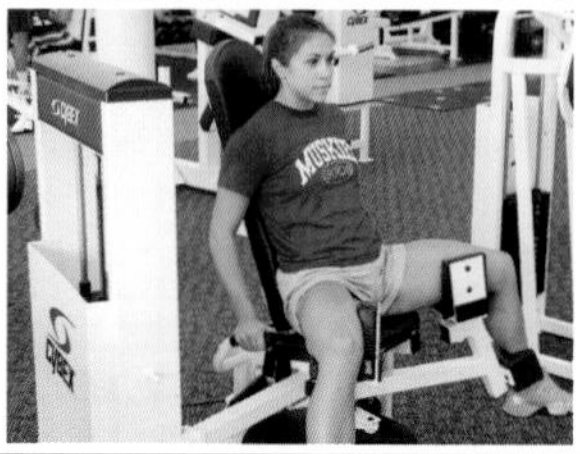	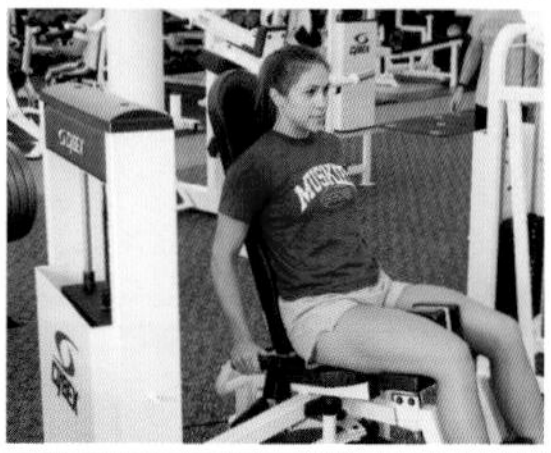
One-arm dumbbell row	Wt / Reps	Notes	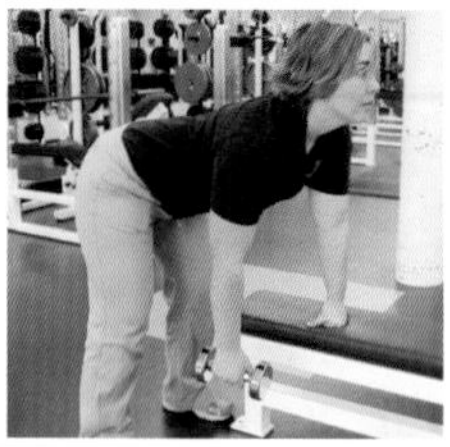	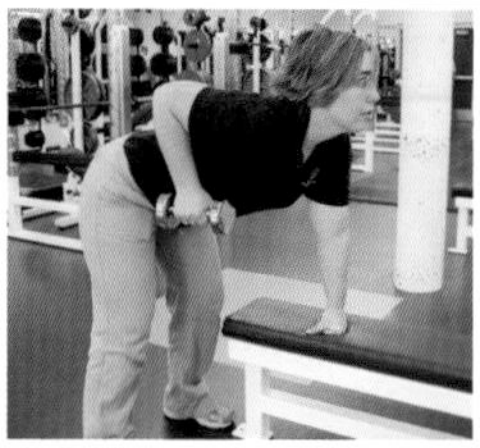
Hanging leg raise/stability ball sit-up	Wt / Reps	Notes	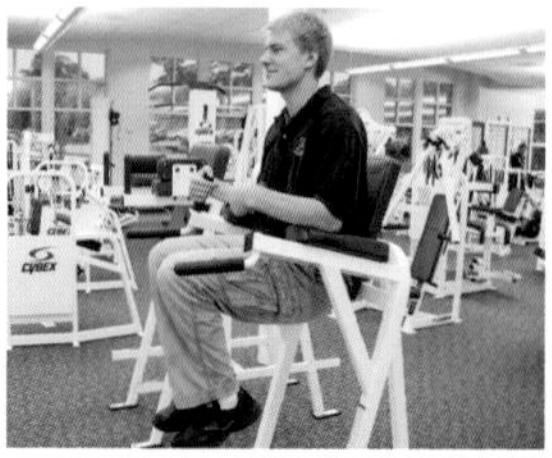	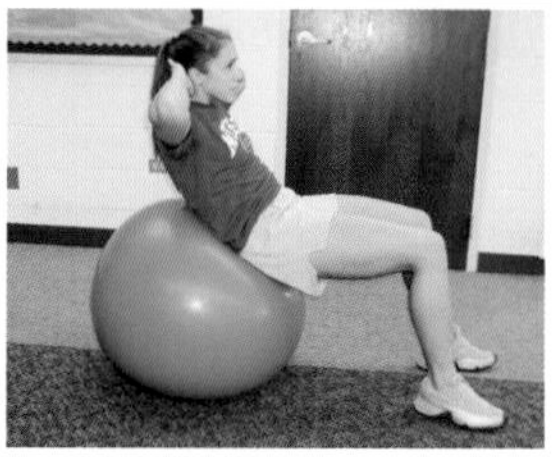
Bench press	Wt / Reps	Notes	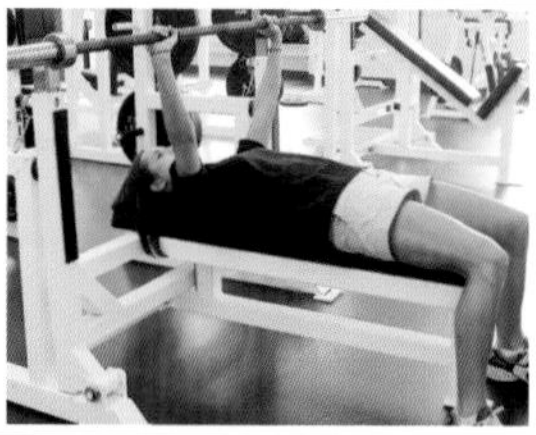	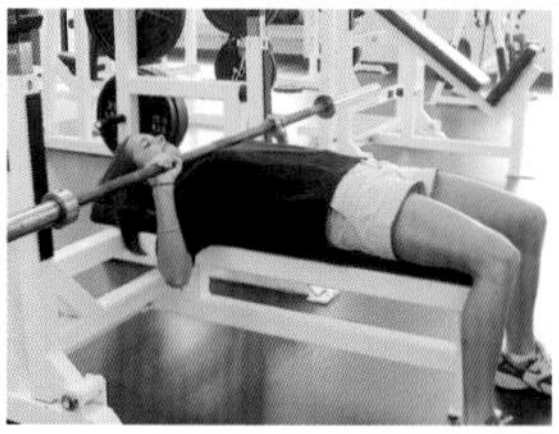
Seated press	Wt / Reps	Notes	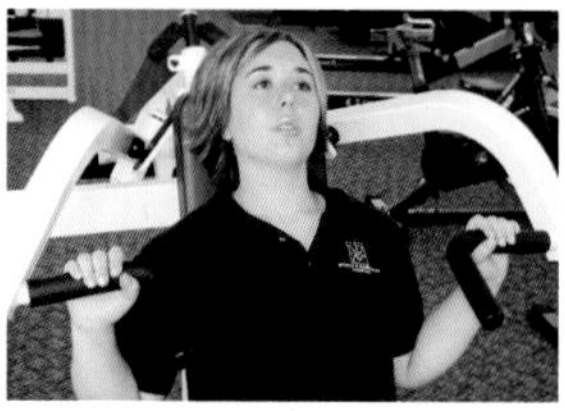	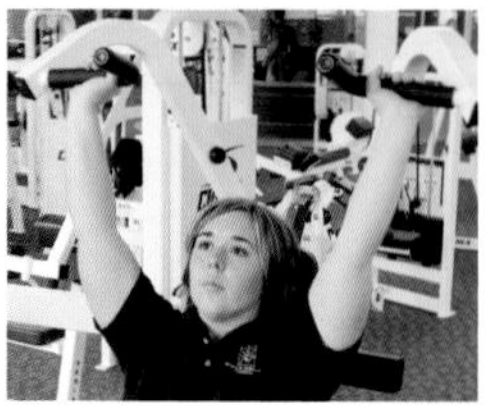

(continued)

FIGURE 6.20   Phase III is almost entirely composed of free-weight exercises.

Phase III: day 1	Sets/effort	Repetitions		Repetition speed	Rest between sets
	1/85-100%	6-9		2/0/2	60-90 s
Seated alternating dumbbell curl	Wt	Notes			
	Reps				
Seated two-arm dumbbell triceps press	Wt	Notes			
	Reps				

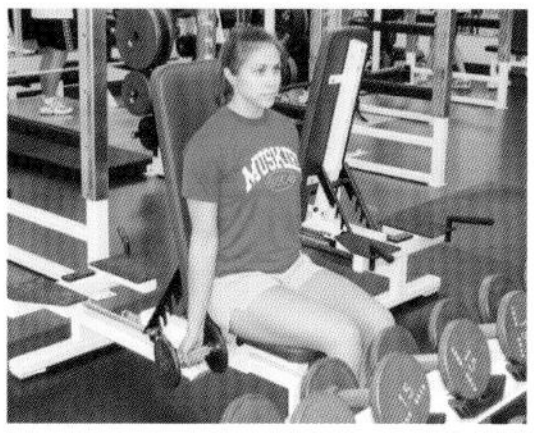

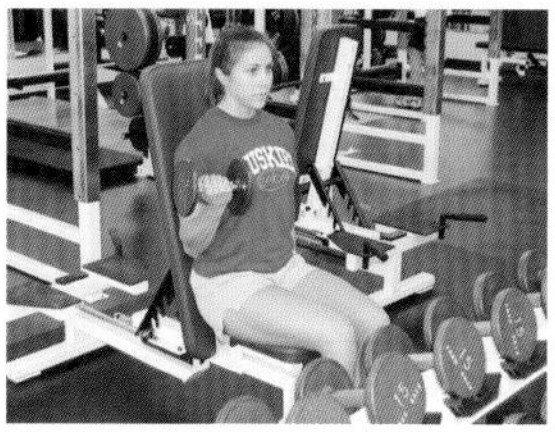

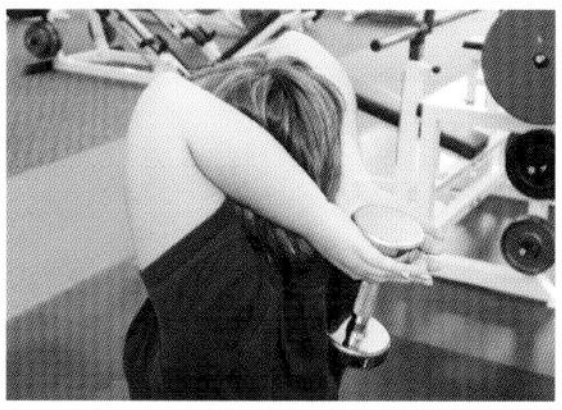

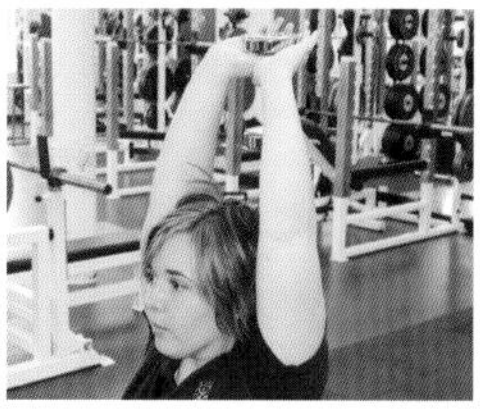

Phase III strength-training program

Weeks 5-6	WEEK 5			WEEK 6		
	Day 1	Day 2	Day 3	Day 1	Day 2	Day 3
Box squat	Wt	Wt	Wt	Wt	Wt	Wt
	Reps	Reps	Reps	Reps	Reps	Reps
Leg adduction	Wt	Wt	Wt	Wt	Wt	Wt
	Reps	Reps	Reps	Reps	Reps	Reps
One-arm dumbell row	Wt	Wt	Wt	Wt	Wt	Wt
	Reps	Reps	Reps	Reps	Reps	Reps
Hanging leg raise/stability ball sit-up	Wt	Wt	Wt	Wt	Wt	Wt
	Reps	Reps	Reps	Reps	Reps	Reps

FIGURE 6.20 *(continued)*

(continued)

Weeks 5-6	WEEK 5			WEEK 6		
	Day 1	Day 2	Day 3	Day 1	Day 2	Day 3
Bench press	Wt	Wt	Wt	Wt	Wt	Wt
	Reps	Reps	Reps	Reps	Reps	Reps
Seated press	Wt	Wt	Wt	Wt	Wt	Wt
	Reps	Reps	Reps	Reps	Reps	Reps
Seated alternating dumbell curl	Wt	Wt	Wt	Wt	Wt	Wt
	Reps	Reps	Reps	Reps	Reps	Reps
Seated two-arm dumbell triceps press	Wt	Wt	Wt	Wt	Wt	Wt
	Reps	Reps	Reps	Reps	Reps	Reps

FIGURE 6.20   *(continued)*

Don't throw these workouts away after you've completed all three phases because you need to repeat them before moving on to an intermediate workout program. After completing 12 weeks of this program, you will be at least 30 percent stronger than when you began. Not too bad for three months of training!

Safety in Strength Training

Resistance training can help you prevent and recover from injuries. If you're not careful, it may also cause injuries—strains and sprains, bumps and bruises, and perhaps worse. Make sure you follow these seven guidelines for weight room safety:

1. **Warm up before you lift.** Warming up increases the amount of blood and oxygen delivered to your muscles, increases the temperature of your muscles and joints, and can enhance your performance by up to 20 percent. Running, biking, and stair-climbing are all examples of good warm-up exercises. They increase circulation (blood flow) throughout the entire body.

2. **Always practice proper form.** Don't let your ego endanger your safety by sacrificing form to lift more weight. Here are some general rules regarding lifting form:

   • Keep your torso firm and your back straight while doing most free-weight exercises.

- Focus on the muscles being worked rather than the weight or number of repetitions.
  - Maintain control of how fast you lift. Force your muscles, not momentum, to move the resistance.

3. **Progress slowly.** Your body does. Using the progression methods outlined in this chapter allows your body to gradually accommodate increasing levels of stress.

4. **Use the equipment properly.** Don't put your fingers where they aren't meant to be. When you work with barbells, make sure the weight is equal on each side, and always use barbell collars.

5. **Always wear shoes; remove your jewelry.**

6. **Use proper breathing technique** (see point–counterpoint discussion on this page).

7. **Have someone spot you on potentially dangerous lifts.** Death is rare in the weight room, but when it happens it's usually when people lift alone. A classic example is bench pressing without a spotter. If you are unable to complete a lift, the bar gets stuck at your chest and can slide down to your neck and suffocate you.

Feeling Pretty Big Lately?

The lyrics of Jean Knight's song "Mr. Big Stuff" describe a man with a large opinion of himself because of his clothing, car, and cash.

So much of people's feelings of strength comes from what or who they compare themselves to. Mr. Big Stuff may have had expensive jewelry, designer clothes, and classic cars, but his knowledge of astronomy was no doubt lacking. Contrast this with King David's reaction when he compared himself to God's creation: "When I consider your heavens, the work of your fingers, the moon and the stars, which you have set in place, what is man that you are mindful of him? The son of man that you care for him" (Psalm 8:3–4)?

Never Hold Your Breath While Lifting?

Most fitness professionals have two recommendations about breathing: 1) Exhale during the most strenuous phase of the lift, and 2) never hold your breath while lifting (National Strength and Conditioning Association, 2000). The first is a good guideline for beginners; however, the second needs to be reconsidered. It is true that holding your breath for an extended time can result in dizziness, disorientation, and even blackouts; but there are some good reasons to hold your breath for brief periods while lifting. Scientific evidence suggests that holding the breath for a brief time has performance and safety advantages (Findley & Keating, 2003; Haykowsky et al., 2001). If someone is asked to pick up a heavy object, he or she will almost always perform what is called a *Valsalva maneuver* just before applying force. A Valsalva maneuver is produced by pressing air from the lungs against a closed glottis. When a person does this, the muscles of the abdomen and rib cage contract, creating a rigid torso. This inner rigidity of the torso supports the vertebral column, which in turn can reduce compressive forces on the vertebral disks during a lift (National Strength and Conditioning Association, 2000; Findley & Keating, 2003). This maneuver has a similar effect to wearing a safety belt while picking up a heavy weight. One word of caution: Hold your breath for no more than two seconds (National Strength and Conditioning Association, 2000).

Next Steps

As this chapter concludes, consider once more the story of Milo to reinforce one last principle. Milo of Croton was unquestionably the most famous athlete of his day—like Shaquille O'Neal, David Beckham, and Tiger Woods all rolled into one. He won five consecutive victories at the Olympics, six at the Pythian Games, nine at the Nemean Games, and ten at the Isthmian Games. Five times he was also granted the title of *Periodonikes*, or quadruple-crown winner, having won at all four festivals in the same cycle. The Greeks worshiped Milo and erected a statue of him inscribed with the words "Neither god nor man can stand against him" (Harris, 1966). And Milo believed it.

Ironically, Milo's belief in his own invincibility led to his demise. One day, while walking through the forest far from the city, he came upon the stump of a tree that had broken off close to the ground and split down the middle. Allured by the challenge to test his strength, he thrust his hands into the wedge in an attempt to tear the stump in half. However, he failed, and when it closed on his fingers, he was trapped. After the sun set, he was killed by wolves (Harris, 1966).

The story of Milo's rise and fall is a reminder that human strength, no matter how great, will one day come to an end. But the Bible says that God's might will last forever: "My flesh and my heart may fail, but God is the strength of my heart and my portion forever" (Psalm 73:26). As you build your physical strength, remember the one whose strength will never be exhausted. Keep in mind that most of the principles and methods in this chapter also apply to building spiritual power.

Key Terms

actin

atrophy

barbell collar

body composition

cardiac muscle

endomysium

epimysium

fascicles

functional capacity

goodness

hypertrophy

isokinetic

isometric

isotonic

lean body mass (LBM)

motor neurons

motor unit

muscular endurance

muscular strength

myofibril

myofilament

myosin

one-repetition maximum (1RM)

osteoblast

osteoclast

osteoporosis

overload principle

perimysium

repetitions

repetition speed

resistance training

rest interval

resting metabolic rate (RMR)

sarcomeres

set

skeletal muscle

smooth muscle

variable resistance

Review Questions

1. Describe four benefits of resistance training.

2. Draw a cross-section of skeletal muscle. Begin with the epimysium and add as much detail as possible.

3. Identify four methods of evaluating muscular strength or endurance.

4. Describe four types of resistance training.

5. Define and describe each of the following items in the strength-training prescription: sets, effort, repetitions, repetition speed, rest interval, method of progression.

6. List seven safety guidelines for resistance training.

Application Activities

1. Grip test

This test requires you to grip a handheld dynamometer as forcefully as possible with the right hand, then the left hand. Prepare for this test by adjusting the grip bar to fit comfortably within your hand. The second joint of the fingers should fit under the handle of the handgrip dynamometer. The proper grip is shown in figure 6.21.

Make sure that the hand dynamometer is set on zero and your arm is parallel to your body. Squeeze the handle as hard as you can. Record your grip strength in kilograms. Reset the dynamometer to zero and repeat the procedure with the opposite hand. Test each hand two more times. Add the highest value from each hand (highest value of left hand plus highest value of right hand). Compare your results to the standards for grip strength on the norm chart in table 6.2 on page 136.

The following are some common testing mistakes for the handgrip test:

- Pushing the dynamometer against the leg while squeezing to gain additional leverage
- Not resetting the dynamometer to zero after each trial
- Squeezing the dynamometer for long periods. It takes only a second to accurately measure grip strength with this device. Squeezing any longer will only cause fatigue and compromise your performance on the second attempt.

2. One-minute push-up test

This test requires you to perform as many push-ups as possible in one minute, using correct form.

Start by lying facedown on a flat surface. Place your hands approximately shoulder-width apart with your feet fully extended. Females should perform this movement with the lower body supported by the knees instead of the feet (see figure 6.22a). Start the one-minute timing device. Keeping your body straight, push your body weight up so that your elbows are fully extended (see figure 6.22b), then lower your body so that your triceps are parallel or slightly below parallel to

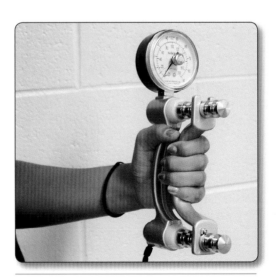

FIGURE 6.21 Grip strength is a good indicator of overall strength.

Table 6.2   Standards for Grip Strength (in lbs.)

Age (yr)	15 – 19		20 – 29		30 – 39		40 – 49		50 – 59		60 – 69	
Gender	M	F	M	F	M	F	M	F	M	F	M	F
Above average	103 – 112	64 – 70	113 – 123	65 – 70	113 – 122	66 – 72	110 – 118	65 – 72	102 – 109	59 – 64	98 – 101	54 – 59
Average	95 – 102	59 – 63	106 – 112	61 – 64	105 – 112	61 – 65	102 – 109	59 – 64	96 – 101	55 – 58	86 – 92	51 – 53
Below average	84 – 94	54 – 58	97 – 105	55 – 60	97 – 104	56 – 60	94 – 101	55 – 58	87 – 95	51 – 54	79 – 85	48 – 50
Poor	≤83	≤53	≤96	≤54	≤96	≤55	≤93	≤54	≤86	≤50	≤78	≤47

Adapted from Dwyer & Davis, 2005.

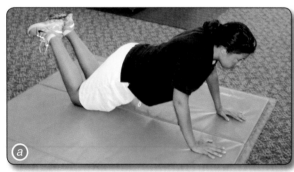

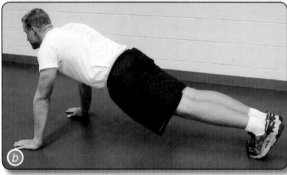

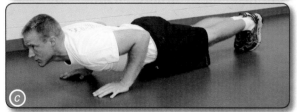

FIGURE 6.22   *(a)* Females should perform the push-up test with the lower body supported by the knees. *(b)* Starting position for the men's push-up test. *(c)* Triceps must be at least parallel to the floor.

the floor (see figure 6.22*c*). You have now completed one repetition. Repeat this movement as many times as you can in one minute. Record the total number of repetitions you complete and compare your results to the norms for one-minute push-ups in table 6.3 on page 137.

The following are some common mistakes participants make on the one-minute push-up test:

- Not keeping the body straight
- Not going through the full range of motion (e.g., arms do not fully extend, triceps are not at least parallel to the surface of the floor)
- Allowing the thighs and abdomen to come into contact with the floor

3. **One-minute sit-up test**

This test requires you to perform as many sit-ups as possible in one minute, using correct form. Begin by lying faceup on a flat surface. Bend your knees to approximately 90 degrees of flexion and place your feet shoulder-width apart. Someone or something will need to keep your feet from moving during this test. Cross your arms and place your hands on your shoulders (figure 6.23*a*). Keep your hands in this position throughout the test. Start the one-minute timing device. Curl your abdomen forward, flexing your upper body until your elbows touch your knees (see figure 6.23*b*). Return to the starting position. This marks the end of one repetition. Repeat this movement as many times as possible in one minute and record the total number of repeti-

Table 6.3   Standards for One–Minute Push-Ups

Age (yr)	15 – 19		20 – 29		30 – 39		40 – 49		50 – 59		60 – 69	
Gender	M	F	M	F	M	F	M	F	M	F	M	F
Excellent	≥52	≥43	≥46	≥40	≥30	≥27	≥22	≥24	≥21	≥21	≥18	≥17
Above average	40 – 51	35 – 42	35 – 45	31 – 39	22 – 29	20 – 26	17 – 21	15 – 23	13 – 20	11 – 20	11 – 17	12 – 16
Average	23 – 39	18 – 35	22 – 35	15 – 30	17 – 21	13 – 19	13 – 16	11 – 14	10 – 12	7 – 10	8 – 10	5 – 11
Below average	18 – 27	12 – 17	17 – 21	10 – 14	12 – 16	8 – 12	10 – 12	5 – 10	7 – 9	2 – 6	5 – 7	1 – 4
Poor	≤17	≤11	≤16	≤9	≤11	≤7	≤9	≤4	≤6	≤1	≤4	≤1

Data from Cooper-Institute for Aerobics Research, 1994.

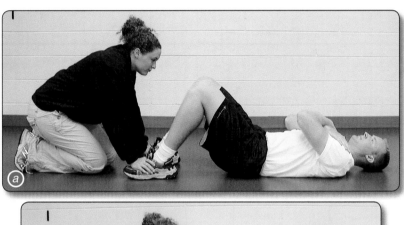

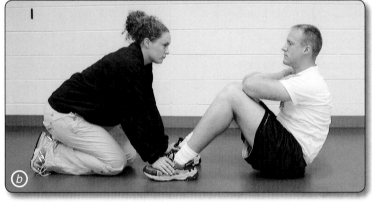

FIGURE 6.23   (a) The beginning position for the sit-up test. (b) Elbows must touch the knees for a complete sit-up to be performed.

tions you complete. Compare your test results to the standards for one-minute sit-ups found in table 6.4 on page 138 to evaluate your muscular endurance.

The following are some common mistakes participants make on the one-minute sit-up test:

- Failing to complete the full range of motion (e.g., not touching the elbows to the knees or not returning to the starting position)
- Swinging the body to gain momentum
- Removing hands from shoulders
- Lifting the hips off the floor

Table 6.4 Standards for One–Minute Sit–Ups

Age (yr)	15 – 19		20 – 29		30 – 39		40 – 49		50 – 59		60 – 69	
Gender	M	F	M	F	M	F	M	F	M	F	M	F
Excellent	≥48	≥42	≥43	≥36	≥36	≥29	≥31	≥25	≥26	≥19	≥23	≥16
Above average	42 – 47	36 – 41	37 – 42	31 – 35	31 – 35	24 – 28	26 – 30	20 – 24	22 – 25	12 – 18	17 – 22	12 – 15
Average	38 – 41	32 – 35	33 – 36	25 – 30	27 – 30	20 – 23	22 – 25	15 – 19	18 – 21	5 – 11	12 – 16	4 – 11
Below average	33 – 37	27 – 31	29 – 32	21 – 24	22 – 26	15 – 19	17 – 21	7 – 14	13 – 17	3 – 4	7 – 11	2 – 3
Poor	≤32	≤26	≤28	≤20	≤21	≤14	≤16	≤6	≤12	≤2	≤6	≤1

Data from Cooper-Institute for Aerobics Research, 1994.

4. Bench press one-repetition maximum (1RM)

This test requires you to lift as much weight as you can for one repetition in the bench press while maintaining proper form. Free weights should be used for this test to be valid, and it is imperative that a spotter be present and alert during the test performance.

Position your body so that your back is on the bench, feet are on the floor, and hands are a little wider than shoulder-width apart on the barbell. Start by removing the weight from the supported uprights to a position in which your arms are fully extended (see figure 6.24a).

Lower the bar to your chest (see figure 6.24b), then push it back up until your elbows are fully extended. It is important to start this test using light weight; lifting only the bar without any additional resistance would be a good place to start for most men. Women can begin by bench pressing 5- or 10-pound dumbbells before moving to a barbell. After warming up with a light weight for 8 to 10 repetitions, increase the weight and try to complete only one repetition. Continue increasing the weight until you can't perform a single repetition at the new weight. Record the highest weight lifted and obtain a body-weight measurement. Calculate your bench press-to-body weight ratio using the formula on the next page, and compare the result to the standards for bench press 1RM in table 6.5 on page 139.

A bench press-to-body weight ratio is determined by dividing the maximum weight lifted in kilograms or pounds by the subject's weight in

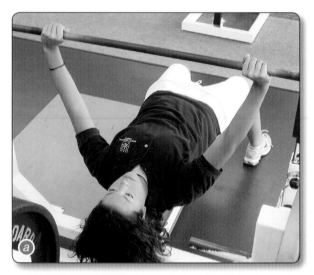

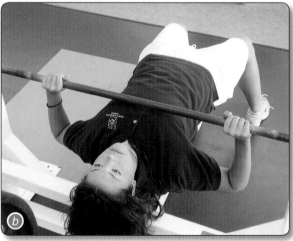

FIGURE 6.24   (a) Starting position for the bench press test. (b) The bar must come in contact with the chest for a successful repetition.

Table 6.5   Standards for Bench Press (One–Repetition Maximum)

Age (yr)	15 – 19		20 – 29		30 – 39		40 – 49		50 – 59		60+	
Gender	M	Fig	M	F	M	F	M	F	M	F	M	F
Excellent	≥1.48	≥0.90	≥1.48	≥0.90	≥1.24	≥0.76	≥1.10	≥0.71	≥0.97	≥0.61	≥0.89	≥0.64
Above average	1.22 – 1.47	0.74 – 0.89	1.22 – 1.47	0.74 – 0.89	1.04 – 1.23	0.63 – 0.75	0.93 – 1.09	0.57 – 0.70	0.84 – 0.96	0.52 – 0.60	0.77 – 0.88	0.51 – 0.63
Average	1.06 – 1.21	0.65 – 0.73	1.06 – 1.21	0.65 – 0.73	0.93 – 1.03	0.57 – 0.62	0.84 – 0.92	0.52 – 0.56	0.75 – 0.84	0.46 – 0.51	0.68 – 0.76	0.45 – 0.50
Below average	0.93 – 1.05	0.56 – 0.64	0.93 – 1.05	0.56 – 0.64	0.83 – 0.92	0.51 – 0.56	0.76 – 0.83	0.47 – 0.51	0.68 – 0.74	0.42 – 0.45	0.63 – 0.67	0.40 – 0.44
Poor	≤0.93	≤0.56	≤0.93	≤0.56	≤0.83	≤0.51	≤0.76	≤0.47	≤0.68	≤0.42	≤0.63	≤0.40

Adapted from Dwyer & Davis, 2005; data from Franklin, 2006.

kilograms or pounds.

For men and women: Bench press (1RM) = maximum weight lifted ÷ body weight

For example, if a person lifts 190 pounds and weighs 185 pounds

Bench press (1RM) = 190 ÷ 185

Bench press (1RM) = 1.02

The following are some common mistakes participants make on this test:

- Failing to lower the weight all the way to the chest
- Bouncing the bar off the chest to gain momentum
- Lifting the hips and legs in an effort to gain a mechanical advantage

5. **Leg press one-repetition maximum (1RM)**

This test requires you to lift as much weight as you can for one repetition in the leg press while maintaining good form. A leg press machine is required for this exam. Data for this exam were originally collected from subjects using a Universal Gym leg press. A comparable leg press, such as the one in figure 6.25, should be used for the test results to be valid.

Sit in the leg press and adjust the seat position so that your knees are bent at a 90-degree angle. Place your feet approximately shoulder-width apart and grasp the handles with your hands (see figure 6.25a). Begin this lift by pushing the foot platform away from your body until your knees are fully extended (see figure 6.25b). Lower the weight to the starting position. This completes one repetition.

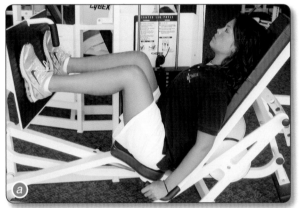

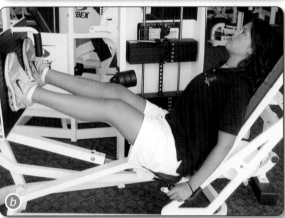

FIGURE 6.25   (a) Starting position for the leg press. (b) Successful completion of the leg press is when both legs are fully extended.

As in the bench press, continue adding resistance until you can't perform a single repetition at the new weight. Record the most weight you pressed for one repetition and obtain an accurate measurement of body weight. Calculate your leg press-to-body weight ratio using the following formula, and compare your results to the standards for leg press in table 6.6.

A leg press-to-body weight ratio is determined by dividing the maximum weight lifted in pounds by the subject's weight in pounds.

For men and women: Leg press (1RM) = maximum weight lifted ÷ body weight

For example, if a person presses 250 pounds and weighs 150 pounds

Leg press (1RM) = 250 ÷ 150

Leg press (1RM) = 1.66

The following are some common mistakes participants make on the leg press (1RM) test:

- Failing to fully extend the legs
- Coming out of the seated position during the test to gain a mechanical advantage
- Using the arms to aid in extending the legs

Table 6.6 Standards for Leg Press (One–Repetition Maximum)

Age (yr)	15 – 19		20 – 29		30 – 39		40 – 49		50 – 59		60+	
Gender	M	F	M	F	M	F	M	F	M	F	M	F
Excellent	≥2.27	≥1.82	≥2.27	≥1.82	≥2.07	≥1.61	≥1.92	≥1.48	≥1.8	≥1.37	≥1.73	≥1.32
Above average	2.05 – 2.26	1.58 – 1.81	2.05 – 2.26	1.58 – 1.81	1.85 – 2.06	1.39 – 1.60	1.74 – 1.91	1.29 – 1.47	1.64 – 1.79	1.17 – 1.36	1.56 – 1.72	1.13 – 1.31
Average	1.91 – 2.04	1.44 – 1.57	1.91 – 2.04	1.44 – 1.57	1.71 – 1.84	1.27 – 1.38	1.62 – 1.73	1.18 – 1.28	1.52 – 1.63	1.05 – 1.16	1.43 – 1.55	.99 – 1.12
Below average	1.74 – 1.90	1.27 – 1.43	1.74 – 1.90	1.27 – 1.43	1.59 – 1.70	1.15 – 1.26	1.51 – 1.61	1.08 – 1.17	1.39 – 1.51	.95 – 1.04	1.30 – 1.42	.88 – .98
Poor	≤1.74	≤1.27	≤1.74	≤1.27	≤1.59	≤1.15	≤1.51	≤1.08	≤1.39	≤.95	≤1.30	≤.88

Adapted from Dwyer & Davis, 2005; data from Franklin, 2006.

References

ACSM. (1998). Exercise in physical activity for older adults. *Medicine and Science in Sports and Exercise, 30*(6): 992

Arendt, E., & Dick, R. (1995). Knee injury patterns among men and women in collegiate basketball and soccer: NCAA data and review of literature. *American Journal of Sports Medicine, 25*: 694-701.

Atlas, C. (2003). Charles Atlas: The world's most perfectly developed man. Retrieved May 31, 2003, from www.cmgww.com/sports/atlas.

Baker, M. (1998). Anterior cruciate ligament injuries and female athletes. *Journal of Women's Health, 7*: 343-349.

Baldo, B. (1996). Grip strength testing. *National Strength and Conditioning Association Journal, 18*(5): 32-35.

Behnke, R. (2006). *Kinetic anatomy.* Champaign, IL: Human Kinetics.

Bompa, T., Di Pasquale, M., & Cornacchia, L. (2002). *Serious strength training.* Champaign, IL: Human Kinetics.

Canadian Physical Activity. (1999). *The Canadian physical activity, fitness & lifestyle appraisal: CSEP's plan for healthy active living.* Ottawa, Ontario: Canadian Society for Exercise Physiology.

Darden, E. (1995). *Living longer and stronger.* New York: Berkley.

Dornemann, T.M. (1997). Effects of high-intensity resistance exercise on bone mineral density and muscle strength of 40-50-year-old women. *Journal of Sports Medicine and Fitness, 37*(4): 246-251.

Dwyer, G.B., & Davis, S.E. (2005). *ACSM's health-related physical fitness assessment manual.* Philadelphia: Lippincott Williams & Wilkins.

Eidelson, S. (2006). Back pain–A universal language. Retrieved October 16, 2006, from www.spineuniverse.com/displayarticle.php/article1457.html.

Fiatarone, A. (2002). Exercise comes of age: Rationale and recommendations for a geriatric exercise prescription. *Journals of Gerontology A: Biological Sciences & Medical Sciences, 54*(5): 262-283.

Findley, B., & Keating, T. (2003). Is the Valsalva Maneuver a proper breathing technique? *National Strength and Conditioning Association Journal, 25*(4): 52-53.

Findley, B., & Keating, T. (2003). Is the Valsalva maneuver a proper breathing technique? *National Strength and Conditioning Association Journal, 25*(4): 52-53.

Fleck, S., & Kraemer, W. (1997). *Designing resistance training programs* (2nd ed.). Champaign, IL: Human Kinetics.

Franklin, B.A., (Ed.). (2006). *ACSM's guidelines for exercise testing and prescription.* Philadelphia: Lippincott Williams & Wilkins.

Gentle, D. (2000). Some amazing feats of grip strength. Retrieved October 6, 2006, from www.naturalstrength.com/history/detail.asp?ArticleID=300.

Guinness World Records. (1957). *Guinness world records 1957.* London: Young.

Guinness Book of World Records (Ed.). (2004). *Guinness world records 2004.* New York: Bantam.

Gwinup, G., Chelvam, P., & Steinberg, T. (1971). Thickness of subcutaneous fat and activity of underlying muscles. *Annals of Internal Medicine, 74*: 408-411.

Harris, H.A. (1966). *Greek athletes and athletics.* London: Indiana Press.

Harris, H.A. (1993). *Sport in Greece and Rome.* Ithaca, NY: Cornell University Press.

Hass, C. (2000). Single versus multiple sets in long-term recreational weightlifters. *Medicine & Science in Sports and Exercise, 32*(1): 235.

Haykowsky, M., Taylor, D., Teo, K., Quinney, A., & Humen, D. (2001). Left ventricular wall stress during leg-press exercise performed with a brief Valsalva maneuver. *Chest, 119*: 150-150.

Hochschuler, S. (1991). *Back in shape: A back owner's manual.* Boston: Houghton Mifflin.

Incledon, L. (2005). *Strength training for women.* Champaign, IL: Human Kinetics.

Jenkins, J. (1975). *A greater strength.* Old Tappan, NJ: Revell.

Katch, F.I., Clarkson, P., Kroll, W., & McBride, T. (1984). Effects of sit-up exercise training on adipose cell size and adiposity. *Research Quarterly for Exercise and Sport, 55*(3): 242-247.

Lauback, L. (1976). Comparative muscle strength of men and women: A review of the literature. *Aviation, Space, Environment and Medicine, 47*: 534-542.

McGlynn, G., & Moran, G.T. (1997). *Dynamics of strength training and conditioning.* (2nd ed.). Chicago: Brown and Benchmark.

National Collegiate Athletic Association. (1994). Injury rate for women's basketball increases sharply. *NCAA News, 31*: 9, 13.

National Osteoporosis Foundation. (2003). Disease facts. Retrieved May 30, 2003, from www.nof.org/osteoporosis/stats.htm.

National Osteoporosis Society. (2003). What is osteoporosis? Retrieved May 30, 2003, from www.nos.org.uk/about.htm.

National Strength and Conditioning Association. (1994). *NSCA's essentials of strength training and conditioning.* Champaign, IL: Human Kinetics.

National Strength and Conditioning Association. (2000). *Essentials of strength training and conditioning.* (2nd ed.). Champaign, IL: Human Kinetics.

Reynolds, J., Stevenson, M., Rutstein, S., & Conte, S. (1990). *Caring for your low back.* San Bruno: Krames.

Rhea, M., Alvar, R., Burkett, B., & Lee, N. (2002). Single versus multiple sets for strength: A meta-analysis to address the controversy. *Research Quarterly for Exercise and Sport, 73*(4): 485-489.

Seung-Houn, L., Sung-Hwan, Y., & Ji-Han Seo, J.M.A.K. (2004). Development of an exercise program to prevent low back pain using an ergonomic approach. *International Journal of Advanced Manufacturing Technology, 24*(5/6): 381-388.

Sharkey, B. (2002). *Fitness and health* (5th ed.). Champaign, IL: Human Kinetics.

Simmons, L. (2005). The regulation of training. *Powerlifting USA, 22*(7): 32-33.

Sinaki, M., Itoi, E., Wahner, H.W., Wallan, P., Gelzcer, R., Mullan, B.P., Collins, D.A., & Hodgson, S.F. (2002). Stronger back muscles reduce the incidence of vertebral fractures: A prospective 10 year follow-up of postmenopausal women. *Bone, 30*(6): 836.

Stone, M.H., Sands, W.A., Pierce, K.C., Newton, R.U., Haff, G., & Carlock, J. (2006). Maximum strength and strength training—A relationship to endurance? *National Strength and Conditioning Association Journal, 8*(3): 44-53.

Strossen, R. (2007). Official list of those certified as closing the No. 4 Captains of Crush gripper. Retrieved September 12, 2001, from www.ironmind.com/ironmind/opencms/ironmind/Main/captainsofcrush4.html.

Westcott, W. (1994). *Strength fitness physiological principles and training techniques.* Boston: WCB/McGraw-Hill.

Wheeler, A.H. (1995). Diagnosis and management of low back pain and sciatica. *American Family Physician*: 1333-1341.

Wipf, J., & Deyo, R. (1995). Low back pain. *Medical Clinics of North America, 79*(2): 231-247.

Suggested Readings

National Strength and Conditioning Association (2000). *Essentials of strength training and conditioning* **(2nd ed.). Champaign, IL: Human Kinetics.**

This is "the" manual for strength-training professionals or anyone desiring to expand their weight-training expertise.

Baechle, T., & Earle, R. (2006). *Weight training: Steps to success* (3rd ed.). **Champaign: Human Kinetics.**

This easy-to-follow resistance training manual is a step-by-step approach for those with little to no strength-training background.

Bompa, T., Di Pasquale, M., & Cornacchia, L. (2002). *Serious strength training.* **Champaign, IL: Human Kinetics.**

Advanced strength-training principles and programs are described and illustrated.

Delavier, F. (2001). *Strength training anatomy.* **Champaign, IL: Human Kinetics.**

If you're curious about which exercises develop particular muscles, this book is for you. A multitude of pictures clearly illustrates the specific musculature trained and most primary strength-training exercises.

Jenkins, J. (1975). *A greater strength.* **Old Tappan, New Jersey: Revell.**

This book documents the life of one of the strongest men who ever lived—Paul Anderson. This modern-day "Samson" has an interesting spiritual journey as well.

Suggested Web Sites

www.nsca-lift.org

The National Strength and Conditioning Association site is for personal trainers and strength coaches.

www.msbn.tv/usavision

The USA Weightlifting site is an excellent source for those interested in recreational or competitive Olympic weightlifting.

www.usapowerlifting.com

The USA Powerlifting site is for those who may be interested in recreational or competitive powerlifting.

www.acefitness.org

The American Council on Exercise (ACE) site is dedicated to developing personal trainers, but it has some excellent information on strength training for consumers.

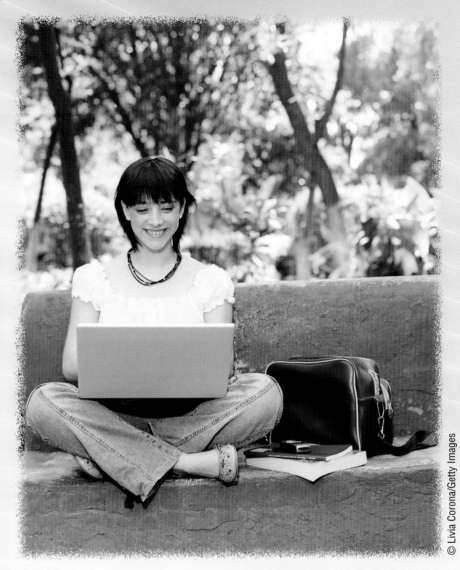

© Livia Corona/Getty Images

Flexibility Assessment and Training

Bob Weathers

After reading this chapter, you should be able to do the following:

1. Describe flexibility.
2. List the factors that affect flexibility.
3. Understand the importance of flexibility.
4. Know your range of motion.
5. Assess your flexibility.
6. Know how to improve or maintain flexibility.

Make Time for Flexibility

It doesn't happen often, but every few months John gets searing pain in his lower back while sitting at his desk or driving a car. For a few days he can barely move, and sitting in a car is almost impossible. The pain is excruciating. He observes that those back pains usually appear when he's been sitting way too much, has been under extra stress, and hasn't taken the time to stretch in the mornings. He usually begins his days with prayer while sitting cross-legged on the floor. After prayer, he usually does a few sit-ups and some stretching exercises. When he misses his prayer time on busy days, he misses his exercises, and that's when the back pain hits. Not taking time to do some flexibility exercises makes him less able to do normal physical bending, and worse than that, debilitates him for several days several times during the year. On the other hand he watches, with a certain degree of envy, a young woman reading a book while she is seated cross-legged on the floor. The book is lying on the floor and her nose almost touches the book. How can she do that?

What Is Flexibility?

Flexibility is defined as the **range of motion (ROM)** that is possible in a joint or group of joints (Corbin, Lindsey, & Welk, 2000). First, **static flexibility** is the ability to hold a stretched position. Second, **dynamic flexibility** is the ability to move slowly and rhythmically through a full ROM. Third, **ballistic flexibility** is the ability to move through a ROM with bobbing, bouncing movements. **Laxity** and **hypermobility** are terms that refer to greater than normal, or excessive, ROM in joints.

When people say they are "stiff as a board," they mean that their joints have limited range of motion. These people may benefit from doing exercises and increasing ROM at key joints in their bodies. You should note that, whether because of nature or nurture, flexibility is highly specific to each joint and type of movement. You or John might have very flexible shoulders while your hips may be quite tight. Likewise, you may have better flexibility at one speed of movement than at another.

Factors That Affect Flexibility

The ROM of a joint may be limited by several characteristics:

- The structure of bones at their points of contact

- The tightness of the joint capsule and the ligaments that hold joints together
- The length and extensibility of surrounding soft tissues, like the muscles acting on the joints and the tendons that attach muscles to bones
- The amount of fat, muscle, and other soft tissues on body segments

Bone Structure

The first characteristic affecting flexibility is bone structure. The elbow is an example of a hinge joint in which bone structure limits ROM. The shapes of the articulating surfaces (where the bones contact each other) permit movement in only one plane, with significant flexion but little or no extension possible beyond returning the joint to 180 degrees. However, the shoulders have ball-and-socket structures that allow movement in three different planes and a large ROM.

Ligament Strength

The second characteristic affecting flexibility has to do with ligament strength. The articulating surfaces of some bones permit varied types and ranges of motion, but the ways in which ligaments hold the joints together prevent ROM in some cases. A stretched ligament is typically called a *sprain,* which is undesirable. It's not wise to walk on the sides of the foot to stretch the ligaments in the ankle.

Muscle and Tendon Elongation

The third characteristic affecting flexibility has to do with muscle and tendon elongation. Proper warm-up before an activity allows tendons (connecting muscle to bone) and muscles to elongate more during activity, preventing injury from exceeding an earlier fixed point. Stretching after activity will help maintain healthy elongation of tendons and muscles and therefore improves flexibility.

Joint Restriction

A fourth characteristic is joint restriction that happens when soft tissue gets in the way. For example, a person's ability to touch the toes may be limited by a large abdomen that contacts the thighs long before other factors inhibit motion.

Scripture teaches that God has given each person specific gifts and abilities that fit the functions he wants him or her to perform within the body of Christ. Likewise, various physical traits affect health and physical fitness. People are different from each other, and for that reason, they can't perform equally. Structures of bones and ligaments and the quantity and nature of muscles, tendons, and other tissues are affected by genetics. The genetic influence is so strong in some individuals that it's difficult or impossible for them to attain normal ROM in certain joints.

You can't change your genetics, but it appears that you have some control over the three other factors that limit flexibility. Research indicates that lower-than-normal flexibility is typically due to poor extensibility (i.e., short length of muscles and tendons) as a result of limited use of a joint through its full ROM. Body temperature is a major factor affecting the extensibility of muscles and tendons; flexibility increases with temperature.

Importance of Flexibility

Some research suggests that increased flexibility might help John avoid back pains, and it's also important for you. The classic book *Hypokinetic Disease* (Kraus & Raab, 1961) associates sedentary living with the inability of muscles to relax and with a variety of medical disorders. Lower-back pain is the chief "tension syndrome" addressed in the Kraus and Raab book. The authors associate tension syndrome with tightness in the muscles that extend the back and the hips.

1 Corinthians 12 speaks metaphorically about the church as a body: "If one part suffers, every part suffers with it; if one part is honored, every part rejoices with it." Back pain from inflexibility is felt in only one body part, but it disables a whole person. The Bible also says in Revelation 21 that the New Jerusalem will be a place without mourning or crying or pain (verse 4). Maintaining flexibility, and thereby limiting painful experiences, allows a taste of a New Jerusalem right now.

Some form of sit-and-reach test is the most common evaluation of flexibility for people who are concerned with health and wellness because of the presumed effect of lower-back and hamstring flexibility on lower-back pain. However, Plowman (1992) and McGill (2001) are among reviewers of the evidence who have some doubts about that relationship. One reason for doubt was a large study of adults that failed to reveal any significant relationship between lower-back pain and performance on the sit-and-reach test (Allen et al., 1998). On the other hand, Grenier, Russell, and McGill (2003) found a relationship between back flexibility and a history of lower-back pain, but sit-and-reach test results had no such relationship.

Wellness can sometimes be affected by sport performance, but the focus in this chapter is on health and the performance of activities required in daily living. Kell, Bell, and Quinney (2001) report that squatting to tie shoes is the activity of daily living that requires the most flexibility. They also report that flexibility in the average person decreases about 20 to 30 percent between 30 and 70 years of age. Hoeger and Hoeger (1999) point out that people, regardless of age, sometimes need to perform rapid or strenuous movements they're not accustomed to, so it may be wise to prepare for activities that are more demanding than they've planned. It will be helpful to keep these occasional demands for ballistic flexibility in mind when reading the later section on improving flexibility. To live the kind of abundant life God wants to give (John 10:10) requires faithfulness to maintaining whole health.

Alter (2004) claims, on the basis of opinion, theory, and equivocal evidence, that the potential benefits of flexibility training go way beyond back health and are "virtually unlimited" (p. 6).

He identifies 11 specific benefits (Alter, 2004, pp. 8-14):

- Union of body, mind, and spirit
- Relaxation of stress and tension
- Muscular relaxation
- Self-discipline and self-knowledge
- Body fitness, posture, and symmetry
- Relief of lower-back pain
- Relief of muscle cramps
- Relief of muscle soreness
- Injury prevention
- Enjoyment and pleasure
- Enhanced sleep

Someone once said that health and fitness are gifts to the young, and after that, you have to earn them. This suggests that flexibility training becomes more important with age, at least among the majority of adults who become progressively less active as they get older. Warburton, Gledhill, and Quinney (2001) emphasize that quality of life is affected by the ability to perform activities of daily living; and the decrease in ROM that is typically seen with aging has been associated with decreased walking speed and reduced ability to use public transport, climb stairs, or get up from a chair. Decreased ROM as a result of aging also brings increased pain and reduced independence, perceived health, social function, mental health, and quality of life. However, the researchers also

The Benefits of Stretching

Conventional wisdom says flexibility is valuable, but it's important to see if there's evidence to support that position. Several recent reviews have been conducted to examine and synthesize research on the relationship between stretching and various benefits. Shrier (1999) concludes that stretching before exercise does not reduce injury risk and observed that stretching before doing other activity is more likely to cause than to prevent injury. Herbert and Gabriel (2002) conclude that stretching before or after exercise should not be counted on to provide protection from muscle soreness. On the other hand, they state that stretching before exercise may provide a little protection from injury, but not enough to be of practical importance. Weldon and Hill (2003) identify four of the better studies that support the position that stretching reduces injury and three studies that do not. Thacker and colleagues at the U.S. Centers for Disease Control and Prevention (2004) found no significant relationship between stretching and total number of injuries, but they conclude, "there is not sufficient evidence to endorse or discontinue routine stretching before or after exercise to prevent injury among competitive or recreational athletes" (p. 371). Shrier (2004a) reports that almost all studies found

athletic performance to be negatively affected by single sessions of stretching before activity, but regular stretching seems to have a positive effect on performance, particularly if stretching follows the activity (Byl, 2004).

All these reviewers lament the poor quantity and quality of research on the value of stretching. Shrier (2004b) faults Thacker and colleagues for combining data from studies of pre- and postexercise stretching for the same analysis. He argues that it is the chronic effect of regular stretching that has value, not the single, acute effect of single stretching sessions, whether before or after exercise.

Witvrouw and colleagues (2004) address another issue in a qualitative analysis of the research on stretching and injury. They propose that contrasting results in the literature can be at least partially explained by the type of activity being studied. Specifically, they believe that stretching is likely to reduce injuries for individuals engaged in bouncing or jumping activities where muscle–tendon units experience high-intensity stretching and shortening cycles. Shrier (2004a), in his analysis of the effect of stretching on performance, supposes that the nature of research prevents the study of competitive performance with appropriate rigor.

point out that considerable reductions in flexibility may exist without noticeable disability.

I mentioned earlier that genetic variation means different levels of flexibility in different individuals. Genetic variation may also mean differences in the significance of flexibility among people of the same age and engaged in the same activities. Not everyone has pain like John's. His may be a result of his genetics or some other factor that makes him vulnerable to such suffering when he doesn't take time to stretch. Some people, on the other hand, may suffer even though they stretch regularly or have great natural flexibility; others may be free of such suffering despite the fact that they never stretch and have below-average flexibility. Because of biological differences, the many ways that people might stretch, and the myriad ways of engaging in physical activity, research findings may never be generalized broadly to all athletes and exercisers.

How Much Flexibility Is Enough?

Corbin, Lindsey, and Welk (2000) state that the optimal amount of flexibility for health is unknown. Norms are available for both sexes at various ages, but little evidence establishes at what levels flexibility becomes excessively high or low. It is clear that some people are able to maintain good flexibility and seem to be well without participating in regular stretching. It is also apparent that people with hypermobility are at greater risk for certain diseases and injuries. Individuals in both of these groups may be among the minority, but as with other areas of life and fitness, more is not necessarily better, and it may be worse.

Protas (2001) provides one table of norms for flexibility and points out that, typically, women have greater flexibility than men and children than adults. Little evidence suggests that most people need more flexibility than most adult males have. Alter (2004) explains that there is controversy regarding the relationship between age and flexibility. The extent to which one's need for or ability to maintain flexibility with age is unclear. However, most authorities seem to believe that it is wise to maintain flexibility within the normal range, especially as people grow older.

You may want only to maintain the flexibility to do the things you need or want to do without feeling restricted by tight muscles or tendons. In the next section of the chapter, I'll help you assess your flexibility and then increase it.

Assessing Your Flexibility

A person can have greater-than-normal flexibility in one joint and at the same time have fairly normal flexibility in a second, and even lower-than-normal flexibility in a third joint. For that reason any single measure of flexibility may not be a good indicator of the person's overall flexibility. Meaningful assessment, then, will either involve measuring dynamic and static flexibility in many joints or measuring a specific type of flexibility in a body segment of particular interest.

As I already mentioned, those interested in assessing health-related fitness have usually employed some type of sit-and-reach test as a measure of flexibility. The American College of Sports Medicine (2006) currently recommends either the Canadian trunk forward flexion test (Canadian Society for Exercise Physiology, 2003) or the YMCA sit-and-reach test (YMCA, 2000), but several other sit-and-reach tests are also in use. For any sit-and-reach test, the ACSM says that you should warm up and do some stretching of the hamstring and back muscles (see the next section of this chapter for information on stretching). Remove your shoes and sit with both knees straight but not locked. Slowly reach forward as far as possible with one hand on top of the other and the tips of the fingers on both hands even. Hold that position for about two seconds. As you bend forward, you should drop your head and exhale, but you should not hold your breath. The better of two trials is your score.

Most sit-and-reach tests appear to have similar validity (Baltaci et al., 2003; Hui et al., 1999; Koen, et al., 2003), being moderately related to flexibility of the hamstrings but poorly related to flexibility of the low back. Therefore, selection of a test can reasonably be based on other considerations. The back-saver test (Meredith & Welk, 2005) is done one leg at a time and has the purported advantages of comparing flexibility in the two legs and reducing risk to spinal discs, ligaments, tendons, and muscles. Although research has not consistently supported the importance of this issue, the modified sit-and-reach test (Hoeger & Hoeger, 1999) was designed to compensate for differences among individuals in relative torso and limb lengths. The back-saver, modified, and Canadian tests all require a special sit-and-reach box. However, the only equipment required for the YMCA test (figure

7.1*a*) is a meter stick, yardstick, or tape measure, giving an advantage in practicality. You simply sit on the floor with your feet about 12 inches (30 cm) apart and slide your fingertips along the measuring stick that is set on the floor between your legs so that it bisects, is perpendicular to, and has its 15-inch (38 cm) mark on a line between your heels. A piece of tape is useful to mark the line between your heels and to hold the ruler in place. See table 7.1 to interpret your results.

Fitnessgram (Meredith & Welk, 2005) is a test battery promoted by the Cooper Institute for Aerobics Research and the American Alliance for Health, Physical Education, Recreation and Dance to assess health-related fitness. In addition to the back-saver sit-and-reach test, the Fitnessgram includes a pass–fail shoulder flexibility test (figure 7.1*b*) that is more related to the ability to perform certain activities of daily living than to organic health. You pass if you can touch your fingertips together behind your back as you reach over the shoulder with one hand and bring the other hand up the back from below.

Improving and Maintaining Your Flexibility

You can maintain or improve flexibility by simply moving joints through their full ROM while going about the business of daily living. However, modern life rarely requires regularly moving all body parts that way. Yoga, tai chi, and Pilates provide benefits for flexibility even if the primary motive for participating in them isn't that. You might prefer to select from a variety of stretching exercises for the specific purpose of maintaining or improving flexibility. Static stretching techniques involve slowly stretching a muscle and then holding the stretch while relaxing the muscles. Dynamic stretching emphasizes movement through a wide ROM, rather than holding a position. Ballistic stretching is a form of dynamic stretching that makes use of the momentum from repetitive bouncing motions. Proprioceptive neuromuscular facilitation (PNF) techniques involve alternately stretching, contracting, and relaxing muscles. PNF should be administered only by trained individuals (American College of Sports Medicine, 2006).

Ballistic stretching was common before the beginning of the fitness boom of the 1970s, but more recently static stretching has generally been preferred over ballistic. Here's why: All muscles have **muscle spindles** that contain stretch receptors that are stimulated when a muscle is stretched. When muscle spindles are stimulated, the muscle contracts reflexively, which is contrary to stretching (Taylor et al., 1990). Although research is not conclusive on the negative effects

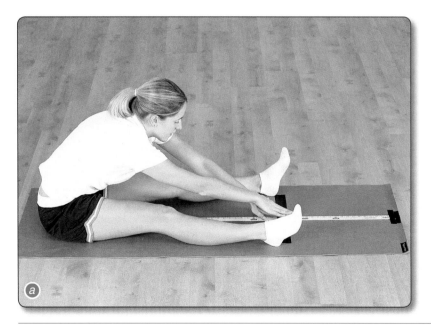
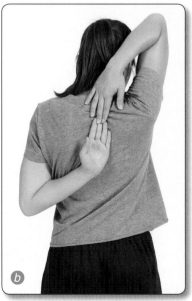

FIGURE 7.1   *(a)* YMCA sit-and-reach test; *(b)* shoulder flexibility test.

Table 7.1 Percentiles by Age and Gender for the YMCA Sit-and-Reach Test in Inches (Centimeters)

	AGE											
	GENDER											
	18–25		26–35		36–45		46–55		56–65		>65	
Percentile	M	F	M	F	M	F	M	F	M	F	M	F
90	22 (56)	24 (61)	21 (53.5)	23 (58.5)	21 (53.5)	22 (56)	19 (48)	21 (53.5)	17 (43)	20 (51)	17 (43)	20 (51)
80	20 (51)	22 (56)	19 (48)	21 (53.5)	19 (48)	21 (53.5)	17 (43)	20 (51)	15 (38)	19 (48)	15 (38)	18 (45.5)
70	19 (48)	21 (53.5)	17 (43)	20 (51)	17 (43)	19 (48)	15 (38)	18 (45.5)	13 33)	17 (43)	13 (33)	17 (43)
60	18 (45.5)	20 (51)	17 (43)	20 (51)	16 (40.5)	18 (45.5)	14 (35.5)	17 (43)	13 (33)	16 (40.5)	12 (30.5)	17 (43)
50	17 (43)	19 (48)	15 (38)	19 (48)	15 (38)	17 (43)	13 (33)	16 (40.5)	11 (28)	15 (38)	10 (25.5)	15 (38)
40	15 (38)	18 (45.5)	14 (35.5)	17 (43)	13 (33)	16 (40.5)	11 (28)	14 (35.5)	9 (23)	14 (35.5)	9 (23)	14 (35.5)
30	14 (35.5)	17 (43)	13 (33)	16 (40.5)	13 (33)	15 (38)	10 (25.5)	14 (35.5)	9 (23)	13 (33)	8 (20.5)	13 (33)
20	13 (33)	16 (40.5)	11 (28)	15 (38)	11 (28)	14 (35.5)	9 (23)	12 (30.5)	7 (18)	11 (28)	7 (18)	11 (28)
10	11 (28)	14 (35.5)	9 (23)	13 (33)	7 (18)	12 (30.5)	6 (15)	10 (25.5)	5 (12)	9 (23)	4 (10)	9 (23)

Reprinted, by permission, from G.B. Dwyer and S.E. Davis, 2005, *ACSM's health-related physical assessment manual* (Philadelphia, PA: Lippincott, Williams, and Wilkins), 83.

of ballistic stretching (Weerapong, Hume, & Kolt, 2004), most researchers will recommend slow, static stretching (Shellock & Prentice, 1985; Smith, 1994) because they believe less stimulation of muscle spindles by avoiding bouncing will make stretching more effective, safer, and less painful.

PNF techniques are based on the actions of **Golgi tendon organs** in tendons. Golgi tendon organs are stimulated by the high tension created in tendons when the related muscles contract with sufficient force or when they are stretched far enough and for sufficient time. With PNF, the muscle is first stretched passively by an outside force, such as when a partner moves one of the limbs. When the limb is moved to the extent of a joint's comfortable ROM, the subject contracts the stretched muscle. When a stretched muscle

contracts forcefully, the result tends to be reflex relaxation of the muscle, allowing it to be stretched to a greater extent. Some PNF procedures involve contraction of **antagonist** muscles immediately after the contraction of the stretched muscle. While research has generally shown PNF to improve flexibility more than other techniques do, it often also produces more muscle soreness, and it usually requires assistance from a trained partner (American College of Sports Medicine, 2006).

ACSM first recommended that people do three to five repetitions of static stretches, holding each stretch to a point of mild discomfort for 10 to 30 seconds. They recommended stretching on at least three days a week and emphasizing the lower back and hip joint (Pollock et al.,1998). Current

Patience

Eugene slipped on the squash court, hit the back of his head on the floor, and was unconscious. At the hospital, doctors thought Eugene would probably miss two weeks of school as he waited for the headaches to subside so he could return to studying. A few months earlier, he had twisted his knee trying to avoid hitting a makeshift referee stand beside a volleyball court. The knee is temporarily supported by braces, but it will require surgery in the future. If he damages the knee again, he will likely have a permanent disability. Yet Eugene goes on, hurting at times, but mostly with a smile in his heart. He trusts that somehow God will use these situations for good. It will just take time.

Proverbs says that a "patient man has great understanding, but a quick-tempered man displays folly" (14:29). However, **patience** in scripture is more than some kind of ethical virtue. It is the ability to be longsuffering, and is a gift from God (2 Corinthians 6:6). I believe Eugene has it. Patience is the first attribute of love in 1 Corinthians 13:4. It is one of a list of items Paul considers he has modeled as a missionary, and it is a characteristic of a "life worthy of the Lord" (Colossians 1:9–13).

God is all-powerful, and yet he is patient with his children. Eugene provides a good model in waiting and gaining strength from the Lord. In contrast, people with a type A personality, in which the adrenaline kicks in over the smallest matter, consider themselves so important, and so right, that they hardly listen to what others are saying.

God provides the opportunity to be long-suffering in serious matters, in unjust situations, and in situations with irritating people. He also provides patience to wait for positive matters, such as achieving physical flexibility and personal wellness. The Lord wants to hear about his children's concerns, irritations, and impatience. Benefits come from being patient while working to make changes over the long haul. There are few quick fixes. Remember that "those who hope in the Lord will renew their strength. They will soar on wings like eagles; they will run and not grow weary, they will walk and not be faint" (Isaiah 40:31; see also Psalm 40:1–3; Psalm 130). That's receiving wellness from patience.

Patience: Is there something you need to be patient with? Memorize Isaiah 40:31 and think of it when you want to give up.

_____

_____

_____

_____

_____

_____

_____

_____

_____

recommendations are similar (American College of Sports Medicine, 2006):

- Warm up for three to five minutes before stretching (with jogging, vigorous walking, dancing, or jumping jacks).
- Do static stretches for the major muscle groups, especially those crossing joints that have limited ROM.

- Stretch at least two days, but ideally five to seven days, each week.
- Stretch to the point of tightness, without causing discomfort.
- Hold each stretch for 15 to 30 seconds.
- Perform two to four repetitions of each stretch.

Some other general guidelines to follow when stretching include the following (Byl, 2004; Harris & Elbourn, 2002):

- Move into the stretch slowly.
- Hold the stretch; do not bounce.
- Feel mild tension in the middle of the stretched muscle.
- If you feel any pain or if the muscle starts shaking, ease off the stretch immediately.
- Relax all other parts of your body, particularly your head, shoulders, and back.
- Don't fight against the muscle; try to relax.
- If you are comfortable and the muscle feels relaxed, try increasing the stretch gently and holding the new position.
- Gently ease out of the stretch.

Most fitness professionals recommend static stretching, but Corbin, Lindsey, and Welk (2000) state that ballistic stretching is important for people who are physically active. Kell, Bell, and Quinney (2001) provide the additional recommendation for people to add resistance training to stretching as a way of increasing flexibility.

McGill (2001) suggests that individuals who are primarily concerned with health and safety, rather than with the enhancement of athletic performance, should limit torso flexibility exercises to those that impose no external load. He also emphasizes that the spine should be cycled slowly and smoothly through the full range of flexion and extension and that care should be taken to keep the spine in a neutral position when doing flexibility exercises for the hips and knees, such as standing hip flexion and lunges. The American College of Sports Medicine (2006) identifies some common high-risk stretching exercises (figure 7.2a) that may not be appropriate for some individuals; they suggest some safer alternatives (figure 7.2b):

High Risk	Alternative
Standing toe touch	Seated toe touch or modified hurdler's stretch
Barre stretch	Seated toe touch or modified hurdler's stretch
Hurdler's stretch	Modified hurdler's stretch
Neck circle	Nontwisting directional stretch
Knee hyper-extension	Kneeling hip and thigh stretch
Yoga plow	Seated toe touch

Think of maintaining good flexibility as a lifelong concern. Unless the activities you are engaging in require movements well beyond their normal range (such as in gymnastics or wrestling), do the flexibility exercises after the activity (or game), not before it (Byl, 2004; Knudson, 1999).

Next Steps

Maintaining flexibility is a gift that you have some control over. Taking time after a warm-up to stretch various muscles and tendons may enhance the joy of movement and quality of life. Take time to assess your current levels of flexibility and then plan and live a life that maintains or enhances your current level of flexibility.

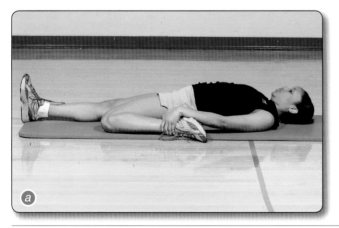
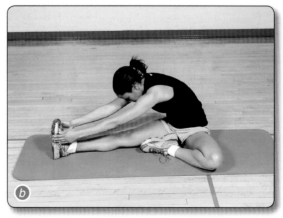

FIGURE 7.2 *(a)* A hurdler's stretch might be harmful for some individuals; *(b)* a modified hurdler's stretch is a safer alternative to the hurdler's stretch.

Key Terms

antagonist

ballistic flexibility

dynamic flexibility

flexibility

Golgi tendon organs

hypermobility

laxity

muscle spindles

patience

range of motion (ROM)

static flexibility

Review Questions

1. Define flexibility.

2. List four factors that affect flexibility.

3. List five documented benefits of flexibility.

4. How does a person determine and measure an optimal level of flexibility?

5. How does a person best improve or maintain flexibility?

Application Activities

1. Perform a sit-and-reach test (or other tests as assigned by your instructor) to determine your back flexibility. Use table 7.1 to compare your score with the norms for your sex and age.

2. What is your mission statement? Is this the same as before? If it is different what did you change and why?

3. Write down your specific flexibility goals in a sentence or two.

   a. In a paragraph or two, assess the behavior and attitudes you are trying to change to improve your flexibility.

   b. Refine your goal with small, realistic, specific, measurable, and concrete steps.

   c. In a paragraph or two, predict and describe two significant obstacles that prevent you from achieving your flexibility goal and describe your plan to overcome those obstacles.

   d. What specific intervention strategies will you have in place to assist you in complying with your plan (the text suggests six; see pages 23-25 in chapter 2)?

   e. How will you evaluate your compliance with your flexibility plan?

   f. How will you measure progress in achieving your flexibility goal?

References

Allen, A.W., Morrow, J.R. Jr., Brill, P.A., Kohl, H.W. III, Gordon, N.F., & Blair, S.N. (1998). Relations of sit-up and sit-and-reach tests to low back pain in adults. *Journal of Orthopaedic and Sports Physical Therapy, 27*: 22-26.

Alter, M.J. (2004). *Science of flexibility* (3rd ed.). Champaign, IL: Human Kinetics.

American College of Sports Medicine. (2006). *ACSM's guidelines for exercise testing and prescription* (7th ed.). Baltimore: Lippincott, Williams & Wilkins.

Baltaci, G., Un, N., Tunay, V., Besler, A., & Gerçeker, S. (2003). Comparison of three different sit and reach tests for measurement of hamstring flexibility in female university students. *British Journal of Sports Medicine, 37*: 59-61.

Byl, J. (2004). *101 fun warm-up and cool-down games.* Champaign, IL: Human Kinetics.

Canadian Society for Exercise Physiology. (2003). *The Canadian physical activity, fitness & lifestyle approach: CSEP—health & fitness program's health-related appraisal & counseling strategy.* Ottawa: Canadian Society for Exercise Physiology.

Corbin, C.B., Lindsey, R., & Welk, G. (2000). *Concepts of fitness and wellness* (3rd ed.). New York: McGraw-Hill.

Dwyer, G.B., & Davis, S.E. (2005). *ACSM's health-related physical assessment manual.* Philadelphia, PA: Lippincott, Williams, and Wilkins.

Grenier, S.G., Russell, C., & McGill, S.M. (2003). Relationships between lumbar flexibility, sit-and-reach test, and a previous history of low back discomfort in industrial workers. *Canadian Journal of Applied Physiology, 28*: 165-177.

Harris, J., & Elbourn, J. (2002). *Warming up and cooling down* (2nd ed.). Champaign, IL: Human Kinetics.

Herbert, R.D., & Gabriel M. (2002). Effects of stretching before and after exercising on muscle soreness and risk of injury: Systematic review. *British Medical Journal, 325*: 468.

Hoeger W.W.K., & Hoeger, S.A. (1999). *Principles and labs for fitness and wellness* (5th ed.). Englewood, CO: Morton.

Hui, A.C., Yuen, P.Y., Morrow, J.R., Jr., & Jackson, A.W. (1999). Comparison of the criterion-related validity of sit-and-reach tests with and without limb adjustment in Asian adults. *Research Quarterly for Exercise and Sport, 70*: 401-406.

Kell, R.T., Bell, G., & Quinney, A. (2001). Musculoskeletal fitness, health outcomes and quality of life. *Sports Medicine, 31*: 863-873.

Knudson, D. (1999). Stretching during warm-up. *Journal of Physical Education, Recreation, and Dance, 70*(7): 24-26.

Koen, A., Lemmink, P.M., Kemper, H.C.G., de Greef, M.H.G., Rispens, P., & Stevens, M. (2003). The validity of the sit-and-reach test and the modified sit-and-reach test in middle-aged to older men and women. *Research Quarterly for Exercise and Sport, 74*: 331-336.

Kraus, H. & Raab, W. (1961). *Hypokinetic Disease.* Springfield, IL: Thomas.

McGill, S.M. (2001). Low back exercises: Prescription for the healthy back and recovery from injury. In Roitman, J.L. (Ed.). *ACSM's resource manual for guidelines for exercise testing and prescription* (4th ed.) (pp.120-130). Baltimore: Lippincott, Williams & Wilkins.

Meredith, M.D., & Welk, G.J. (2005). *Fitnessgram test administration manual* (3rd ed.). Champaign, IL: Human Kinetics.

Plowman, S.A. (1992). Physical activity, physical fitness, and low back pain. *Exercise and Sport Sciences Reviews, 20*: 221-242.

Pollock, M.L., Gaesser, G.A., Butcher, J.D., Després, J-P., Dishman, R.K., Franklin, B.A., & Graber, C.E. (1998). The recommended quantity and quality of exercise for developing and maintaining cardiorespiratory and muscular fitness and flexibility in healthy adults. *Medicine and Science in Sports & Exercise, 30*: 975-991.

Protas, E.J. (2001). Flexibility and range of motion. In Roitman, J.L. (Ed.), *ACSM's resource manual for guidelines for exercise testing and prescription* (4th ed.) (pp. 120-130). Baltimore: Lippincott, Williams & Wilkins.

Shellock F., & Prentice, W. (1985). Warming up and stretching for improved physical performance and prevention of sports-related injuries. *Sports Medicine, 2*: 267-278.

Shrier, I. (1999). Stretching before exercise does not reduce the risk of local muscle injury: A critical review of the clinical and basic science literature. *Clinical Journal of Sports Medicine, 9*: 221-227.

Shrier, I. (2004a). Does stretching improve performance? A systematic and critical review of the literature. *Clinical Journal of Sport Medicine, 14*: 267-273.

Shrier, I. (2004b). Meta-analysis on preexercise stretching (letter to editor). *Medicine & Science in Sports & Exercise, 36*: 1832.

Smith, C. (1994). The warm-up procedure: To stretch or not to stretch. A brief review. *Journal of Orthopaedic and Sports Physical Therapy, 19*: 12-17.

Taylor, D., Dalton, J., Seaber, A., & Garrett, W. (1990). Viscoelastsic properties of muscle-tendon units: The biomechanical effects of stretching. *American Journal of Sports Medicine, 18*: 300-309.

Thacker, S.B., Gilchrist, J., Stroup, D.F., & Kimsey, C.D., Jr. (2004). The impact of stretching on sports injury risk: A systematic review of the literature. *Medicine & Science in Sports & Exercise, 36*: 371-378.

Warburton, D.E.R., Gledhill, N., & Quinney, A. (2001). Musculoskeletal fitness and health. *Canadian Journal of Applied Physiology, 26*: 217-237.

Weerapong, P., Hume, P., & Kolt, G. (2004). Stretching: Mechanisms and benefits for sport performance and injury prevention. *Physical Therapy Reviews, 9*: 189-206.

Weldon, S.M. & Hill, R.H. (2003). The efficacy of stretching for prevention of exercise-related injury: A systematic review of the literature. *Manual Therapy, 8*: 141-150.

Witvrouw, E., Mahieu, N., Danneels, L., & McNair, P. (2004). Stretching and injury prevention: An obscure relationship. *Sports Medicine, 34*: 443-449.

YMCA. (2000). *YMCA fitness testing and assessment manual* (4th ed.). Champaign, IL: YMCA.

Suggested Readings

Alter, M.J. (2004). *Science of flexibility* **(3rd ed.). Champaign, IL: Human Kinetics.**

Consult sections of interest (sciences of, clinical considerations of, principles of, anatomy of, and specific sport applications of flexiblity) in this book to gain a greater understanding of flexibility.

Anderson, B. (2000). *Stretching: 20ᵗʰ anniversary revised edition.* **Bolinas, CA: Shelter Publications.**

One of the most popular fitness books in the world, this book provides a summary of 200 different stretches with routines and stretching programs for over 20 sports.

Nelson, A.G., & Kokkonen J. (2007). *Stretching anatomy.* **Champaign, IL: Human Kinetics.**

See inside every stretch—and maximize flexibility. *Stretching Anatomy* will arm you with the knowledge to increase range of motion, supplement training, enhance recovery, and maximize efficiency of movement. You'll also gain a detailed understanding of how each stretch affects your body.

Suggested Web Sites

www.gsu.edu/~wwwfit/flexibility.html

Georgia State University Exercise and Physical Fitness page has photographs of a model doing 10 common stretches.

www.nia.nih.gov/HealthInformation/ Publications/ExerciseGuide/chapter04c.htm

The National Institute on Aging at the U.S. National Institutes of Health provides general guidelines and illustrates (some animated) stretches from the chapter on stretching.

www.rice.edu/~jenky/stretch.html

The Rice University Sports Medicine Web site gives advice about flexibility and illustrates stretches.

www.bath.ac.uk/~masrjb/Stretch/stretching_ 1.html#SEC1

The University of Bath site includes nine chapters by Bradford Appleton, dancer and martial artist, at the University of Bath (posted in 1994).

Understanding Your Behaviors

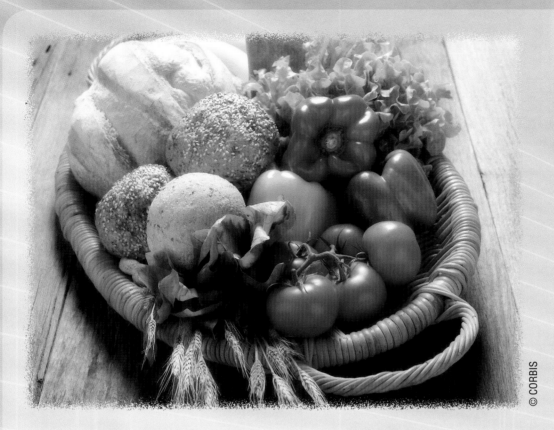

© CORBIS

Nutritional Health and Wellness

Peter Walters

After reading this chapter, you should be able to do the following:

1. Outline the digestive process.
2. Understand the function of six major nutrient categories.
3. Understand fundamental principles and strategies for healthy eating.
4. Realize the benefits and challenges of being a vegetarian.
5. Appreciate the value of fasting.

Anyone who has ever ridden a seesaw quickly realizes that it is easier to be up or down than balanced in between. Balance requires patience and hard work; even so, it might be the most important principle in developing a healthy diet.

Humans need to consume the right amount of more than 40 essential nutrients. If you do not get enough vitamin C, your gums will become inflamed and start to bleed. If you take too much, fatigue, diarrhea, and nausea will follow. An excess amount of protein causes increased calcium loss and kidney stones, but too little leads to muscles' wasting. Death can be caused not only by dehydration but also by drinking too much water. Almost every nutrient has a proper dosage, which varies depending on a person's age, sex, size, activity level, and ethnicity.

Fortunately, God has equipped human bodies with mechanisms that do a tremendous amount of the homeostatic work. If you get out of bed in the morning and go for a 20-minute jog, your heart rate, blood pressure, and respiration rate respond to the challenge. If you cut your finger, your blood and skin cells jump into action to stop the bleeding and restore the wounded tissue. When you lie down at night, your body instinctively moves through five stages of sleep to restore mental, emotional, and physical stability.

Although much of human physiology functions involuntarily, we play a vital role in either helping or hindering the process. We seek shelter and wear clothes to assist the thermoregulatory system maintain a core temperature of about 98 °F (37 °C). The digestive system performs most of the heavy lifting by assimilating and distributing nutrients to the cells, but we play a fundamental role by determining what food—and how much of it—to consume. These decisions have both physical and moral consequences.

The principle of moderating food intake described in practically every major nutrition textbook is also supported by scripture. When God directly and supernaturally fed the entire nation of Israel during their exodus through the Egyptian desert, he said this:

> "Each one is to gather as much as he needs. Take an omer for each person you have in your tent." The Israelites did as they were told; some gathered much, some little. And when they measured it by the omer, he who gathered much did not have too much, and he who gathered little did not have too little. Each one gathered as much as he needed. (Exodus 16:16–18)

Taking enough to satisfy your needs is what God commanded in the Old Testament. The principle is seen again in the New Testament teachings of Jesus. In the Gospel of Matthew, Christ responded to the worries of his followers by reminding them that God was committed to meeting their needs for food, clothing, and shelter (Matthew 6:25–34).

It seems that whatever standard God establishes, humans in their sinfulness can misconstrue trough ascetic rejection or selfish indulgence. Throughout history religious zealots have attempted to win the special approval of God through extreme self-denial. These individuals believed that they would more fully realize spiritual blessings by refusing their personal needs.

During the fourth century, Saint Ascepsimas wore so many chains that he had to crawl around on his hands and knees. A monk by the name of Basarion would not give in to his body's desire to lie down when he slept—so he slept standing for more than 40 years of his life. Simon the Stylite lived atop a narrow pillar for 34 years (Tan, 1982).

Although self-renunciation has appealed to a handful of spiritual zealots, a more common subversion has been to overindulge in what God created as good. The apostle Paul describes enemies of the cross as those who have made a "god of their stomach" by consuming food with reckless abandon (Philippians 3:18–19). Thomas Aquinas joined other spiritual leaders by placing gluttony in the list of the seven most deadly sins, alongside pride, covetousness, lust, anger, envy, and sloth (Pegis, 1997). Even though gluttony is mentioned more often than tithing in the Bible, it is not a very popular topic in most churches.

The apostle Peter illustrates how a disciple of Jesus can miss the mark of receiving God's gifts through staunch rejection or unfettered acceptation:

> Jesus knew that the Father had put all things under his power, and that he had come from God and was returning to God; so he got up from the meal, took off his outer clothing, and wrapped a towel around his waist. After that, he poured water into a basin and began

to wash his disciples' feet, drying them with the towel that was wrapped around him. He came to Simon Peter, who said to him, "Lord, are you going to wash my feet?" Jesus replied, "You do not realize now what I am doing, but later you will understand." "No," said Peter, "you shall never wash my feet." Jesus answered, "Unless I wash you, you have no part with me." "Then, Lord," Simon Peter replied, "not just my feet but my hands and my head as well!" Jesus answered, "A person who has had a bath needs only to wash his feet; his whole body is clean. And you are clean, though not every one of you." (John 13:3–10)

After being rebuked for his refusal, Peter asked for a complete bath. Neither extreme, however, was part of the Master's plan, and the same holds true for people's nutritional well-being.

In summary, the goal is to receive every type of grain, fruit, vegetable, and meat from the Maker with thanksgiving while being careful not to squander any of his bountiful provisions.

Studies suggest eating habits change for the worse during the collegiate years, despite a student's good intentions. One longitudinal study conducted by Tufts University (Food Service Director, 2002) found that 59 percent of college freshmen's diets change for the worse after leaving home. One of the biggest changes is that, away from their parents, students stop eating fruits and vegetables—70 percent report not eating the recommended amounts. What replaces the quick and healthy snacks of broccoli, carrots, bananas, and apples? The top five snack foods are listed in figure 8.1 (Food Institute Report, 2002).

Fundamentally, **nutrition** is the science of how food affects the body. A broader definition includes the social, economic, cultural, and psychological aspects of eating (Whitney & Rolfes, 2002). It is through the science of nutrition that you will understand the digestive process, the role of macro and micro nutrients, and practical methods for ensuring nutritional balance.

The Digestive System

The **digestive system** operates as an assembly line in reverse, taking whole foods and breaking them down into their chemical components. As you can see in figure 8.2, digestion begins in the mouth and ends some 27 feet (8 m) later at the rectum. Whenever we swallow, our digestive system goes on "auto pilot." Because we are not in control of most of the digestive process, it is easy to overlook how much work our body does.

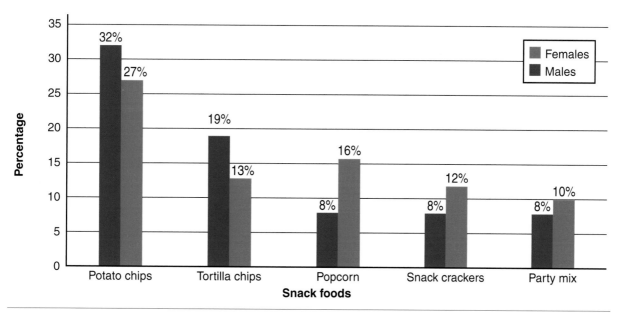

FIGURE 8.1 Comparison by sex of what college students snack on the most.

Data from Food Institute Report, 2002.

The 30-Day Experiment

Perhaps a group of college students took their inspiration from Morgan Spurlock's 30-day experiment of eating nothing except what he could buy at McDonald's. The experiment later became the basis of the critically acclaimed documentary *Super-Size Me* (Spurlock, 2007). The college freshmen decided to spend the same stretch of time consuming nothing but pizza (Hales, 2005). Despite remarkable creativity and variety in the types of pizza they ate, by the second week most of them cringed at the mere sight of another cardboard delivery box. They reported feeling bloated, undergoing severe and constant headaches, and experiencing a general sense of fatigue that would not go away. One student was actually convinced he had scurvy, the same disease brought on by vitamin C deficiency that used to afflict sailors on long voyages. As committed as they were, not one of these students made it for the full 30 days.

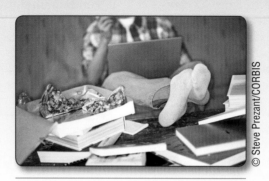

© Steve Prezant/CORBIS

Eating nothing but pizza for 30 days was more than a group of college students could endure.

Perhaps a metaphor can help. Imagine a river that begins in the North Pole and zigzags its way to every continent before ending in the South Pole. On each continent, the main river branches into several smaller rivers and streams so that all six billion people on the planet can receive fresh water. In addition to water, these rivers carry every food imaginable—including watermelon, peanuts, turkey, and rice—so that the nutritional needs of the entire world can be met.

Such a river exists in our bodies. With the help of the circulatory system, the digestive system gets just the right amount of water, protein, fat, carbohydrate, vitamins, and minerals to each of the one hundred trillion cells in our bodies—then picks up waste products for disposal and elimination on its return trip.

Digestion begins in the mouth. When you take a bite of food, your teeth and tongue begin to mechanically break it down into smaller units. Saliva not only bathes your food with water, but it also allows you to taste because your taste buds work only when moisture is present. When the food has been reduced to a soft, moist mass, called a **bolus**, your tongue pushes it to the back of your mouth and into the pharynx, where it is swallowed. For the fraction of a second it takes to

swallow, your respiratory tract is closed, and you can neither breathe nor talk. After you swallow, the rest of the digestive process is involuntary. For the next two or three seconds, powered not by gravity but by muscular contractions called **peristalsis**, the bolus travels down your **esophagus** to the **stomach**.

A circular muscle called the **esophageal sphincter** separates the esophagus and the stomach. When you swallow, this muscle relaxes, forming an opening through which the food can pass. The rest of the time it is closed, to keep the food from moving in the opposite direction. It is the first of several muscular valves to regulate the passage of food. The stomach, contrary to popular belief, is not behind the navel but higher up, just below the diaphragm. This saclike structure is shaped like a capital J when empty and like a boxing glove when full. When food is present, the stomach expands and contracts about three times per minute to churn the food and bathe it in gastric juices. These fluids, secreted by thousands of glands in the stomach lining, consist of water, **hydrochloric acid (HCL)**, and an enzyme called **pepsin**. Hydrochloric acid not only breaks down the food, but it also kills many of the harmful microorganisms in food. The stomach would literally digest itself if it weren't for its mucus lining. The major cause of gastric ulcers is **Helicobacter pylori** bacteria, which interferes with the production of the mucus lining and leaves the lining of the stomach unprotected from hydrochloric acid. A perforated ulcer is when the acid of the stomach has completely penetrated the stomach wall. Fortunately, in most cases this harmful bacterium can be managed through medical treatment.

About one hour after a meal, the food that has been processed by the stomach, called **chyme**, begins to pass a little bit at a time through the **pyloric sphincter** into the **duodenum**, the first section of the small intestine. Most digestion and absorption occurs in the small intestine. This narrow, twisting tube, about 1 inch (2.5 cm) in diameter and 20 feet (6 m) long, fills most of the lower abdomen. For three to six hours, peristalsis moves the chyme through the other two sections: the **jejunum** and the **ileum**. The liver secretes bile and the pancreas secretes pancreatic enzymes into the small intestine. Bile breaks down large

fat globules into small ones; pancreatic enzymes break down sugar and starch into simple sugars, fat into fatty acids and glycerol, and protein into amino acids. Additional glands in the intestinal walls secrete other enzymes that break down other nutrients as well. In this form, they can be absorbed. The small intestine's capacity for absorption is greatly increased by millions of tiny fingerlike projections called **villi** that line its walls (see figure 8.3).

Each villus, about 0.02 to 0.06 inches (0.05 to 0.15 cm) long, is covered by even tinier **microvilli**. One square inch (2.5 square cm) of small intestine contains some 20,000 villi and 10 billion microvilli. They dramatically increase the surface area of the small intestine. As a matter of fact, if you were to flatten out the small intestine completely, it would be roughly the size of a tennis court! Beneath the villi's single layer of cells are capillaries, where simple sugars and amino acids enter the bloodstream and fatty acids and glycerol enter the lymphatic system. What remains unabsorbed—a

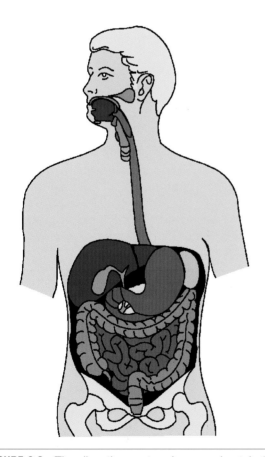

FIGURE 8.2 The digestive system is approximately 27 feet (8 m) in length.

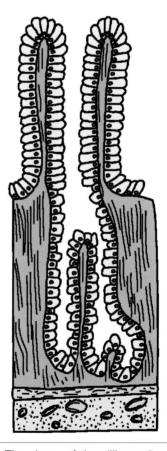

FIGURE 8.3 The shape of the villi greatly expand the surface area of the small intestines.

watery residue of indigestible food and digestive juices—passes through, again by peristalsis, to the large intestine, where it spends the next 12 to 24 hours. The large intestine, about 2.5 inches (6.4 cm) in diameter and 5 to 6 feet (1.5 to 1.8 m) long, is shaped like an inverted U. It performs several important functions: It absorbs water (about 1.6 gallons [6.1 L] daily) and dissolved salts from the small intestine's residue, and its bacteria promote the breakdown of undigested materials. What remains is moved toward the **rectum**, the final 6 to 8 inches (15 to 20 cm) of the **alimentary canal**. The rectum stores feces until elimination.

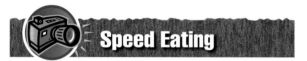

Speed Eating

For the fifth straight year, Takeru Kobayashi, who weighs 144 pounds (65 kg) and stands 5 feet 7 inches tall (170 cm), wins the coveted Mustard Yellow Belt. This belt goes to the person who can eat the most hot dogs (bun included) in 12 minutes. In the following photograph, Kobayashi won for gobbling a nauseating 49 dogs in the time allowed. This missed the mark of his own world record of 53, set in 2004 (Nathan's Web site, 2005).

Six Major Nutrient Groups

Nutrients are substances the body can use for growth, maintenance, and repair. The body needs to take in about 43 different nutrients to function properly. Nutrients can be grouped into six categories: carbohydrate, protein, lipid (fat), water, vitamins, and minerals (see table 8.1).

These six nutrients are further classified according to size and energy. Carbohydrate, protein, and fat are **macronutrients**, because they make up the bulk of your diet. Vitamins and minerals are **micronutrients**, because they are required in much smaller amounts. For example, the average person consumes about 2.5 gallons (9.5 L) of food and water per day, but only an eighth of a teaspoon of that is vitamins and minerals. This does not mean they are unimportant, however. The ignition key is only a small part of a car, but it's hard to get the car started without it! A deficiency in B_{12}, just one of the eight B vitamins, can result in anemia, hypersensitive skin, and degeneration of peripheral nerves resulting in paralysis (Whitney & Rolfes, 2002). You may have noticed the omission of water as a macronutrient. People definitely need a large supply of water; however, water is a micronutrient because it does not contain energy.

Food energy is measured in calories. You may recall from high school chemistry that a **calorie** is the amount of energy necessary to raise one kilogram of water by one degree Celsius. When

Table 8.1 **Primary Functions of the Six Major Nutrients**

Nutrient	Primary functions
Water	Dissolves and carries nutrients, removes waste, and regulates body temperature
Protein	Builds new tissues, antibodies, enzymes, hormones, and other compounds
Carbohydrate	Provides energy
Fat	Provides long-term energy, insulation, and protection
Vitamins	Facilitate use of other nutrients; involved in regulating growth and manufacturing hormones
Minerals	Help build bones and teeth; aid in muscle function and nervous system activity

Nutrient Density

The phrase *empty calories* is used to describe high-sugar, low-nutrient foods. Foods that contain an abundance of nutrients relative to the energy they provide may be referred to as having "packed calories." In either case, the determination is made through a method known as **nutrient density**, which calculates the nutritional value of food compared to the number of calories it contains.

Figure 8.4 illustrates a comparison of the nutrient density of a typical 12-ounce (355 ml) glass of soft drink and the same amount of fat-free milk.

To calculate the nutrient density of any food, divide the amount of a selected nutrient by the calories the food provides. For example, an 8-ounce (240 ml) glass of orange juice contains 125 milligrams of vitamin C and 111 calories, and a generic brand of orange drink usually contains 84 milligrams of vitamin C and 128 calories for the same serving size. Divide 125 milligrams by 111 calories to calculate a nutrient density of 1.12 for vitamin C in the serving of orange juice, and divide 84 milligrams by 127 calories to calculate a nutrient density of 0.65 for vitamin C in the serving of orange drink.

Orange juice contains twice the nutritional power of vitamin C as a typical orange drink. Although there is a significant difference in the amount of vitamin C, there are even more dramatic variations of other nutrients. Orange juice is a "packed calorie" food because it contains more than 5 times the magnesium, 7 times the folate, and 18 times the vitamin A of a typical orange drink.

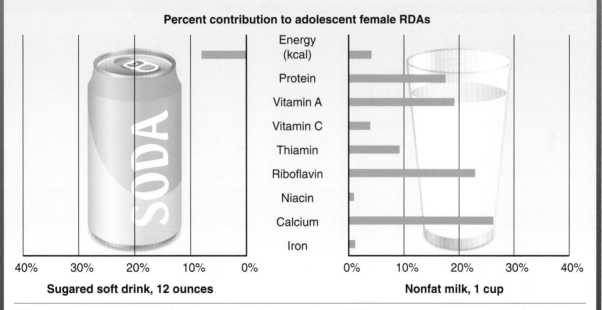

Percent contribution to adolescent female RDAs

Energy (kcal), Protein, Vitamin A, Vitamin C, Thiamin, Riboflavin, Niacin, Calcium, Iron

40% 30% 20% 10% 0%   0% 10% 20% 30% 40%

Sugared soft drink, 12 ounces   **Nonfat milk, 1 cup**

FIGURE 8.4   A comparison of the nutrient density of a 12-ounce (355 ml) soft drink to an equal serving of nonfat milk.

Adapted from G. Wardlaw and J. Hampl, 2007, *Perspectives in nutrition,* 9th ed. (New York: The McGraw-Hill Companies), 42. With permission of the McGraw-Hill Companies.

discussing nutrition and exercise, however, calorie usually means **kilocalorie**, 1,000 calories, or the amount of energy necessary to raise a liter of water by one degree Celsius. To avoid confusion, when calorie is used in this text it will be used in the conventional manner.

Phytochemicals

Although 99.9 percent of food is made up of the six major nutrient groups, some compounds in food are not in any nutrient group. For example, phytochemicals are nonnutrient compounds found primarily in plant-derived foods. They help the body destroy carcinogens, which are cancer-causing agents (Whitney & Rolfes, 2002). Foods that are particularly high in phytochemicals are cruciferous vegetables—vegetables of the cabbage family—such as cabbage, broccoli, brussels sprouts, sprouts, kale, and cauliflower.

The energy nutrients are carbohydrate, protein, and fat; the nonenergy nutrients are water, vitamins, and minerals.

Carbohydrate

Carbohydrate is fuel for the body and brain. Carbohydrate comes in three types: **simple carbohydrate**, **complex carbohydrate**, and **fiber**. Simple carbohydrate is further divisible into **monosaccharides**, which contain only one type of sugar—such as **glucose** (blood sugar), **fructose** (fruit sugar), and **galactose**—and **disaccharides**, which are made up of glucose combined with another sugar. The three primary disaccharides are **maltose**, **lactose**, and **sucrose**, and those are what most people mean by sugar. Complex carbohydrate, or starch, is a **polysaccharide**, which contains long chains

Terms for the Carbohydrate Conscious

Low-carbohydrate diets come into fashion periodically. In a 2004 survey, 30 to 40 million American adults (16% of the adult population at the time) said they were trying to control their weight by counting grams of carbohydrate instead of calories. Manufacturers introduced 930 low-carbohydrate foods in the United States between 1999 and 2004 (Consumer Reports, 2004). Three relatively new terms—glycemic index, glycemic load, and net carbohydrate—have crept into the vocabulary of those who are carbohydrate conscious.

Low-carbohydrate diets are based, in part, on the effect that carbohydrate has on blood sugar and insulin levels, which rise and fall after the consumption of carbohydrate. Some foods have a quick and dramatic effect on glucose and insulin levels, while others have a slower, more moderate effect. **Glycemic index** (GI) is one measure of how foods affect the level of blood sugar. GI is determined by consuming 50 grams of carbohydrate from a particular food and measuring the effect on blood sugar during the two hours after consumption. The resulting value is compared to an index in which a reference food (most often glucose) is given a 100-point value. High-GI foods have

a measure greater than 70, foods with a value between 55 and 69 are considered intermediate, and those below 55 are considered low. Table 8.2 illustrates the glycemic index of some common foods.

A more comprehensive list of glycemic measures can be found in an article titled "International Tables of Glycemic Index and Glycemic Load Values," which was published in the *American Journal of Clinical Nutrition* (Powell, Holt, & Brand-Miller, 2002).

Foods that are high in sugar and low in fat generally elevate blood sugar and insulin rapidly. Chronically large doses of insulin outputs have been found to be related to a sluggish feeling, a reduced rate at which calories are burned, increased hunger, elevated blood triglycerides, increased fat synthesis and storage, and increased risk for developing diabetes (Miller, 2003).

One major drawback of the glycemic index is that the values are based on the consumption of 50 grams of carbohydrate rather than on a typical serving size. You would have to consume more than 4 cups (950 ml) of whole milk to get 50 grams of carbohydrate. Only 2 ounces (56 g) of jellybeans, however, have

(continued)

(continued)

Table 8.2 Glycemic Index and Load for Various Foods

	Serving size	Glycemic index	Carbohydrate (g)	Glycemic load
Apple	1 medium	38	22	8
Baked beans	1 cup (253 g)	48	54	26
Banana	1 medium	55	29	16
Chocolate	1 oz (28 g)	49	18	9
Honey	1 tsp (5 ml)	73	6	4
Ice cream	1 cup (132 g)	61	31	19
Milk, nonfat	1 cup (240 ml)	32	12	4
Milk, whole	1 cup (240 ml)	27	11	3
Orange	1 medium	44	15	7
Potato chips (crisps)	1 oz (28 g)	54	15	8
Potato, baked	1 cup (227 g)	85	57	48
Spaghetti	1 cup(140 g)	41	40	16
Vanilla wafers	5 cookies	77	15	12
White bread	1 slice	70	10	7
Whole-wheat bread	1 slice	69	13	9

Adapted from Powell, Holt, & Brand-Miller, 2002.

50 grams of carbohydrate. As a result, many health professionals look at **glycemic load**, which takes into account the glycemic index along with the actual amount of carbohydrate consumed (Donatelle, 2006). To calculate the glycemic load, the grams of carbohydrate are multiplied by the glycemic index and then divided by 100. A small bagel that contains 30 grams of carbohydrate would be multiplied by the glycemic index (72) and divided by 100 to result in a glycemic load of 22:

$$(30 \times 72) \div 100 = 22$$

Most consumers simply count the number of grams of carbohydrate they consume rather than look at glycemic index tables or calculate the glycemic load of their diets. Therefore, many manufacturers are doing everything they can to lower the grams of carbohydrate in the food they sell.

One recent strategy has been to use a term called **net carbohydrate** (commonly called net carbs). Although the term has no agreed-on definition, it generally refers to the total grams of carbohydrate per serving minus the grams of sugar alcohols and fermentable fiber. These sugar alcohols (erythritol, hydrogenated starch hydrolysates, isomait, lactitol, maititol, mannitol, sorbitol, xylitol) are not digested in the small intestine but instead pass to the large intestine where they are digested by fermentation. They do not elevate blood sugar and insulin levels nearly as much as regular sugar does.

Manufacturers are subtracting these particular types of carbohydrate because they do not have as much absorbable energy as regular carbohydrate does. They do contain calories, however, ranging from 0.2 calorie to 3 calories per gram—nearly as much as a normal carbohydrate.

(continued)

(continued)

What can science offer regarding the effectiveness of low-carbohydrate diets? One of the few long-term studies indicates that low-carbohydrate dieters lose weight faster than low-fat dieters (Foster, 2003). But although the low-carbohydrate dieters lost an average of 8.4 pounds (3.8 kg) more than the low-fat dieters did during the first six months, the gap between the two groups narrowed to a statistically insignificant amount by the end of a year.

Why do low-carbohydrate diets work? A study that tracked the calorie consumption of low-fat and low-carbohydrate dieters reported that during a six-month trial the low-carbohydrate dieters cut an average of 189 more calories per day than the low-fat dieters did (Samaha, 2003). This reduction would be more than enough to account for the extra 8.4 pounds (3.8 kg) that low-carbohydrate dieters lost in the study cited earlier. Despite all the impressive terminology, weight management always seems to come back to calorie intake and expenditure.

of glucose molecules bonded together. Because the body must break these bonds to release the chemical energy stored in them, complex carbohydrate takes longer to digest and therefore allows for a more sustained energy release than simple carbohydrate does. In some cases these bonds cannot be broken down by human digestion; that is the case with fiber. Unlike animals, humans lack the necessary enzymes to break down the energy in fiber. Fiber comes in two types: soluble and insoluble. **Soluble fiber** dissolves in water to form a gel, and it can help lower blood cholesterol and control blood sugar levels. **Insoluble fiber** does not dissolve, and it can help prevent constipation and other bowel disorders. Each of the three types of carbohydrate and their subcategories and primary functions are listed in table 8.3.

The 2005 dietary guidelines published by the U.S. Department of Health and Human Services (DHHS) and the U.S. Department of Agriculture (USDA) recommend that 45 to 65 percent of total calorie intake come from carbohydrate—at least 130 grams of carbohydrate per day (U.S. Department of Health and Human Services, U.S. Department of Agriculture, 2005). This minimum is required to supply the brain with an adequate amount of glucose. It is a fairly moderate recommendation, considering that the average American adult male consumes 220 to 330 grams and the average American adult female consumes 180 to 230 grams of carbohydrate daily (Institute of Medicine, 2002). According to the Institute of Medicine (2002), an agency that works with DHHS and USDA to establish nutritional guidelines, an adequate intake of fiber is 14 grams for every 1,000 calories.

Table 8.3 Categories and Functions of Carbohydrate

Carbohydrate	Subcategories	Primary sources
Simple	Monosaccharides, disaccharides	Processed sugar, fruit, dairy
Complex	Polysaccharides, starches	Breads, fruits, vegetables, nuts, legumes
Fiber	Soluble, insoluble	Bran, vegetables, fruits, nuts, oats, legumes

Protein

Nothing can match protein's power for physical growth and repair. **Protein** is made up of **amino acids**, which are the building blocks of cell membranes, muscle tissues, and enzymes. There are 20 amino acids, 9 of which are essential. Foods that contain all nine, such as meat, eggs, and dairy products, are called **complete proteins**. Americans get about 70 percent of their protein from these animal products. Most fruits, grains, and vegetables, with the notable exception of soy, are incomplete proteins.

Although it contains four calories per gram, protein is not usually a major source of energy—rarely does it contribute more than 10 percent of daily

Is Sugar Bad for You?

Sugar isn't really bad for you. Sugar is in fruits, grains, vegetables, and nearly everything you eat. And the chemical structure of "refined" sugar is no different from that of "natural" sugar. Despite what you may have heard, sugar's only proven health risk is tooth decay (U.S. Department of Health and Human Services & U.S. Department of Agriculture, 2005). But the problem is quantity. Virtually all major health organizations currently recommend reducing the amount of sugar in the diet because, according to the USDA, the yearly sugar intake of the average American has continually risen over the last 99 years, from 4 pounds (1.8 kg) in 1900 to 90 pounds (41 kg) per person in 1999 (Kanton, 1999)(see figure 8.5).

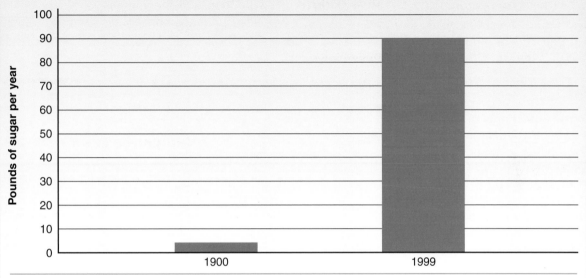

FIGURE 8.5 Change in average annual intake of sugar per person in the United States.

Adapted from Kanton, 1999.

Do Athletes Need More Protein?

One of the ongoing debates among coaches and athletes is whether those who participate in vigorous sports and exercise need additional protein. Although the available research does not provide a definitive answer concerning the exact amount of protein a particular athlete needs, the weight of the evidence does suggest that individuals involved in vigorous physical activity can benefit by increasing dietary protein beyond the recommended dietary allowance (RDA) suggestion of 0.8 to 1.0 grams per kilogram of body weight. Existing science seems to indicate that endurance athletes can benefit from dietary intake of 1.2 to 1.6 grams of protein per kilogram of body weight and strength athletes should get 1.6 to 1.8 grams per kilogram of body weight (American College of Sports Medicine, 2000; Lemon, 1995).

To illustrate how to calculate protein needs, consider the case of a 140-pound (63.6 kg) college-age male who wants to gain muscle weight. He is willing to begin resistance training, get adequate rest, and change his diet to meet his objectives. How much protein would you recommend he consume per day? The RDA for this male would be between 51 and 64 (63.6 kg multiplied by 0.8 and 1.0) grams of protein per day. However, based on the evidence concerning protein and strength training, he should consume between 102 and 115 (63.6 kg multiplied by 1.6 and 1.8) grams of protein per day.

caloric expenditure. An exception to this rule is for people such as marathon runners who train exceptionally hard while on a low-calorie diet. In this case the body begins to draw on protein stored in muscle tissue for energy (Sharkey, 2002).

Most American adults get between 14 and 18 percent of their calories from protein, thus falling well within the range of the 10 to 35 percent recommended by the *Dietary Guidelines for Americans 2005* (U.S. Department of Health and Human Services & U.S. Department of Agriculture, 2005).

Fat

Contrary to popular belief, **fat** is a vital ingredient in a healthy diet. Besides being the most energy-rich nutrient (nine calories per gram), fat is needed to transport vitamins A, D, E, and K; conduct nerve impulses efficiently; and cushion vital organs. It also serves as a thermal regulator and makes up a large portion of bone marrow and brain tissue. People like fat because it enhances the flavor and texture of food.

There are three primary types of fatty acids: **saturated**, **monounsaturated**, and **polyunsatu-**

rated. Although most of what you eat contains a mixture of all three types, usually one type predominates. For example, margarine has between 40 and 75 percent polyunsaturated, 10 to 50 percent saturated, and 5 to 25 percent monounsaturated fatty acids. Therefore, it is classified as a polyunsaturated fat (see table 8.4).

Table 8.4 Grams of Fatty Acids Per 100 Grams of Food Weight

	Saturated	Monounsaturated	Polyunsaturated
Coconut oil	85	6.6	1.7
Butter	54	20	2.6
Palm oil	45	42	8
Lard	41	44	9
Cottonseed oil	26	21	48
Margarine	16	21	41
Soybean oil	15	23	57
Olive oil	14	70	11
Corn oil	13	25	58
Sunflower oil	12	20	63
Safflower oil	10	13	72
Rapeseed oil	7	57	32

Each fat is classified according to its most predominant fatty acid.

Four Key Questions You Should Answer When Reading Food Labels

Examine figure 8.6 and try to answer the next few questions before proceeding.

1. How many servings and calories am I actually eating?
2. What nutrients should I limit and which should I be sure to obtain?
3. What is relevant about the food label footnote?
4. How can I tell if a % Daily Value is high or low?

U.S. Food and Drug Administration, 2004.

1. How many servings and calories am I actually eating? Serving size is one of the easiest items to overlook when examining a food label. Many people assume that nutritional values represent the entire contents of a package or container. If you did that with a package of macaroni and cheese, you would be underestimating the calorie and nutritional content by 50 percent.

More important than the serving size printed on the box is the actual quantity of food you eat. This is what determines your calorie consumption. A general guide to the low-, moderate-,

(continued)

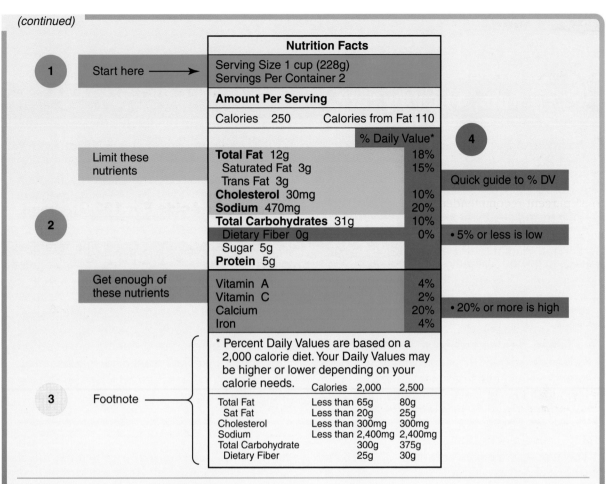

FIGURE 8.6 Typical food label for macaroni and cheese.
From U.S. Food and Drug Adminisration, 2004.

and high-calorie foods follows (values based on a 2,000-calorie diet):

- 40 calories or fewer is considered low,
- 100 calories is considered moderate (5 percent of total intake),
- 400 calories is considered high (20 percent of total intake).

These values are based upon a 2,000 calorie diet.

2. What nutrients should I limit and which should I be sure to obtain? Four nutrient values need to be limited: saturated fat, *trans* fat, cholesterol, and sodium. The goal is to get no more than 100% of the daily values for these nutrients each day. There is not a reference daily value for trans fat, but experts recommend limiting the amount of trans fat in your diet as much as possible. Studies show that trans fat is highly correlated with an increased risk of heart disease because it increases blood cholesterol levels by altering the way cholesterol is removed from the blood. Therefore, the Institute of Medicine recommends keeping intake of trans fatty acids to an absolute minimum (Institute of Medicine, 2002).

Consumers can use the food label not only to help them limit particular nutrients but also to encourage the intake of nutrients that are often neglected in the diet such as dietary fiber, vitamin A, vitamin C, calcium, and iron.

3. What is relevant about the food label footnote? The footnote points out that the percent daily values is based on a 2,000- or 2,500-calorie diet. In addition, a column that says "less than" reminds consumers to be careful of overconsumption of some nutrients.

4. How can I tell if a % Daily Value is high or low? Foods that contains 5 percent or less of a person's daily values are considered low. On the other hand, foods that contain 20 percent or more of a person's daily values are considered high. You can use this 5/20 guide as a quick reference to nutrient quantity.

Nuts: A Healthy Fat?

"A handful a day may help reduce the risk of heart disease," is the claim boldly written on some new peanut containers, but should you try to include nuts in your daily diet? This new health claim is among the first to be permitted by the Food and Drug Administration in the United States because more than 30 studies have indicated that nuts help reduce cholesterol levels. Nuts are relatively good sources of vitamin E and are rich in monounsaturated fat and soluble fiber, both of which tend to lower LDL (bad) cholesterol.

During one controlled trial, researchers randomly assigned 27 people with high cholesterol to eat almonds daily for a month as part of various low-fat diets. The study, published in the American Heart Association Journal *Circulation* (Jenkins et al., 2002), found that almonds reduced LDL cholesterol by as much as 9.4 percent. In two large-population studies from Harvard University, people who ate nuts often had lower risks of sudden cardiac death and heart attacks than those who rarely or never ate nuts had (Albert et al., 2002).

Adding a handful of nuts to your diet is a good idea. Note that this particular claim is allowed on package labels for almonds, peanuts, pecans, pistachios, hazelnuts, walnuts, and some pine nuts. It cannot be used on labels for Brazil nuts, cashews, macadamias, and some other pine nuts, which have a bit too much saturated fat.

The average American consumes 32.7 percent of calories from fat, of which approximately 20 percent is saturated (Briefel & Johnson, 2004; U.S. Department of Health and Human Services & U.S. Department of Agriculture, 2005). The latest guidelines regarding dietary fat recommend consuming 20 to 35 percent of calories from fat, of which 10 percent or less comes from saturated sources.

Vitamins

Most vitamins and minerals are measured in milligrams (a thousandth of a gram) or micrograms (a millionth of a gram) instead of in grams, because humans need only very small doses of **vitamins** to maintain health. Even so, a prolonged deficiency in just one of the many vitamins can lead to severe health effects. For example, the deficiency of vitamin B_1 (thiamine) results in a disease called beriberi that produces general fatigue, muscular atrophy, paralysis, and eventual heart failure. Insufficient levels of folic acid (another B vitamin) increase the risk of neural tube defects such as spina bifida, which can result in the spinal cord's protruding from the spinal column. Vitamins are critical to blood coagulation and the production of energy, hormones, enzymes, and antibodies.

Vitamins are classified according to the substrate they are soluble in. Vitamin C and the B-complex vitamins are water-soluble vitamins. Vitamins A, D, E, and K are fat soluble. A mnemonic phrase to help you remember the fat-soluble vitamins is "**a**ll **d**ogs **e**at **k**ittens." After you've memorized the fat-soluble vitamins, you can simply remember that all the rest are water soluble (see table 8.5). You may think it would be simpler to remember that vitamins C and the B-complex vitamins are water soluble, but there are eight B vitamins.

Table 8.6 identifies symptoms associated with vitamin deficiencies and excess along with foods that contain substantial amounts of each vitamin people need.

Table 8.5   **The 13 Essential Vitamins**

Fat soluble	Water soluble
A	B_1 (thiamin)
D	B_2 (riboflavin)
E	B_3 (niacin)
K	Biotin
	Panothenic acid
	B_6
	Folate
	B_{12}
	C

Table 8.6 Fat-Soluble and Water-Soluble Vitamins

Fat soluble	Major functions	Important sources	Signs of deficiency	Effects of megadoses
Vitamin A	Maintains eyes, vision, skin, linings of the nose, mouth, digestive and urinary tracts, immune function	Liver, milk, butter, cheese, carrots, spinach, cantaloupe, other orange or dark green vegetables or fruits	Night blindness, dry skin, increased susceptibility to infection, loss of appetite, anemia, kidney stones	Headache, vomiting and diarrhea, dryness of mucous membranes, vertigo, double vision, bone abnormalities, liver damage, increased risk of miscarriage and birth defects, convulsions, coma, respiratory failure
Vitamin D	Aids in calcium and phosphorus metabolism, promotion of calcium absorption; develops and maintains bones and teeth	Fortified milk and margarine, fish liver oils, butter, egg yolks, exposure to sunlight	Rickets (bone deformities) in children; bone softening, loss, and fractures in adults	Calcium deposits in kidneys and blood vessels, causing irreversible kidney and cardiovascular damage
Vitamin E	Protects and maintains cellular membranes	Vegetable oils, whole grains, nuts and seeds, green leafy vegetables, asparagus, peaches; smaller amounts widespread in other foods	Red blood cell breakage and anemia, weakness, neurological problems, muscle cramps	Relatively nontoxic, but may cause excess bleeding or formation of blood clots
Vitamin K	Blood clotting; maintains bone metabolism	Greens, cereals, fruits, meats, milk products	Hemorrhage	Jaundice, inability to clot

Water Soluble	Major functions	Important sources	Signs of deficiency	Effects of megadoses
Vitamin B$_1$ (thiamin)	Converts carbohydrate into usable forms of energy; maintains appetite and nervous system function	Yeast, whole-grain and enriched breads and cereals, organ meats, liver, pork, lean meats, poultry, eggs, fish, beans, nuts, legumes	Beriberi (symptoms include edema or muscle wasting, mental confusion, anorexia, enlarged heart, abnormal heart rhythm, muscle degeneration and weakness, nerve changes)	None reported
Vitamin B$_2$ (riboflavin)	**Energy metabolism;** maintains skin, mucous membranes, and nervous system structures	Dairy products, whole-grain and enriched breads and cereals, lean meats, poultry, green vegetables, liver	Cracks at corners of mouth, sore throat, skin rash, hypersensitivity to light, purple tongue	None reported

(continued)

Table 8.6 *(continued)*

Fat soluble	Major functions	Important sources	Signs of deficiency	Effects of megadoses
Vitamin B₃ (niacin)	Converts carbohydrate, fat, and protein into usable forms of energy; essential for growth; supports skin, nervous system, and digestive health	Eggs, chicken, turkey, fish, milk, whole grains, nuts, enriched breads and cereals, lean meats, legumes	Pellagra (symptoms include weakness, diarrhea, dermatitis, inflammation of mucous membranes, mental illness)	Flushing of the skin, nausea, vomiting, diarrhea, changes in metabolism of glycogen and fatty acids, low blood pressure
Biotin	Energy metabolism use, synthesizes fat, amino acid metabolism	Widespread in foods	Abnormal heart action, muscle pain, fatigue, weakness	None reported
Panothenic acid	Used in energy metabolism	Widespread in foods	Vomiting, insomnia, fatigue	Water retention (uncommon)
Vitamin B₆ (pyridoxine)	Enzyme reactions involving amino acids and the metabolism of carbohydrate, fat, and nucleic acids	Green leafy vegetables, eggs, poultry, whole grains, nuts, legumes, liver, kidney, pork	Anemia, convulsions, cracks at corners of mouth, dermatitis, nausea, confusion	Neurological abnormalities and damage, depression, loss of reflexes, weakness, restlessness
Folate	Amino acid metabolism; synthesizes RNA and DNA; synthesizes new cells	Green leafy vegetables, yeast, oranges, whole grains, legumes, liver	Anemia, gastrointestinal disturbances, decreased resistance to infection, depression	Diarrhea, reduction of zinc absorption, possible kidney enlargement and damage
Vitamin B₁₂	Synthesizes red and white blood cells; other metabolic reactions	Eggs, milk, meat, liver	Anemia, fatigue, nervous system damage, sore tongue	None reported
Vitamin C	Maintains and repairs connective tissue, bones, teeth, and cartilage; promotes healing; aids in iron absorption	Peppers, broccoli, spinach, brussels sprouts, citrus fruits, strawberries, tomatoes, potatoes, cabbage, other fruits and vegetables	Scurvy (weakening of collagenous structures resulting in widespread capillary hemorrhaging), anemia, reduced resistance to infection, bleeding gums, weakness, loosened teeth, rough skin, joint pain, poor wound healing, hair loss, poor iron absorption	Urinary stones in some people, acid stomach from ingesting supplements in pill form, nausea, diarrhea, headache, fatigue

Antioxidants

Free radicals are released during metabolism and stimulated by pollution, smoking, radiation, and stress. Free radicals run throughout the body attacking cells in the brain, heart, bloodstream, and immune system. **Antioxidants** help minimize the damage caused by these free radicals. Vitamins are among the most powerful antioxidants, along with carotenoids, flavonoids, and selenium.

Minerals

Minerals are in many ways linchpins to health. A linchpin is a pin placed crosswise at the end of an axle to keep a wheel from coming off. Although relatively simple in design and insignificant in size, a linchpin is paramount in its supportive role. The same is true of minerals. Minerals are present in all living cells and maintain the body's delicate acid and base balances, enable muscular contraction to occur, and aid in the production of both hormones and enzymes.

Minerals are classified as major minerals or **trace minerals**. The body needs more than five grams a day of the major minerals, which include sodium, potassium, calcium, phosphorus, magnesium, sulfur, and chlorine. Trace minerals (the body needs less than five grams a day of these) include iron, iodine, copper, fluorine, and zinc. Although 31 minerals have been found in the human body, only 24 are currently known to be essential.

Table 8.7 lists the major functions and food sources of all of the major minerals and some of the trace minerals and the symptoms associated with excesses and deficiencies.

Water

Although it contains no energy or vitamins and trace amounts of minerals, water is the most important nutrient in the body. Despite its lack of nutritional value, water is necessary for the absorption of vitamins, minerals, and nutrients in food. It is also used for energy production, temperature regulation, and elimination. It lubricates joints, helps with digestion, and contributes to sweat production. The body is 50 to 70 percent water (exactly how much depends on age and body composition). Muscle contains a higher concentration of water than many other tissues do—right around 70 percent. Therefore, males, who proportionally have greater muscle mass than females do, also have more water. Greater muscle mass is also why a young adult has more water than a senior citizen.

Many brands and varieties of bottled water are on the market, but the evidence seems to indicate that none of them is significantly safer or healthier than regular tap water. A study by a consumer advocacy group found that, of the 1,000 bottles and 103 brands tested in the United States, about one-third were contaminated with bacteria, arsenic, or synthetic organic chemicals, and at least one-fourth were drawn directly from the tap (Natural Resources Defense Council, 1999). In the final analysis, the FDA concluded that bottled water, on average, was not safer or more pure than regular tap water. Despite this, 1 in 15 American households spends between 250 and 10,000 times more for water by choosing to purchase bottled water (U.S. Food and Drug Administration, 1999).

It is difficult, but not impossible, to drink too much water. Most of the time the body will eliminate through urination the water it doesn't need. But if you are not getting enough, your body will let you know through thirst. A rough, one-size-fits-all recommendation is eight cups (1.9 L) per day. You can get a more accurate recommendation by dividing your body weight in pounds by 2. That number is how many ounces of water you should drink per day. (So if you weigh 140 pounds, you should drink 70 ounces.) Perhaps the simplest method to use to evaluate whether you're getting enough water is to check the frequency of urination and color of your urine. When you're urinating frequently and the color of your urine is pale yellow, you are probably well hydrated (Clark, 2003). This method may be less accurate if you take vitamin supplements, because they can darken the color of your urine. Keep in mind that these recommendations do not take into account two very important variables: heat and activity level. If you are working hard in a hot climate, you will need a lot more water.

Table 8.7 Essential Major Minerals and Trace Minerals

Major minerals	Major functions	Important sources	Signs of deficiency	Effects of megadoses
Sodium	Body water balance, acid–base balance, nerve function	Salt, soy sauce, salted or cured foods, table and sea salt.	Muscle weakness, loss of appetite, nausea, vomiting; sodium deficiency is rarely seen	Edema, hypertension in sensitive people
Chloride	Aids in digestion; regulates waters in body	Salt, cured foods, pickles	Muscle cramps, apathy, poor appetite	Vomiting
Potassium	Nerve function and body water balance	Squash, lima beans, tomatoes, bananas, milk, meats	Muscular weakness, nausea, drowsiness, paralysis, confusion, disruption of cardiac rhythm	Irregular heartbeat, heart attack
Calcium	Maintains bones and teeth, blood clotting; maintains cell membranes; controls nerve impulses and muscle contraction	Milk and milk products, tofu, fortified orange juice and bread, green leafy vegetables	Stunted growth in children, bone mineral loss in adults	Nausea, vomiting, hypertension, constipation, urinary stones, calcium deposits in soft tissues, inhibition of absorption of certain minerals
Phosphorus	Energy formation, component of teeth and bones	Milk, chicken, seeds, nuts, salmon	Nausea, weakness, confusion, loss of bone calcium	Muscle spasms
Magnesium	DNA and protein synthesis, blood clotting, muscle contraction, ATP production	Cheese, sesame seeds, almonds, halibut, spinach, yogurt	Neurological disturbances, impaired immune function, kidney disorders, nausea, weight loss, growth failure in children	Nausea, vomiting, central nervous system depression, coma; death in people with impaired kidney function
Iron	Component of hemoglobin (carries oxygen to tissues), myoglobin (in muscle fibers), and enzymes	Lean meats, legumes, enriched flour, green vegetables, dried fruit, liver; absorption is enhanced by the presence of vitamin C	Iron-deficiency anemia, weakness, impaired immune function, cold hands and feet, gastrointestinal distress, pale appearance	Iron deposits in soft tissues, causing liver and kidney damage, joint pains, sterility, and disruption of cardiac function
Zinc	Enzyme reactions, including synthesis of proteins, RNA, and DNA; wound healing; immune response; ability to taste	Whole grains, meat, eggs, liver, seafood (especially oysters)	Growth failure, reproductive failure, loss of appetite, impaired taste acuity, skin rash, impaired immune function, poor wound healing, night blindness	Vomiting, impaired immune function, decline in serum HDL levels, impaired magnesium absorption
Iodine	Regulates energy production and growth, component of thyroid hormone	Iodized salt, milk, seaweed, seafood, bread	Goiter, mental retardation, hearing loss, and growth failure in newborns	Pimples, goiter, decreased thyroid function

Major minerals	Major functions	Important sources	Signs of deficiency	Effects of megadoses
Selenium	Antioxidant with vitamin E	Seafood, meat, eggs, grains	Muscle pain and tenderness, heart failure, Keshan disease (impairs the structure and function of the heart)	Hair and fingernail loss, weakness, irritability
Copper	Metabolizes iron; aids in brain development and utilization of glucose, cholesterol, and immunity	Bread, potatoes, beans, nuts, seeds, seafood (especially oysters)	Seizures, anemia, growth retardation	Wilson's disease (accumulation of copper in kidneys and liver), tremors, liver disease
Manganese	Forms body fat and bone (specifically builds cartilage)	Wheat germ, pineapple, blackberries, tea, sweet potatoes, broccoli	Impairs energy metabolism, produces bone abnormalities	Toxicity is a greater threat than deficiency. Irritibility, hallucinations, severe lack of coordination
Fluoride	Promotes calcium growth; inhibits bacterial activity on tooth surface; inhibits tooth decay and loss of tooth enamel	Water, mouthwash, toothpaste	Tooth decay	Fluorosis (mottled discoloration and pitting of tooth enamel)
Chromium	Aids in use of glucose, energy metabolism	Liver, whole grains, meat, beer, wine, legumes	Weight loss, poor glucose control	Skin and kidney damage
Molybdenum	Aids in oxygen transfer from one molecule to another	Dried beans, grains, dark green vegetables, milk	Rapid heartbeat, nausea, vomiting, coma	Joint pain, growth failure, anemia, gout

Can You Drink Too Much Water?

Most people who drink too much water are simply inconvenienced by frequent trips to the bathroom. But in rare cases, too much water can lead to serious consequences. At the 2000 Houston Marathon, for example, 21 runners developed a condition known as **hyponatremia** (low sodium levels in the blood due to overconsumption of water). Of those runners, 14 had to be hospitalized (Mulvihill, 2001). If left untreated, hyponatremia can lead to death. Although there are other causes, the primary reason people develop this condition is that they limit their sodium intake while consuming large amounts of water. Combined with long periods of exercise, typically lasting four or more hours, this creates a serious sodium deficiency. Take these steps to avoid the condition (Clark, 2003):

- Eat salty foods the week before a long-distance endurance event.
- Stop drinking water during exercise if your stomach is sloshing.
- During extended exercise (exercise that lasts more than four hours) in the heat, consume a sport drink that contains sodium.

Death By Dehydration

If someone wanted to lose weight very rapidly, vigorous exercise (especially in the heat) without rehydrating would be one way of accomplishing that objective. It is also very dangerous. In 1977, 3 collegiate wrestlers died of dehydration while trying to make it into a lower weight category for competition (Sharkey, 2002). An average-sized person has about 11 gallons (41.63 L) of water in his body when fully hydrated. During vigorous exercise, a person can lost 1 pint (0.47 L) to a little over a gallon (3.78 L) of water per hour. If a person were losing one half gallon (1.89 L) of water per hour, it would take less then six hours to reach a fatal level of water loss (see table 8.8).

Table 8.8　Effects of Water Loss

Percentage of water loss in the body	Physical effect
1	Thirsty
5	Slight fever
8	Glands stop producing sweat, skin turns blue
15	Trouble walking
20	Death

Nutritional Guidelines and Principles

The year 1929 marked the beginning of the Great Depression, the longest and worst economic downturn in the history of the modern industrialized world. During that time, when families lost their entire life savings in a couple of days, and when up to a quarter of the workforce was unemployed, Americans had to stand in the government bread lines to stay fed. Out of concern for vitamin and mineral deficiencies, the United States federal government publicized the dietary guidelines shown in figure 8.7, graphically represented by a circle containing seven food groups.

By the 1950s and '60s, those deficiencies were no longer a problem, but concern was growing about declining levels of physical fitness, especially among children. In 1956, President

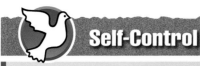

Self-Control

Probably everyone has experienced a time when they lost control, or when someone else lost control in anger against them. Some may have occasionally been a victim to one who has lost control; for others it may have occurred often. These experiences usually cut deeply, and the resulting wounds often leave lifelong scars. For both the perpetrator and victim, this lack of self-control brings pain, not healing or wellness. The same is true of people who lose control to food and allow it to allure them into eating too much or too little. Allow God to control and direct your life and your eating. Don't let negative images of self portrayed in the media or emotional satisfaction from food have control. To be **self-controlled** is to let God be in charge of your life.

Asceticism was prevalent in the thinking of Classical Greece and Hellenism. Ascetics believe it is possible to achieve a high spiritual or intellectual state by renouncing worldly pleasures. I remember a girl who ground up egg shells each day and ate them. She didn't like doing that, but it was an act of self-discipline, self-control. Scripture does not encourage asceticism. Writers of scripture appreciated far too much the beauties of creation and the hands of its Creator (and perhaps a properly cooked egg!) to encourage eating egg shells and pursuing an ascetic lifestyle.

It's important to recognize humans' powerlessness over things. As Alcoholics Anonymous' literature says, people need to depend on a power greater than themselves. "For God did not give us a spirit of timidity, but a spirit of power, of love and of self-discipline" (2 Timothy 1:7). Being self-controlled will minimize the things you might destroy and help you enjoy and nurture all creation.

Self-control: How would your diet change if you had unlimited will power?

_____

_____

_____

_____

_____

_____

_____

_____

_____

_____

Eisenhower founded the President's Council for Physical Fitness and Sports to encourage schoolchildren to strive for particular fitness objectives. A major element of the program was nutrition; the campaign's slogan was "Food for Fitness." During these decades, the U.S. Department of Agriculture revised the dietary guidelines and reduced the seven food groups to "the basic four" (see figure 8.8).

The four basic food groups persisted, with slight modifications, until the introduction of the Food Guide Pyramid in 1992. In addition to reclassifying food into six groups, the pyramid recognized that people need more servings of some food groups than of others (see figure 8.9). For example, it recommended 6 to 11 daily servings of bread and cereals but only 2 or 3 of meat and dairy. This is the scheme that most of today's college students were taught in school.

Thirteen years later, in 2005, the U.S. Department of Agriculture and the U.S. Department of Health and Human Services published a document titled *Dietary Guidelines for Americans 2005*. The recommendations and guidelines established in this document came after an extensive review of the nutritional science literature. Because of the significance of many new discoveries, a decision was made to develop a new food guide system

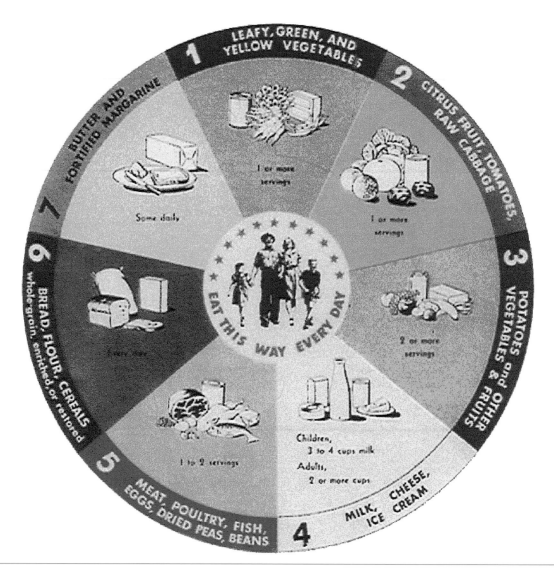

FIGURE 8.7   The first graphical representation of dietary recommendations by the U.S. Department of Agriculture.

From USDA. Available: www.mypyramid.gov/professionals/index.html. Click MyPyramid—USDA's New Food Guidance System.

that reflected the best of what nutritionists know today. Therefore, the New Food Guide reflects a culmination of work on the part of two of the most influential health organizations in the United States (see figure 8.10).

Six Principles That Support the New MyPyramid

The new MyPyramid is based on six principles: activity, variation, proportionality, moderation, personalization, and gradual improvement (U.S. Department of Agriculture, 2007, www.mypyramid.gov/professionals/index.html; click MyPyramid—USDA's New Food Guidance System; see slide number 36).

Activity is a new principle added to the pyramid and is represented by a person on the left-hand side climbing stairs. This addition is included because growing evidence demonstrates the positive role physical activity plays in people's overall well-being. Given overwhelming evidence that physical activity is critical to health, the dietary guidelines recommend 30 minutes a day of exercise for adults and 60 minutes a day for children.

Variety is another key principle. No single food or food group can meet all the body's nutritional needs. The dietary guidelines recommend eating "a variety of nutrients within and among food groups" (U.S. Department of Health and Human Services & U.S. Department of Agriculture, 2005). The different colored bands indicate a need for

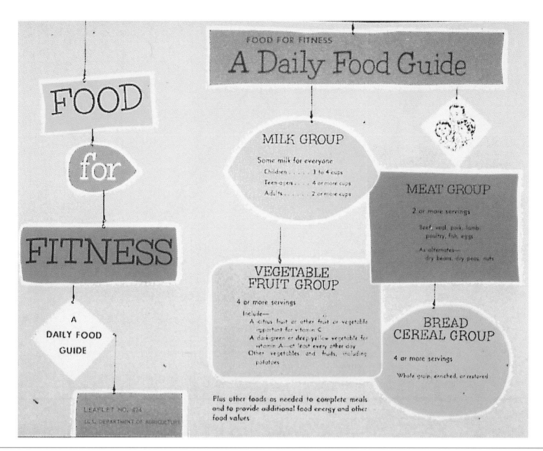

FIGURE 8.8 "Food for Fitness" was the President's Council for Physical Fitness and Sports slogan when the council was first created in 1956 by President Eisenhower.

From USDA. Available: www.mypyramid.gov/professionals/index.html. Click MyPyramid—USDA's New Food Guidance System.

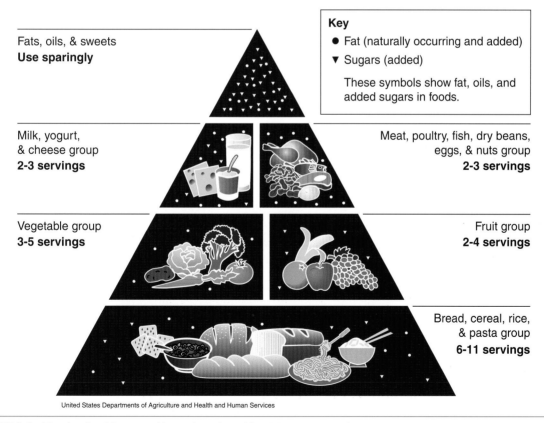

FIGURE 8.9 The food guide pyramid was introduced in 1992.

Reprinted from USDA. Available: www.mypyramid.gov/professionals/index.html. Click MyPyramid—USDA's New Food Guidance System.

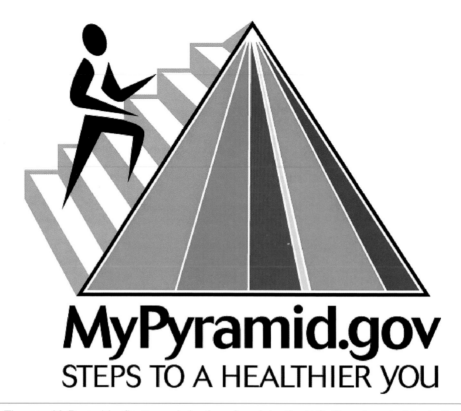

FIGURE 8.10 The new MyPyramid reflects a culmination of work by the U.S. Department of Agriculture and the U.S. Department of Health and Human Services.

Reprinted from www.mypyramid.gov/professionals/index.html. Click MyPyramid—USDA's New Food Guidance System.

No Wonder We Are Getting Larger

In as little as two decades, portion sizes have tripled in caloric value in some cases (see table 8.9). This rapid expansion has led to a corresponding epidemic growth in obesity.

Little wonder that one of the fastest shrinking minorities in America are individuals who are at a healthy body weight.

Table 8.9 Changes in Portion Sizes From 1985 to 2005

	CALORIES PER PORTION	
Food item	20 years ago	Today
Bagel	140 calories (3 in. [7.6 cm] diameter)	350 calories (6 in. [15.2 cm] diameter)
Fast-food cheeseburger	333 calories	590 calories
Spaghetti and meatballs	500 calories (1 cup of spaghetti with sauce and 3 small meatballs)	1,025 calories (2 cups of spaghetti and 3 large meatballs)
Bottle of soda	85 calories (6.5 oz [29.6 ml])	250 calories (20 oz [591.5 ml])
Fast-food French fries	210 calories (2.4 oz [70.1 ml])	610 calories (6.9 oz [204.1 ml])
Turkey sandwich	320 calories	820 calories

Adapted from National Heart, Lung, and Blood Institute, 2005, *Portion distortion quiz.* Available: www.nhlbi.nih.gov.

each of the six food groups represented. It is also important to remember to include variety within each of the food groups.

Proportionality is communicated by the varying widths of the food group bands. This size difference is meant to suggest that a person should eat more foods from the larger wedges and fewer from the smaller.

Moderation is perhaps the least obvious principle illustrated in the pyramid. The narrowing bands from bottom to top are meant to illustrate moderation. The 2005 guidelines suggest limiting the amount of added fat and sugar to foods. Foods within groups can vary in the amount of added fat and sugar. The bottom, wider portion of each band represents foods that are lowest in fat and sugar content. The top, which is narrower, represents foods within each group where fat and sugar have been added. For example, an apple would be at the bottom of the fruit band, sweetened applesauce higher in the band, an apple pie toward the top. The core idea here is that moderation should be maintained especially with regard to high-fat and high-sugar foods.

Gradual improvement is portrayed by the slogan "Steps to a Healthier You." This phrase helps communicate that behavioral change typically occurs slowly, one small step at a time. This is reinforced by the image doing exactly what the slogan says.

The name MyPyramid and the image of just one person climbing steps represents the principle of personalization. The principles of creating a healthy diet are the same for all, but when it comes to caloric intake, energy expenditure, and nutritional choices, people do vary. Fortunately, the new food guide pyramid has tools that allow each person to get personalized recommendations based on particular needs. In the next section, you will discover how to do this.

Your Personal Pyramid

The real power of the food guide pyramid is realized when you go to the Web site, put in your individualized information, and receive a personalized report. In this section, you will be guided through this process. The first step is to log on to the U.S. Department of Agriculture's Web site: MyPyramid. gov. This particular Web page is illustrated in figure 8.11.

This home page displays lots of interesting information you can explore later, but for right now go to the top right-hand portion of this Web

page to the section called MyPyramid Plan and click Go Now. When the new page resolves, enter your age, height, weight, sex, and activity level. To illustrate this process, I will enter data for a hypothetical person—an 18-year-old female college freshman who is physically active 30 to 60 minutes most days of the week (see figure 8.12). In addition, her body weight is 142, and her height is 5 feet, 7 inches (if you want to enter these values, you may). Let's call her Jacinda.

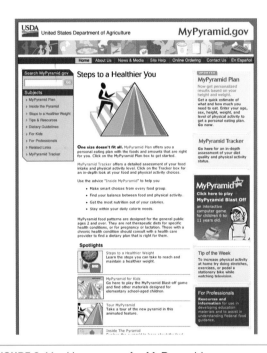

FIGURE 8.11   Home page for MyPyramid.gov.

From USDA. Available: www.mypyramid.gov.

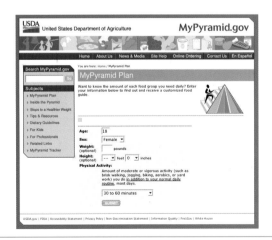

FIGURE 8.12   Personalize your pyramid by age, sex, and activity level.

From USDA. Available: www.mypyramid.gov.

After entering your personalized information, as I've done for Jacinda, click Submit. When the next page loads (this may take a few moments), your individualized recommendations will appear. This page has information specifically tailored to you (see figure 8.13).

The first piece of personalized information you will see is an estimate of your daily caloric expenditure. Jacinda's estimate is 2,000 calories per day. The recommendation notes that this figure is only an estimate that needs to be monitored to determine accuracy. In other words, if Jacinda begins carefully consuming 2,000 calories per day and begins to lose weight, the formula used to calculate her caloric expenditure may be underestimating her requirements. On the other hand, if she begins to gain weight, her caloric requirements may be overestimated. Although minor adjustments may be necessary, this formula used by the Institute of Medicine should come close to accurately estimating calorie needs (Institute of Medicine, 2002).

Below this estimate are specific recommendations for food from each of the five food groups: grains, vegetables, fruits, milk, and meat and beans. The new MyPyramid no longer uses the term "servings" because that led to confusion about how much a serving actually is. For one person, a serving of breakfast cereal may be more than two cups, for another it may be less than one. The original pyramid had a long list of equivalents; the new pyramid simplifies the picture by listing everything in cups and ounces.* For additional assistance with food portions, the new pyramid gives several examples of common sizes in each of the five food groups. Click Grains (see figure 8.14). If you select the "Learn More" button, several common foods in this food group can be explored.

Return to the page with your individualized recommendations and notice that just below the food groups is a recommendation that nearly half the grains you eat should be whole grains. According to the National Health and Nutrition Examination Survey (NHANES), which measures consumption norms, Americans are currently consuming most of their grains from refined sources (National Health and Nutrition Examination Survey, 2002). Refined grains are processed in such a way that many of the nutrient-rich vitamins and minerals have been removed.

The next recommendation is to "Vary Your Veggies." This reinforces the principle of variation by recommending various amounts of particular vegetable categories, such as dark green, orange, and high starch. According to the NHANES (2002), consumption patterns for most Americans differ greatly from these recommended levels. The NHANES reported that middle-age females con-

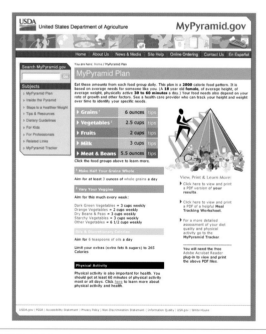

FIGURE 8.13 Personalized recommendations are part of the pyramid.

From USDA. Available: www.mypyramid.gov.

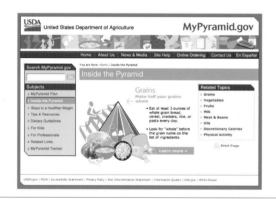

FIGURE 8.14 Information on each food group can be individually selected.

From USDA. Available: www.mypyramid.gov.

*For those less familiar with cups and ounces, you can easily convert these measures to metric by multiplying ounces by 28.34 to get grams and cups by 236.58 to get milliliters.

sumed, on average, one cup of dark green vegetables, approximately two-thirds cup of orange vegetables, and less than a cup of legumes per week. Each of these examples is less than half of what the 2005 guidelines recommended.

The final personalized recommendations are the number of teaspoons of oil and the amount of discretionary calories you should aim to take in each day. Jacinda needs six teaspoons of oil per day. Oils, like vegetable oil, canola oil, and corn oil, are liquid at room temperature. Most oils, with the exception of coconut and palm oils, are high in monounsaturated and polyunsaturated fat and low in saturated fat and cholesterol.

Finally, you'll get a recommendation for **discretionary calories**. A discretionary calorie is a new concept in the revised food guide pyramid. These calories are like having luxury calories. Before you spend them you need to understand exactly how they are calculated. Back to Jacinda: She has been given a dietary plan based on 2,000 calories, of which 265 calories are discretionary. It is important to realize that the 265 discretionary calories are included in the 2,000-calorie allotment. Health experts who designed the new food guide pyramid are assuming that your food choices within each of the five food groups will be low in added fat and sugar. If Jacinda does this consistently in each of her food selections, her intake per day should be around 1,735 calories. Now she has 265 calories left to choose from among some options:

- Eat more foods from any food group.
- Eat higher-calorie forms of foods—those that contain solid fat or added sugar. Examples are whole milk, cheese, sausage, biscuits, sweetened cereal, and sweetened yogurt.
- Add fat or sweeteners to foods. Examples are sauces, salad dressings, sugar, syrup, and butter.
- Eat or drink items that are mostly fat, calorie sweeteners, or alcohol, soda, wine, and beer.

Canadian Food Guide

As you might expect, most industrialized countries have developed nutritional recommendations and visual graphics to help their citizens make wise nutritional choices. Figure 8.15 shows the Web page for Canada's Food Guide recommendations. Similar to MyPyramid, a personalized dietary plan

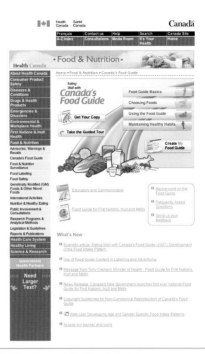

FIGURE 8.15   Canada's Food Guide.

Reprinted, by permission, from Health Canada, 2007. Available: www.hc-sc.gc.ca/fn-an/food-guide-aliment/index_e.html.

is recommended after demographic information and particualr food selections are identified.

Here is a summary of the dietary guidelines for Canadians:

- Enjoy a variety of foods.
- Emphasize cereals, breads, other grain products, vegetables, and fruit.
- Consume no more than 30 percent of your calories from fat and no more than 10 percent as saturated fat.
- Consume at least 55 percent of your total calories from carbohydrate.
- Reduce sodium intake.
- No more than 5 percent of your calories should come from alcohol, or two drinks per day (whichever is less). Consume no alcohol during pregnancy.
- Consume no more caffeine than the equivalent of four regular cups of coffee per day. Consume water containing no less than 1 milligram per liter of fluoride.

You can usually find information about a particular country's nutritional habits and recommendations by doing a Google search for dietary guidelines for the country you're interested in. If you choose to compare the models in this chapters to others, you will most likely find that there are many more similarities than differences. Whether you are a Canadian, German, French, American, or from another country, letting national guidelines direct your nutritional decisions is one way to ensure you are getting all the nutrients your body needs. As you practice using food guides like the ones discussed in this chapter you will soon be able to categorize foods according to the nutrient group, accurately estimate serving sizes, and evaluate menu selections according to their nutritional contribution. Using these tools will not only expand your knowledge but will also improve your health.

Vegetarian Alternative

Interest in vegetarian cuisine has dramatically risen, as evidenced by changes in restaurants and on college campuses. A survey by the National Restaurant Association found that 20 percent of its customers wanted a vegetarian option (Wardlaw & Hampl, 2007). In another study, 15 percent of college students said they selected vegetarian options at lunch or dinner on any given day (Johnston & Sabate, 2006). It would be erroneous to conclude that one in every nine college students is a vegetarian because they are merely interested in vegetarian cuisine. The study shows, however, that curiosity about the background, rationale, and method of vegetarian consumption is significant. About 7.5 million Americans (1 in every 40 adults) and 1.4 million Canadians (1 in every 25 adults) identify with one of the four vegetarian classifications identified in table 8.10 (Wardlaw & Hampl, 2007).

Table 8.10 **Four Major Vegetarian Subgroups**

Group	Dietary restrictions
Vegan	Strictest vegetarian; diet consists of plant foods only
Lacto-vegetarian	Diet consists of plant and milk products
Ovo-vegetarian	Diet consists of plant and egg products
Lacto-ovo-vegetarian	Diet consists of plant, milk, and egg products

Background

Historically, vegetarianism has been linked with philosophies and religions. Around 600 BC, the prophet Daniel, along with three of his friends, refused to eat meat from the King of Babylon's table in order to obey God's Old Testament law (Daniel 1:5–21). In the sixth century BC, Pythagoras advocated a meatless diet for its physical health and its ecological, religious, and philosophical benefits (Johnston & Sabate, 2006). Traditional Hindus and Trappist monks adopt vegetarian diets as a practice of their faith. However, most vegetarians today (with notable exceptions such as the Seventh-Day Adventists) do not list religious faith as the rationale for their diet. Two of the most common reasons given now are health and ecology.

Rationale

Numerous studies show that the death rates from cardiovascular disease, hypertension, cancer, type 2 diabetes, and obesity are lower for vegetarians than for nonvegetarians (Berkow & N.D., 2005; Gardner, 2005; Hu, 2003; Johnston & Sabate, 2006; Lejeune, 2005; Newby, 2005). The lower rates of death and disease may be due in part to the fact that vegetarian diets tend to be lower in saturated fat and cholesterol and higher in complex carbohydrate, dietary fiber, folate, vitamin C, vitamin E, carotenoids, and phytochemicals (Leitzmann, 2005). The lower incidence of chronic disease is not solely due to the diet of vegetarians but to the fact that they tend to be more educated, more physically active, wealthier, and more health conscious than nonvegetarians (BBC News, 2006; Gale et al., 2006; Millet & Dewitte, 2007).

It also makes sound ecological sense to eat primarily plant foods, because food sources require different amounts of energy for their production. The least amount of energy is needed to produce grains—about one-third of the caloric output (total amount of calories harvested) is spent to produce each calorie of grain. Animal products, however, require 10 to 90 calories for each calorie of edible food (Whitney & Rolfes, 2002). Figure 8.16 illustrates how much less fuel vegetarian diets require than meat-based diets.

Around 40 percent of the world's grain products are currently used to raise meat-producing animals, and although some of these grain products are inedible for humans, most of them are consumable products (Wardlaw & Hampl, 2007). Eating for ecological reasons is wise.

Planning a Vegetarian Diet

Vegetarians who include milk and egg products in their diets can meet recommendations for most nutrients almost as easily as nonvegetarians can (Whitney & Rolfes, 2002). However, people who follow a strict vegetarian diet consisting exclusively of plant products need to pay more careful attention to get the right amount of nutrients. Getting enough protein is not the problem that it was once thought to be for vegetarians. Studies show that those on plant-based diets are unlikely to develop protein deficiencies if their energy intakes are adequate (Whitney & Rolfes, 2002). At the forefront of nutritional concerns for vegans (strict vegetarians) are potential deficiencies of vitamin D, vitamin B$_{12}$, iron, zinc, and calcium (Johnston & Sabate, 2006). With a little planning, however, vegans can compensate for these deficiencies (see table 8.11).

Some slight modifications to the MyPyramid food plan allow vegetarians to consume sufficient nutrients (see table 8.12).

For more information on consuming a vegetarian diet, visit the Web sites listed at the end of the chapter.

The meat eater consumes a typical U.S. diet of meat, other animal products, and plant foods:

The lacto-ovo-vegetarian eats a diet that excludes meat, but includes milk products and eggs:

The vegan eats a diet of plant foods only:

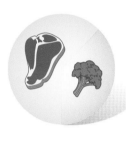
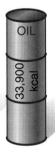
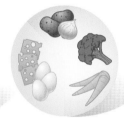
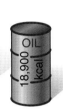
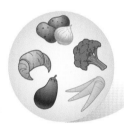

| Meat and animal products 2,000 kcal | Plant foods 1,300 kcal | Fuel required to produce this food 33,900 kcal | Animal products 1,000 kcal | Plant foods 2,300 kcal | Fuel required to produce this food 18,900 kcal | Plant foods 3,300 kcal | Fuel required to produce this food 9,900 kcal |

FIGURE 8.16   Amounts of fuel required to feed individuals consuming food from three different sources, each providing 3,300 calories a day. Note the fossil fuels necessary to produce each of these diets is based on U.S. conditions.

Adapted from Pimentel, 1980.

Table 8.11   Food Sources of Potential Dietary Pitfalls for Vegetarians

Vitamin D	Vitamin D-fortified products like ready-to-eat cereals, soy or rice milk, or from a supplement. One other nondietary solution is to spend 5 to 15 minutes a day in the sun.
Vitamin B$_{12}$	Fortified foods such as ready-to-eat-cereals, soy beverages, meat substitutes, special yeast products, and from supplements
Iron	Whole grains, dried fruits, green leafy vegetables, nuts and seeds, beans, soy, and fortified breads and breakfast cereals
Zinc	Whole grains, nuts, beans, and soy products
Calcium	Legumes, dark green leafy vegetables, nuts, and fortified orange juice, soy milk, tofu, bread, and other foods

Table 8.12 Modifications to MyPyramid Food Group Serving Requirements for Vegetarians

Group	Lacto-vegetarian	Vegan	Key nutrients supplied
Grains	6 – 11	8 – 11	Protein, thiamin, niacin, folate, vitamin E, zinc, magnesium, iron, and fiber
Beans and other legumes	2 – 3	3	Protein, vitamin B_6, zinc, magnesium, and fiber
Nuts, seeds	2 – 3	3	Protein, vitamin E, and magnesium
Vegetables	3 – 5 (include one dark green or leafy variety daily)	4 – 6 (include one dark green or leafy variety daily)	Vitamin A, vitamin C, and folate
Fruits	2 – 4	4	Vitamin A, vitamin C, and folate
Milk	3	—	Protein, riboflavin, vitamin D, vitamin B_{12}, and calcium

This meal plan is based on a diet of 1,600 to 1,800 calories per day and contains about 75 to 100 grams of protein.

Adapted from G. Wardlaw and J. Hampl, 2007, *Perspectives in nutrition,* 9th ed. (New York: The McGraw-Hill Companies), 261. With permission of the McGraw-Hill Companies.

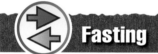

Fasting

In the book *Celebration of Discipline*, Richard Foster writes the following:

> The list of Biblical personages who fasted reads like a Who's Who of scriptures: Moses the lawgiver, David the king, Elijah the prophet, Esther the queen, Daniel the seer, Anna the prophetess, and Paul the apostle. (Foster, 1998, p. 48)

Pastor and author Mark Buchanan notes the following (Buchanan, 2006, p. 36):

> You can't read very far in any direction in the Bible without realizing that fasting was part of the natural rhythm of life for the people of God. They expected and planned to fast as naturally as they expected and planned to eat. To them, fasting was woven into the rhythm of life like day and night, summer and winter, sowing and reaping, waking and sleeping. There were times you ate and times you fasted.

Although Jesus resisted the Pharisees' rigid rules regarding fasting, he fasted himself and indicated that fasting was expected of his followers, particularly after his ministry on earth was completed.

> When you fast, do not look somber as the hypocrites do, for they disfigure their faces to show men they are fasting. I tell you the truth, they have received their reward in full. But when you fast, put oil on your head and wash your face, so that it will not be obvious to men that you are fasting, but only to your Father, who is unseen; and your Father, who sees what is done in secret, will reward you. (Matthew 6:16–18)

They said to him, "John's disciples often fast and pray, and so do the disciples of the Pharisees, but yours go on eating and drinking." Jesus answered, "Can you make the guests of the bridegroom fast while he is with them? But the time will come when the bridegroom will be

(continued)

(continued)

taken from them; in those days they will fast." (Luke 5:33–35)

Clearly, the Bible supports fasting, but going without food for a long time does bring some negative health effects. Following are a number of wellness concerns associated with long-term fasting:

- Decreased metabolic function
- Decreased mental activity
- Potential for the creation of disordered eating (specifically anorexia)
- Increased muscle wasting
- Decreased bone mineral density
- Increased risk for menstrual dysfunction

A classic nutritional deprivation study was first published in the book *The Biology of Human Starvation* (Keys, 1950). In the study, Dr. Ancel Keys carefully documented the effects of chronic energy restriction on a group of 32 men. The experiment was designed to mimic the starvation among prisoners of war in World War II. For six months, the caloric intake of the men was cut in half. As you might expect, each subject had significant weight loss. Yet in addition to weight reduction, several other psychosocial concerns emerged. The men grew increasingly depressed, self-centered, and apathetic, losing interest in almost every-

thing except food. The subjects began reporting an extreme preoccupation with food. They spent their days talking about the flavor and texture of food. Before meals they chatted about food preparation and taste. At night the men dreamed about food. They became increasingly protective of the food that they were rationed, secretly stowing away morsels of food for later consumption. As the experiment continued, the men became increasingly isolated, withdrawing from individuals with whom they had previously shared friendships. Six of the men developed character neuroses, while two others developed mild psychoses.

Although extreme in terms of duration, this study provided a revealing window into the physiological and psychological hardship of food scarcity.

In light of biblical admonitions and scientific evidence, is it advisable to fast? Do some research and form an opinion about whether the scientific evidence is strong enough to warrant the discontinuation of fasting.

There are no specific rules for fasting, but here are five scriptural motives for fasting:

- To hear from God (Acts 13:2)
- To intercede for others (Psalm 35:13)
- As an act of repentance (Joel 1:13–14)
- For strength and direction (Acts 14:23)
- As an act of worship (Luke 2:37)

Next Steps

I have covered a lot of nutritional ground in this chapter, and I will end as I started with a warning about extremes. Some view the Dietary Guidelines, Dietary Reference Intakes, and the meal plan at MyPyramid.gov as the "right" way to eat. Others see the information in this chapter as another bombardment of messages from nutritional experts who cannot seem to go two weeks without announcing yet another food that causes cancer or increased blood pressure. These reactions occupy two extremes: dogged adherence and mindless neglect.

At first glance, dogged adherence seems superior. Unwavering commitment to a detailed dietary

regimen was en vogue when Jesus walked the planet. The dietary system included more than 200 laws designed to prevent disease and demonstrate to the world that the Israelites were set apart by God. Yet it was Jesus who caused a stir by breaking many of these sacred dietary regulations. He gathered food when he wasn't supposed to, dined with inappropriate company, and consumed foods and drink so freely that his critics call him a glutton and drunkard (Matthew 11:19). Jesus simply refused dogmatic adherence to the "dietary line".

The other extreme is disregard for any level of discipline, structure, or order. People become too tired of counting grams of fat, number of calories, and ounces of water; so they decide to follow the mantra, "Let us eat and drink, for tomorrow we die" (1 Corinthians 15:32).

Is there a better way? Indeed there is. In his letter to his young apprentice Timothy, Paul talks about how to guard against extremes:

> The Spirit clearly says that in later times some will abandon the faith and follow deceiving spirits and things taught by demons. Such teachings come through hypocritical liars, whose consciences have been seared as with a hot iron. They forbid people to marry and order them to abstain from certain foods, which God created to be received with thanksgiving by those who believe and who know the truth. For everything God created is good, and nothing is to be rejected if it is received with thanksgiving, because it is consecrated by the word of God and prayer.

(1 Timothy 4:1–5)

In an interview published in *Christianity Today*, John Stott comments about this portion of Paul's letter to Timothy (Stott, 1996, p. 24):

> Paul avoids both extremes: Asceticism is a rejection of the good gifts of the good Creator. Its opposite is materialism—not just possessing material things, but becoming preoccupied with them. In between asceticism and materialism is simplicity, contentment, and generosity, and these three virtues should mark all of us.

Living between the extremes is wonderful advice not only for your spirit, but also for your nutritional health.

Key Terms

alimentary canal

amino acids

antioxidants

asceticism

bolus

calorie

carbohydrate

chyme

complete proteins

complex carbohydrate

digestive system

disaccharides

discretionary calories

duodenum

energy metabolism

esophageal sphincter

esophagus

fat

fiber

free radicals

fructose

galactose

glucose

glycemic index

glycemic load

Helicobactor pylori

hydrochloric acid (HCL)

hyponatremia

ileum

insoluble fiber

jejunum

kilocalorie

lactose

macronutrients

maltose

micronutrients

minerals

monosaccharides

monounsaturated fat

net carbohydrate

nutrient density

nutrition

pepsin

peristalsis

polysaccharides

polyunsaturated fat

protein

pyloric sphincter

rectum

saturated fat

self-controlled

simple carbohydrate

soluble fiber
stomach
sucrose
trace minerals

variety
villi and microvilli
vitamins

Review Questions

1. Describe how nutritional imbalances affect the world people share (environment, economy, culture, religion, and health).

2. Diagram the digestive system.

3. Identify the specific contributions each of the six major nutrients makes to health.

4. Using MyPyramid or Canada's Food Guide, outline a healthy diet for an 18-year-old female who is getting less than 30 minutes of vigorous activity each day.

5. What changes would you need to make in the diet you developed in the answer to the previous question if that individual were a vegetarian?

Application Activities

1. Search for the dietary guidelines of a country that isn't the United States. Compare and contrast those guidelines offered by MyPyramid.

2. Assess your existing diet by going to www.mypyramidtracker.gov.

3. Outline a dietary plan that is in line with the personalized recommendations at Mypyramid.gov.

References

Albert, C.M., Gaziano, J.M., Willett, W.C., & Manson, J.E. (2002). Nut consumption and decreased risk of sudden cardiac death in the physicians' health study. *Archives of Internal Medicine, 162*(12): 1382.

American College of Sports Medicine. (2000). Position paper: Nutrition and athletic performance. *Journal of the American Dietetic Association, 100*: 1543-1556.

BBC News. (2006). High IQ link to being vegetarian. Retrieved December 19, 2006, from http://news.bbc.co.uk/2/hi/health/6180753.stm.

Berkow, S.E., & N.D., B. (2005). Blood pressure regulation and vegetarian diets. *Nutrition Reviews, 63*(1): 1-8.

Briefel, R.R., & Johnson, C.L. (2004). Secular trends in dietary intake in the United States. *Annual Review of Nutrition, 24*: 401-431.

Buchanan, M. (2006). *The rest of God: Restoring your soul by restoring Sabbath.* Waco, TX: Word Publishing Group.

Clark, N. (2003). *Sports nutrition guidebook* (3rd ed.). Champaign, IL: Human Kinetics.

Consumer Reports. (2004). The truth about low-carb foods. *Consumer Reports* (June): 12.

Donatelle, R. (2006). *Access to health* (9th ed.). San Francisco: Pearson.

Food Institute Report (2002). When, why, and on what are college students snacking on. *The Food Institute Report*: 4.

Food Service Director. (2002). Freshmen college student dining habits. *Food Service Director, 15*(3): 1.

Foster, G. (2003). A randomized trial of low carbohydrate diet for obesity. *New England Journal of Medicine, 348*(21): 2082-2090.

Foster, R.J. (1998). *Celebration of discipline: the path to spiritual growth.* San Francisco: Harper.

Gale, C.R., Deary, I.J., Schoon, I., Batty, G.D., & Batty, G.D. (2006). IQ in childhood and vegetarianism in adulthood: 1970 British cohort study. *British Medical Journal, 334*(7587): 245.

Gardner, C.D. (2005). The effect of a plant-based diet on plama lipids in hypercholesterolemic adults. *Annals of Internal Medicine, 142*: 725-733.

Hales, D. (2005). *An invitation to health* (11th ed.). Belmont, CA: Wadsworth.

Health Canada. (2007). Canada's food guide. Retrieved June 1, 2007, from www.hc-sc.gc.ca/fn-an/food-guide-aliment/index_e.html.

Hu, F. (2003). Plant-based foods and prevention of cardiovascular disease: An overview. *American Journal of Clinical Nutrition, 78*(suppl.): 544S.

Institute of Medicine. (2002). *Dietary reference intakes for energy, carbohydrate, fiber, fat, fatty acids, cholesterol, protein, and amino acids.* Washington, DC: Institute of Medicine.

Jenkins, D.J., Kendall, C.W., Marchie, A., Parker, T.I., Connelly, P.W., Qian, W., Haight, J.S., Faulkner, D., Vidgen, E., Lapsley, K.G., & Spiller, G.A. (2002). Dose response of almonds on coronary heart disease risk factors: Blood lipids, oxidized low-density lipoproteins, lipoprotein(a), homocysteine, and pulmonary nitric oxide: A randomized, controlled, crossover trial. *Circulation, 106*(11): 1327-1332.

Johnston, P.A., & Sabate, J. (Eds.) (2006). *Nutritional implications of vegetarian diets.* Philadelphia: Lippincott, Williams & Wilkins.

Kanton, L.S. (Ed.). (1999). *A comparison of the US food supply with the food guide pyramid recommendations.* Washington, DC: United States Department of Agriculture.

Keys, A.B. (1950). *The biology of human starvation.* Minneapolis: University of Minnesota Press.

Lejeune, M.P. (2005). Additional protein in-take limits weight regain after weight loss in humans. *British Journal of Nutrition, 93*: 281-289.

Leitzmann, C. (2005). Vegetarian diets: What are the advantages? *Forum of Nutrition, 57*: 147.

Lemon, P. (1995). Do athletes need more protein and amino acids? *International Journal of Sports and Nutrition, 5*: S39-S61.

Miller, B.J. (2003). Glycemic load and chronic disease. *Nutritional Review, 61*(5): S49.

Millet, K., & Dewitte, S. (2007). IQ and vegetarianism: Non-conformity may be hidden driver behind relation. *British Medical Journal, 334*(7589): 327-328.

Mulvihill, K. (2001). Runners beware: Too much water can be dangerous. Reuters News. Retrieved June 27, 2007, from www.womenrunners.com/training_hyponatremia.htm.

Nathan's Web site. (2005). Hot dog contest results 2005. Retrieved August 5, 2006, from www.nathansfamous.com/nathans/contest/hot_dog_contest_2005_results.php.

National Health and Nutrition Examination Survey. (2002). Report: National health and examination survey. Retrieved June 1, 2007, from www.cdc.gov/nchs/nhanes.htm.

National Heart, Lung, and Blood Institute. (2005). Proportion distortion quiz. Retrieved 2005, from www.nhlbi.nih.gov.

Natural Resources Defense Council. (1999). *Bottled water: Pure drink or pure hype?* New York: NRDC.

Newby, P.K. (2005). Risk of overweight and obesity among semivegetarian, lactovegetarian, and vegan women. *American Journal of Clinical Nutrition, 81*: 1267.

Pegis, A. (Ed.). (1997). *Basic writings of St. Thomas Aquinas.* Indianapolis: Hackett.

Pimentel, D. (1980). *Food, energy, and the future of society.* Boulder, CO: Associated University Press.

Powell, K.F., Holt, S., & Brand-Miller, J. (2002). International tables of glycemic index and glycemic load values. American *Journal of Clinical Nutrition, 62*: 5-56.

Samaha, F. (2003). A low carbohydrate as compared with a low-fat diet in severe obesity. New *England Journal of Medicine, 348*(21): 2074-2081.

Sharkey, B. (2002). *Fitness and health* (5th ed.). Champaign, IL: Human Kinetics.

Spurlock, M. (2007). 30 days. Retrieved June 1, 2007, from http://tv.yahoo.com/tvpdb?d=tvi&cf=0&id=18 08702629.

Stott, J. (1996). Basic Stott: An interview by Roy McCloughry. *Christianity Today, 40*(1): 24.

Tan, P.L. (1982). *Encyclopedia of 7,700 illustrations.* Rockville, MD: Assurance.

U.S. Department of Health and Human Services, & U.S. Department of Agriculture. (2005). Dietary guidelines for Americans 2005. Retrieved from www.health.gov/dietaryguidelines.

U.S. Department of Agriculture. (2007). MyPyramid. Retrieved June 1, 2007, from www.mypyramid.gov.

U.S. Food and Drug Administration. (1999). Water sold state to state safe to drink. United States Food and Drug Administration (July/August).

U.S. Food and Drug Administration. (2004). How to understand and use the nutrition facts label. Retrieved August 8, 2006, from www.cfsan.fda.gov/~dms/foodlab.html.

Wardlaw, G., & Hampl, J. (2007). *Perspectives in nutrition* (9th ed.). Boston: McGraw-Hill.

Whitney, E.N., & Rolfes, S.R. (2002). *Understanding nutrition.* Belmont, CA: Wadsworth/Thomson.

Suggested Readings

Duyff, R. (2002). *ADA: Complete food and nutrition guide* **(2nd ed.). Chicago: American Dietetic Association.**

This comprehensive book from the American Dietetic Association is packed with simple, practical tips and flexible guidelines to help you choose nutritious, flavorful, and convenient foods that suit your needs and lifestyle—no matter your age or stage of life.

Selkowitz, A. (2000). *The college student's guide to eating well on campus.* **Bethesda, MD: Tulip Hill Press.**

Targeted toward college students, this guidebook describes how to avoid gaining "the freshman fifteen" and how to make healthy food choices while in college.

Sizer, F., & Whitney, E.N. (2006). *Nutrition concepts and controversies* **(10th ed.). Belmont, CA: Wadsworth/Thomson.**

The biological foundations of nutrition are covered without assuming any previous knowledge. This nutrition textbook helps students gain a nutritional background that will assist them in making healthy food choices.

Wardlaw, G., & Hampl, J. (2007). *Perspectives in nutrition* **(9th ed.). Boston: McGraw-Hill.**

The text places special emphasis on the application of nutrition principles in everyday life by exploring the health consequences of nutrition practices.

Whitney, E.N., & Rolfes, S.R. (2002). *Understanding nutrition.* **Belmont, CA: Wadsworth/Thomson.**

This student-focused textbook presents the major concepts in nutrition including the body's use of food nutritents and diet planning throughout the life cycle.

Suggested Web Sites

www.ivu.org

Web site supported by the International Vegetarian Union.

www.vrg.org

An informative Web site on vegetarianism by the Vegetarian Resource Group.

www.eatright.org

Web site for the American Dietetic Association, one of the most respected sources of dietary information in the United States.

www.health.gov/dietaryguidelines

Web site that provides the 2005 version of dietary guidelines for Americans.

www.mypyramid.gov

Detailed information about the new food pyramid.

www.hc-sc.gc.ca/hpfb-dgpsa/onpp-bppn/food_guide_rainbow_e.html

Canada's Food Guide, with dietary reference intakes, healthy weights, nutrition labeling, food programs, and resources.

www.cfsan.fda.gov/label.html

A detailed description of what U.S. food labels mean.

www.nal.usda.gov/fnic/foodcomp/search

The USDA nutritional database provides a search tool to find the nutritional contents of a particular food.

http://fnic.nal.usda.gov/nal_display/index.php?info_center=4&tax_level=1

U.S. Food and Nutrition Center site with food guide information for various ethnic and cultural groups.

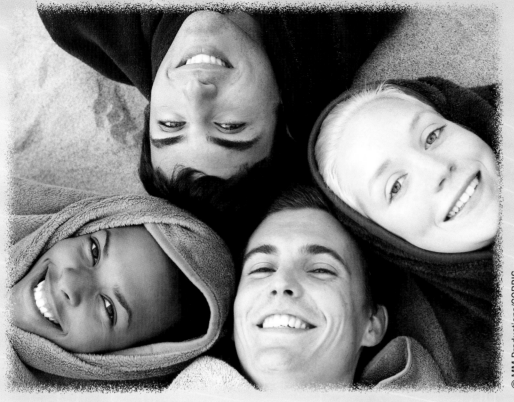

© MM Productions/CORBIS

Emotional Health and Wellness

Peter Walters • Doug Needham • Bud Williams

After reading this chapter, you should be able to do the following:

➊ Appreciate the mind–body connection.

➋ Learn the ABCs of stress.

➌ Identify how stress can help or hinder.

➍ List three principles for becoming stress hardy.

➎ Identify the primary symptoms and causes of depression.

➏ Learn strategies for treating depression.

➐ Understand the fundamental factors that contribute to happiness.

Intelligence quotient (IQ) has long been considered a leading predictor of a person's potential for achievement. More recently, psychologists have determined that a different type of intelligence, called *emotional intelligence* or *emotional quotient* (EQ), makes an even greater difference in personal and professional success than IQ does (Goleman, 1995).

According to the author of the international bestseller *Emotional Intelligence*, Dr. Daniel Goleman of Harvard University, EQ involves the ability to know one's own emotions, manage them appropriately, and recognize the emotional states of others. More than a decade of research has shown that people with these skills are more productive at work and are happier at home. They're also less prone to stress, depression, and anxiety, and they bounce back quicker from serious illnesses (Goleman, 1995; Goleman, 2002; Matthews, 2002).

According to Dr. Travis Bradberry, who has surveyed more than 500,000 men and women about their emotional intelligence, only 36 percent can accurately identify their emotions when they occur. Approximately 70 percent reported not being able to handle stress effectively, and only 15 percent said they felt respected by others at work (Bradberry, 2003). A survey of more than 1,000 students attending Christian colleges across America found that the "ability to communicate feelings" ranked dead last among their relational abilities (Walters et al., 2006). The students—both male and female—rated themselves better at listening, self-understanding, honesty, conflict resolution, assertiveness, and trustworthiness than they rated themselves at being able to communicate feelings.

The good news is that, while IQ barely budges over a lifetime, you can boost your emotional intelligence. Psychologist John Mayer, PhD, of the University of New Hampshire, is one of the pioneers in EQ research. He likens emotional intelligence to skill in algebra (Hales, 2007). Mayer suggests that just as people can learn to solve algebraic equations through a step-by-step process, they also can learn the skills that enhance emotional intelligence.

This chapter teaches theoretical principles and specific skills to expand emotional aptitude in two specific areas, stress and depression. A Kansas State study conducted over a 13-year period reported that the nature of mental health issues on college campuses changed between 1988 and 2001. At the beginning of the study most students were seeking help with relational challenges;

stress and anxiety topped the list toward the end of the study (Benton et al., 2003). According to the National College Health Assessment survey (National College Health Association, 2006), which involved 47,202 students from 74 campuses across the United States, 15 percent of students reported being diagnosed with depression, up from 10 percent in 2000.

Stress and depression are major health issues for students, and they can become serious if left untreated. Therefore the aim of this chapter is to will teach you to understand, detect, and know how to get help for these common issues.

A large portion of this chapter is focused on heavy emotions, but we don't want that to be its only focus. For that reason, the chapter concludes with a discussion about happiness. Several scientific studies have identified traits that increase the likelihood of experiencing happiness. We'll explore the results of those studies.

Stress and the Mind–Body Connection

The Canadian medical researcher Hans Selye was examining the effects of an ovarian extract that had recently been isolated on a group of laboratory rats. During the testing Selye noticed that the rodents' adrenal glands had enlarged, their immune glands had shrunk, and their stomachs had developed bleeding ulcers (Sapolsky, 2004). Selye was alarmed by these results, but he didn't want to jump to conclusions so he repeated the study. The second time he included a control group that had been injected with a neutral saline solution instead of with the extract. To his amazement, the rats in the control group developed the same symptoms. Wracking his brain for another explanation, Dr. Selye realized that he wasn't exactly adept at handling the rats. As he tried to inject them, they would often squirm out of his grasp and he would have to chase them around the lab with a broom. The poor creatures were seriously stressed out! Further experiments confirmed this hypothesis, and Selye extended it beyond rats. His prediction—that sufficient levels of stress can cause physical illness in humans—since then has been thoroughly investigated and upheld by a new brand of medical research called **psychoneuroimmunology (PNI)**, the study of the mind's healing and harmful effects on the body (Sapolsky, 2004).

Many studies report the negative and positive consequences related to varying states of mind. In one study college students were tested for salivary

IgA (S-IgA), an antibody that fights infection, five days before, the day of, and two weeks after final exams. The results showed their S-IgA levels were lowest on the days of the exams (Brain Mind Bulletin, 1989), suggesting a compromised immune system. In another study with S-IgA, researchers induced positive moods among their subjects by asking them to imagine a situation in which they experienced "care and compassion". When researchers measured levels during these positive states, they found S-IgA to have increased (Rein, Atkinson, & McCraty, 1995).

Mind–body medicine has flourished recently because Americans report higher levels of stress than ever before. According to a recent survey, 75 percent of U.S. adults feel "great stress" at least one day a week, and some feel it almost daily (American Institute of Stress, 2002). Adults aren't the only ones feeling more stress. The Cooperative Institutional Research Program reports that students, specifically college freshmen in the United States, are feeling more overwhelmed than ever before (Sax, 1999). According to their findings, almost one third (30.2 percent) of first-year students described themselves as "frequently overwhelmed". That may sound normal for freshmen, but the revealing part of this data is that the percentages increased over time. Figure 9.1 illustrates from 1985 to 1999 that the number of first-year students who said they were frequently overwhelmed doubled (Sax, 1999).

How stressed are you? It is easy to underestimate how much stress you have and overestimate how much you can endure. A stress test in the application activities at the end of this chapter can help you identify your existing stress load, or you can take the fun test in the box on this page.

The ABCs of Stress

A common definition of **stress** is "any specific or nonspecific response of the body to any demand made upon it" (Ellison, 2002). This definition is

Quick Stress Test

You are under too much stress if

- there are teeth marks on your textbooks;
- you don't have an ulcer, you have a black hole;
- you put posters on your walls to cover your fingernail scratches; or
- you fall asleep counting things on your to-do list.

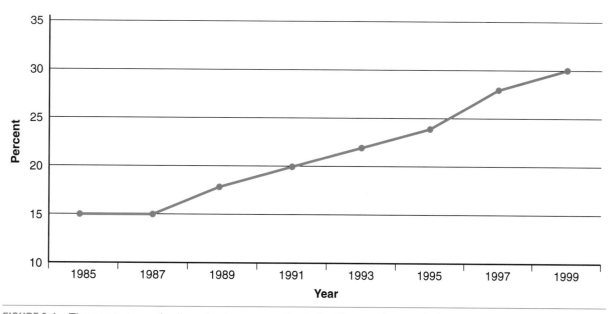

FIGURE 9.1   The percentage of college freshman reporting being "frequently overwhelmed" doubled between 1985 and 1999.

Sax, 1999.

quite broad. To gain a better understanding of exactly what stress is, we need to analyze stress more specifically. Noted psychologist Dr. Albert Ellis did just that. He stated that at least three components must exist for stress to occur (see figure 9.2). He called these the "ABCs of stress" (Ellis et al., 1997).

A = Activating Events

An **activating event, or stressor**, is any event or condition that triggers a stress response. Thomas Holmes, psychiatrist at the University of Washington School of Medicine, and Richard Rahe, a scientist for the United States Military, were some of the first to scientifically examine stressors (Holmes & Rahe, 1967). They examined the medical records of 5,000 patients who had recently suffered illness. Then they asked the patients whether they had experienced any stressful life events preceding their illness. If so, patients were then asked to rate the severity of that stressful event (measured on a 100-point scale). What they reported was a positive correlation between stress events and illness. In other words, as stress increases so does illness. Table 9.1 presents the results of their research.

As you can see, death of a spouse was considered the most stressful life experience. It is also interesting to note that events generally viewed as positive and enriching, such as getting married, receiving a job promotion, and entering retirement, rank fairly high as stressors. If you can't relate to many of the life changes identified by Holmes, a scale specific to college students was adapted from Holmes' original work and is listed in table 9.2 (Anderson, 1972).

Life changes are only one of three categories of stressors. The second is catastrophes. Natural disasters, war, rape, assault, torture, and other events like those can so traumatize people that they later develop **post-traumatic stress disorder (PTSD).** People with this condition tend to have vivid nightmares or flashbacks in which they relive the awful experience again and again.

Epidemiologists report that most people will experience a traumatic event in their lives, and that up to 25 percent of them will develop PTSD (Kessler, 2000).

The third category, which is less intense but still important, is what researcher Richard Lazarus terms "daily hassles" (Lazarus, 1984). After questioning many adults, he concluded that most people identify relatively minor annoyances as their main sources of stress and tension. These are some of the more common daily hassles:

• Misplacing and losing things
• Dealing with troublesome people
• Concern over physical appearance
• Anxiety over financial matters
• Feeling overwhelmed by too many things to do

What is stressing you out? The list below identifies how 1,077 students from Christian Colleges ranked their leading stressors (Walters et al., 2006).

1. **Academic work:** Men and women both rated the tension of keeping up with academic responsibilities significantly higher than any other life stressor. Perhaps this is no surprise given the primary task of students.

2. **Future concerns:** These include concerns regarding choosing a major, fears about how successful they will be in college, finding a soul mate, and determining a career ranked second.

3. **Spiritual matters:** This particular stressor seems to be unique to students attending private Christian institutions. Specific issues in this category included determining personal beliefs, establishing consistency of spiritual disciplines, experiencing a crisis of beliefs, and feelings of inferiority

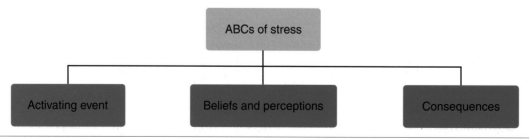

FIGURE 9.2   Three ingredients essential for stress to occur.

Ellis et al., 1997.

Table 9.1   Intensity of Common Stressful Events

Life change units	Event	Life change units	Event
100	Death of spouse	29	Change in responsibilities at work
73	Divorce	29	Son or daughter leaving home
65	Marital separation	29	Trouble with in-laws
63	Jail term	28	Outstanding personal achievement
63	Death of close family member	26	Spouse begins or stops work
53	Personal injury or illness	25	Change in living conditions
50	Marriage	24	Revision of personal habits
47	Fired at work	23	Trouble with boss
45	Marital reconciliation	20	Change in work hours or conditions
45	Retirement	20	Change in residence
44	Change in health of family member	19	Change in recreation
40	Pregnancy	19	Change in church activities
39	Sex difficulties	18	Change in social activities
39	Gain of new family member	17	Mortgage or loan for lesser purchase (car, TV, and so on)
39	Business readjustment	16	Change in sleeping habits
38	Change in financial state	15	Change in number of family get-togethers
37	Death of close friend	15	Change in eating habits
36	Change to different line of work	13	Vacation
35	Change in number of arguments with spouse	12	Christmas
31	Mortgage or loan for major purchase (e.g., home)	11	Minor violations of the law
30	Foreclosure of mortgage or loan		

Adapted from *Journal of Psychosomatic Research, 11,* T. Holmes and R. Rahe, The social readjustment rating scale, p. 213-218. Copyright 1967 with permission from Elsevier.

toward people who seem to have a better relationship with God than they have.

4. **Interpersonal relationships:** College is a unique time of relational transition. Students leave the familiar family environment—not just for the day, but for weeks and months at a time—and venture off into new relationships. Dealing with roommates and peers with different perspectives and trying to maintain a balance between social involvement and academic success can be challenging.

5. **Financial matters:** College is expensive. According to the U.S. Department of Education, the average cost of a four-year private college education was $23,940 per year in 2002-2003 (U.S. Department of Education, 2006). Over four years, tuition will be a total of approximately $100,000—not exactly "small change."

Examining exposure to life change, catastrophic events, and daily life hassles can help identify potential stressors. But it is important to

Table 9.2   Intensity of Common Stressful Events Among College Students

Life change units	Event (adapted for college students)	Life change units	Event (adapted for college students)
87	Death of a spouse	50	Change to a different line of work
77	Marriage	50	Change to a new school
77	Death of a close family member	48	Major change in social activities
76	Divorce	47	Major change in responsibilities at work
74	Marital separation	46	Major change in the use of alcohol
68	Death of a close friend	45	Revision of personal habits
68	Pregnancy or fathering a child	44	Trouble with school administration
65	Major personal injury or illness	43	Work at a job while attending school
62	Fired from work	42	Trouble with in-laws
60	Broken marital engagement or steady relationship	42	Change in residence or living conditions
58	Sex difficulties	41	Change in or choice of a major field of study
58	Marital reconciliation	41	Change dating habits
57	Major change in usual type and/or amount of recreation	40	Outstanding personal achievement
57	Major change in self-concept or self-awareness	38	A lot more or a lot less trouble with your boss
56	Major change in the health of a family member	36	Major change in church activities
54	Engaged to be married	34	Major change in sleeping habits
53	Major change in financial state	33	Trip or vacation
52	Mortgage or loan for purchase of less than $10,000	30	Major change in eating habits
50	Enter college	26	Major change in the number of family get-togethers
50	Gain a new family member	22	Found guilty of minor violations of the law
50	Major conflict in or change in values		

Reprinted from G.E. Anderson, 1972, *College schedule of recent experience* (Fargo, ND: North Dakota State University). By permission of G.E. Anderson.

remember that the same event may affect different people in different ways. For example, one person might find driving home from work very stressful, while another might find it relaxing. A person's beliefs and perceptions about those events have an enormous effect on how stress is internalized and expressed.

B = Beliefs or Perceptions

The following well-known story illustrates that the way a person construes or interprets an event affects the response to it:

On an airplane flying from New York to Boston, a middle-aged man was quickly losing patience with the family next to him. The two toddlers were standing in their seats, crawling around on the floor, making a lot of noise, and otherwise misbehaving. Their mother, however, was doing nothing to control them. She just sat staring blankly into space, oblivious to the commotion. Finally, unable to take it any more, the man demanded, "Lady, can't you do something about your kids?" Startled, as if awakened from a deep sleep, she quickly reprimanded her children, fastened them in their seats, and gave them toys to occupy them. Then she turned to the man sitting next to her and quietly apologized. "I'm sorry, sir. I guess I was distracted. Three hours ago I received a phone call and was told that my husband had been seriously injured in an automobile accident. They said to get there as soon as I could, because he might not make it."

Knowing about that phone call changed the gentleman's characterization of the woman from her being a negligent mother to her being a grieving spouse. This may not have completely eliminated the gentleman's frustration, but it probably helped him be more understanding of the situation.

Most people respond to stressors without thinking about how their perceptions and beliefs affect them. As we develop and mature, the environment and experiences mold our beliefs. At a certain point, however, beliefs about self, others, and the world begin to solidify, and rather than think afresh about every new event, people respond based on previous experiences and interpretations of them. Increasingly, people see what they believe, rather than believe what they see.

Albert Ellis said that the space between stimulus (activating event) and response (consequences) determines how effectively a person deals with stress. Thought patterns, attitudes, and world view can either help a person remain calm and joyful or create a life filled with anxiety and tension. In this section we'll quickly explore four thought patterns that can destroy serenity and one that can restore it.

Just a handful of beliefs can chain you to the dungeon of distress. Dr. Burns, psychologist and author of the best-selling book *Feeling Good*, identifies several of what he calls common forms of "distorted thinking" (Burns, 1989). Here are some of his examples:

1. **All-or-nothing thinking:** Looking at things in absolute, black-and-white categories.

2. **Mental filtering:** Dwelling on the negatives and ignoring the positives.

3. **Emotional reasoning:** Reasoning from how you feel. "I feel lousy, therefore things are lousy."

4. **Labeling:** Identifying with your shortcomings. Instead of saying "I made a mistake," you tell yourself, "I'm a jerk, a fool, a loser."

You may find this list uncomfortably familiar. It describes self-destructive thinking that typically results in inner turmoil and tension-filled relationships. The good news is that it's possible to change thought patterns. Psychologists call this **cognitive restructuring, or reframing.** Sometimes it takes a little creativity to reframe a stressful event but it can be done, as the following story illustrates:

After being away from her parents for almost three months with no communication, Julie, a college freshman, sent a letter home. In her letter she described that a fire burned down her dorm during the second week of school. She was hospitalized with minor burns, but nothing too serious. Because of the fire she was forced to relocate off campus where she met her new boyfriend. He had dropped out of college the previous year but had found work at a local convenience store. Unfortunately, she found out two days ago that she is pregnant. Julie signed the letter and included a postscript to "see other side." On the back side of the letter she said that nothing on the other side was true, but she was failing Biology 231. (Cialdini, 2000)

Now that's reframing! But is cognitive reconditioning just being thankful that, even though something didn't go as planned, the results weren't as bad as they could have been? That sounds like just another version of positive thinking, where you try to look on the bright side. Reframing really does mean something different for a disciple of Christ. Jesus said, ". . .the truth will set you free" (John 8:32). Scripture is filled with biblical examples that help combat common distortions. A few are listed here:

1. **All-or-nothing thinking:** Scripture teaches that although people were created in the image of God, they possess a nature that opposes him. Even after someone makes a definite choice to submit to Christ, a paradoxical state of holy and unholy intentions and behavior exists. The apostle Paul describes this struggle in Romans 7:21–25. People

are a mixed bag, wanting to do what's right but often falling short.

2. **Mental filtering:** It would have been hard not to laugh along with Abraham and Sarah at God's promise to give them a child (Genesis 17:17, 18:12). Sarah was well past childbearing years and Abraham was about to reach the century mark. Yet despite the impossibility of their circumstances, scripture records that Abraham believed God and eventually received the son he was promised.

3. **Emotional reasoning:** Imagine you are in a small boat in the middle of the night. Waves from a raging storm are swamping your tiny vessel. The boat is beginning to sink. You have no life vest, and if the ship goes down you most assuredly will drown. After bailing water with all your might, you realize your best efforts are fruitless; the boat is sinking. Can you relate to the disciples' emotional outcry, "Don't you care if we drown?" to their sleeping leader who led them into the eye of the storm (Mark 4:35–40)? Jesus got up and rebuked the wind and his followers for their emotional, rather than spiritual, reasoning.

4. **Labeling:** John the Baptist is locked in a prison cell waiting—waiting until Herod will eventually have his head on a platter. John begins to question if Jesus really is the true Messiah. Plagued by his doubts, he finally asks one of his followers to go ask Jesus if he really is who he says he is. Jesus' response is amazing. First he tells John's messenger of the works he is doing, then he says, "I tell you, among those born of women there is no one greater than John" (Luke 7:28a). If you wonder if Jesus labels his children as doubters and disbelievers when they honestly question the truth, he doesn't.

These examples are just a sampling of how thinking from a broader worldview can significantly alter the impact of events that one typically sees from a negative perspective.

C = Consequences

Whether the response is logical or not, the body will react almost immediately when the brain registers a potential threat. Walter Cannon, noted physiologist at Harvard Medical School, was the first to use the term *fight-or-flight response* for the physiological changes that occur when danger is perceived (Cannon, 1932). Researchers have learned much about how the body responds to stressors since Cannon's original observations.

Now we know the nervous system activates the endocrine system to release a number of stress-related hormones. Some of the more notable ones are cortisol, epinephrine, and nonepinephrine. These hormones are responsible for the host of physiological responses to stress, some of which include the following:

- Pupils dilate to admit extra light for more sensitive vision.
- Mucous membranes of the nose and throat shrink, while muscles force a wider opening of passages to allow easier airflow.
- Secretion of saliva and mucous decreases, intestinal muscles stop contracting, and digestion is halted.
- Bronchi dilate to allow more air into lungs.
- The liver releases sugar into the bloodstream to provide energy from muscles and the brain.
- The bladder relaxes. Emptying the bladder contents reduces excess weight, making it easier to flee.
- Endorphins are released to block distracting pain.
- Hearing becomes more acute.
- Heart rate and stroke volume increase blood flow.
- The spleen releases more red blood cells to meet an increasing demand for oxygen and to replace any blood loss from injuries.

As uncomfortable and strange as these symptoms may seem, they are essential for survival. Without them we would be ill prepared for life-threatening emergencies. The problem is that we often mistake annoyances and frustrations for major emergencies.

Pros and Cons of Stress

Is stress good or bad? The answer is complex. First, we must point out that stress is one of the biggest contributors to a broader phenomenon, **arousal**. Arousal simply means a state of physiological and emotional activation (Weinberg & Gould, 2003). Because stress is highly related to arousal, it's possible to make some cautious inferences to stress by examining the literature pertaining to arousal.

Drive Theory

One of the first relevant discoveries related to arousal was that it has a positive impact on performance: The greater the arousal, the greater the performance. Originally, scientists thought that the relationship was linear. This was known as the **drive theory** and is illustrated in figure 9.3 (Hill, 1957; Spence & Spence, 1996).

Inverted-U Theory

Later studies clearly demonstrated that the relationship between arousal and performance was *not* always a linear relationship. Two researchers, Yerkes & Dodson (1908), reported that arousal does enhance performance but only up to a certain level. There is a point at which continual increases in arousal decreases, rather than increases, performance. They illustrated this theory in what is commonly referred to at the **inverted-U theory** of arousal. As you can see in figure 9.4, low to moderate levels of stress enhance performance, but extremely high levels of arousal decrease performance.

Individual Zones of Optimal Functioning

More recently, another model concerning arousal and performance has received consid-erable attention. It is called the **individualized zones of optimal functioning (IZOF)**. Yuri Hanin, a noted Russian psychologist, suggested that people have a zone of optimal arousal, rather than a specific point of optimal arousal as presented in the inverted-U model (Hanin et al., 1986). Hanin also argued that the optimal level of arousal doesn't always occur at the midpoint of the continuum but instead varies from individual to individual. That is, some individuals have a zone of optimal functioning at the lower end of the continuum, some in the midrange, and others at the upper end. Figure 9.5 illustrates this hypothesis, which has since been supported by other investigators (Gould & Tuffey, 1996).

These models don't tell the whole story, though, because they only deal with the effects of arousal over a very short period of time. What happens when you are chronically aroused? Consider some modern examples: You're frustrated at your inability to avoid procrastination, distressed over a relational conflict that seems impossible to resolve, or discouraged because you continually fall short of living a life pleasing to God. Imagine what it would be like to live with issues such as these for weeks, months, or even years. Persistent stress can become debilitating.

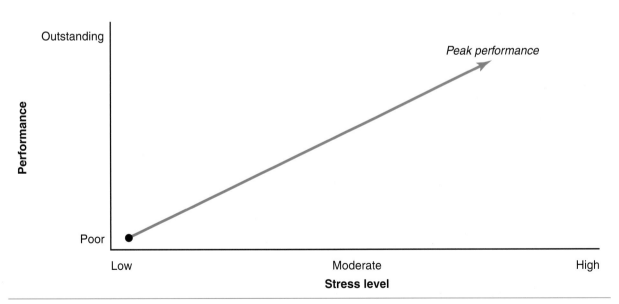

FIGURE 9.3 The relationship between performance and stress level according to the drive theory.

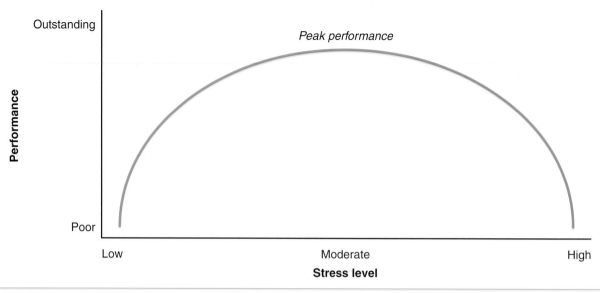

FIGURE 9.4   The inverted-U model of the relationship between performance and stress level.

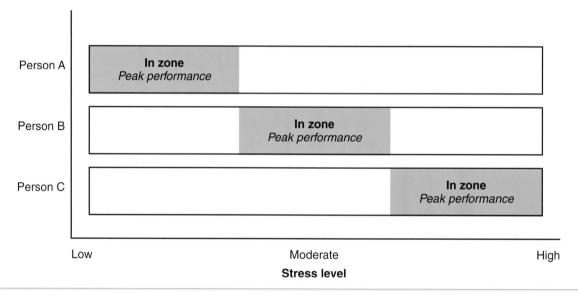

FIGURE 9.5   The individualized zones of optimal functioning theory of the relationship between performance and stress level.

Based on D. Gould and S. Tuffey, 1996, Zones of optimal functioning research, *Anxiety, Stress, and Coping, 9:* 53-68.

When Stress Turns Ugly

Hans Selye, whom we introduced at the beginning of the chapter, proposed a three-stage model describing how people deal with chronic stress (see figure 9.6). This model is called the **general adaptation syndrome (GAS).**

1. The first stage is the alarm reaction, the fight-or-flight response we described earlier. Here homeostasis, or a state of equilibrium, is disrupted.

2. In the second resistance stage, the body seeks to self-correct, drawing on available resources to restore equilibrium.

3. Exhaustion, the final stage, occurs if equilibrium can't be regained.

Unrelieved or unmanaged stress eventually destroys a person. Dr. Fred Goodwin of the National Institute of Mental Health says that humans have a fairly robust capacity to withstand even massive doses of acute stress. The downfall is the inability to mobilize for recurrent stressful episodes (Greenberg, 2002). Legendary U.S. World War II General George Patton stated Goodwin's conclusions more succinctly: "Fatigue makes cowards of us all" (Miner & Rawson, 1997, p. 189). The most challenging life experiences are those stressful situations that are not quickly resolved. Parenting a child with a severe birth defect, caring for a friend who has mental illness, or loving an aged spouse who has Alzheimer's disease are examples of the challenges that require

deep inner strength. Those challenges slowly erode even the best intentions.

So we ask again: Is stress good or bad? The simple answer is that stress can be helpful up to a point; but if it's too intense or if it's too prolonged, trouble can occur. Therefore, it's a good idea to have some strategies and techniques that can help us manage stress even during the most troubling times.

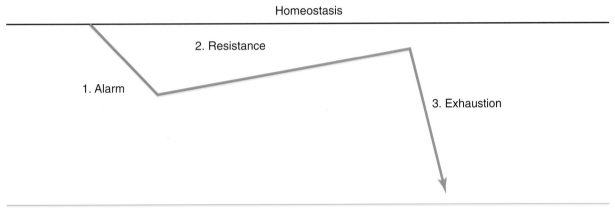

Homeostasis

1. Alarm

2. Resistance

3. Exhaustion

FIGURE 9.6 Sustained stress eventually results in exhaustion.

Is There Such a Thing as "Righteous Worry"?

The disciples of Jesus knew that worry was not Jesus' way. During one hillside chat, Christ told his followers,

> Do not worry about your life, what you will eat or drink; or about your body, what you will wear. Is not life more important than food, and the body more important than clothes? Look at the birds of the air; they do not sow or reap or store away in barns, and yet your heavenly Father feeds them. Are you not much more valuable than they? Who of you by worrying can add a single hour to his life? (Matthew 6:25–27)

He repeats this admonition as he foresees a time in which his followers will be rejected by their communities, disowned by family, and arrested for being a follower of "the way":

> Whenever you are arrested and brought to trial, do not worry beforehand about what to say. Just say whatever is given you at the time, for it is not you speaking, but the Holy Spirit. (Mark 13:11)

Not only did Jesus warn against worry, he exemplified the antithesis of worry during crisis. The boat he and his disciples were in was sinking, and he was sound asleep (Matthew 8:23–25). An angry mob was ready to stone a woman to death, and Jesus calmly wrote in the sand, dispersing the crowd (John 8:1–11). Before a Roman judge who claimed to have the power to crucify or release Jesus, Christ calmly refused to reply to accusations or questions (Mark 15:3–5).

Clearly, Jesus had enormous inner peace during times of testing. On the other hand,

(continued)

(continued)

some events and circumstances seemed to weigh heavily on his heart. Perhaps the most dramatic example came right before his trial: While praying on the Mount of Olives, he "sweat as if it were great drops of blood" (Luke 22:44).

In addition to stories of Jesus, scripture records how the apostle Paul seemed frequently concerned and at other times anxious. In a lengthy record of his specific difficulties, Paul concludes by acknowledging his daily pressure:

> I have worked much harder, been in prison more frequently, been flogged more severely, and been exposed to death again and again. Five times I received from the Jews the forty lashes minus one. Three times I was beaten with rods, once I was stoned, three times I was shipwrecked, I spent a night and a day in the open sea, I have been constantly on the move. I have been in danger from rivers, in danger from bandits, in danger from my own countrymen, in danger from Gentiles; in danger in the city, in danger in the country, in danger at sea; and in danger from false brothers. I have labored and toiled and have often gone without sleep; I have known hunger and thirst and have often gone without food; I have been cold and naked. Besides everything else, I face daily the pressure of my concern for all the churches. (2 Corinthians 11:23–28)

In Paul's letter to the Church at Philippi, he foresees that his anxiety will be alleviated by the safe return of Epaphroditus:

> But I think it is necessary to send back to you Epaphroditus, my brother, fellow worker and fellow soldier, who is also your messenger, whom you sent to take care of my needs. For he longs for all of you and is distressed because you heard he was ill. Indeed he was ill, and almost died. But God had mercy on him, and not on him only but also on me, to spare me sorrow upon sorrow. Therefore I am all the more eager to send him, so that when you see him again you may be glad and I may have less anxiety. (Philippians 2:25–28)

What is your reaction? I can almost hear your reply: "It's OK to be concerned, but not worried." One of the problems with that response is that, according to Merriam-Webster Dictionary, one of the definitions of worry is "to feel or experience concern" (Merriam-Webster, 2007). What, then, is your distinction between being worried and concerned? Here are some other questions to consider as you grapple with this issue:

When does concern transfer into worry?

Is it ever appropriate to worry?

What does worry say about my faith in God and my concern for his agenda?

Managing Stress

Various studies in Canada have highlighted the enormous cost of managing stress.

- According to the Canadian Mental Health Association, about 20 percent of the average company's payroll goes toward dealing with stress-related problems, such as absenteeism, employee turnover, disability leaves, counseling, medicine, and accidents (Canadian Mental Health Association, 2006).

- Health Canada reported that "work–life conflict"—stress that arises when work and family clash—costs Canadian business $4.5 billion to $10 billion a year (Health Canada, 2006).

- Mental health problems—stress, depression and addiction—are a $33-billion-a-year drain on Canada's economy, according to the corporate-sponsored Global Business and Economic Roundtable on Addiction and Mental Health (Riga, 2006).

Given the high cost of treating individuals living in the exhaustion phase of Selye's model, people's learning effective stress management techniques would not only increase serenity but save money. Here is an abbreviated list of some of the low-cost, more popular, stress management methods:

• **Deep breathing.** Take a deep breath, inhaling through your nose. Hold the air you have inhaled for five to seven seconds before slowly exhaling. As you release your breath, focus not only on exhaling all your air but also on releasing muscle tension. Repeat three or four times. It is amazing how something this simple can have a dramatic effect on acute levels of stress. Musicians and athletes have used this technique for years to quiet their nerves before a concert or sporting event.

• **Refocus.** Continuing to brood over unpleasant, uncontrollable situations only increases your anxiety. Refocusing your mind on "whatever is true, whatever is noble, whatever is right, whatever is pure, whatever is lovely, whatever is admirable" (Philippians 4:8) is a pathway out of the dark valleys of the mind. Refocusing your thoughts sounds easier than it actually is, but a change of mind can liberate you from the chains of anxiety, fear, doubt,

and discouragement. See the box titled "The Power of Refocusing" on this page.

Reality Checks

Everyone can benefit from an occasional reality check. When you need one, ask yourself the following questions:

- How important will this current situation be a year from now?
- On a scale of 1 to 10, 10 being a worldwide catastrophe, where would I rate my problem?
- What difference will this make when I am standing before God in heaven?

Viewing your crisis from a larger perspective has a way of diminishing its effect.

The Power of Refocusing

Tom had been dating Emily for two years. During that time his love for and commitment to her had grown to a point that he was convinced she was "the one." Tom had tried hard to follow God's will in the manner in which he related to Emily socially, physically, and spiritually. One day, though, Emily sheepishly told Tom she didn't have peace about their relationship. She quickly added that it wasn't anything that Tom had done; it was simply an unsettled feeling she couldn't shake. After another week, she told Tom she couldn't see him anymore. Tom was floored. In his words, "it was like a divorce."

Tom was consumed with questions:
What could I have done differently?
What's wrong with me?
How did I miss God's leading?
What is the future of this relationship?

From the moment he got up in the morning until he went to bed at night, Tom couldn't think about anything other than his broken relationship with Emily. He continued to attend class, but he merely occupied a seat because his mind was on his pain. Two weeks passed and assignments and papers were beginning to pile up. Because he was so hurt, all Tom's conversations were about Emily. About three weeks after the breakup, one of Tom's friends bluntly said, "You've got to get on with your life. You can't change your circumstances, but you can change your reaction." That was the moment the light began to dawn. Although it was hard, Tom began trying to replace thoughts of Emily with scripture, schoolwork, and other social relationships. Looking back on this event, Tom acknowledged, "The power of taking responsibility for your thoughts is the path of deliverance."

• **Exercise.** When you think about it, exercise actually increases physical stress (at least temporarily). Yet, after the body responds to the initial increase in heart rate, blood pressure, and energy expenditure, the floodgates of stress fly open. Exercise pulls the plug on stress. Researchers have discovered that even mild forms of exercise substantially reduce an individual's stress level. Ornstein and Sobel (1989) reported that walking one mile at a moderate pace significantly lowered subjects' anxiety levels. The cathartic effect of exercise has a long and robust history, both in the United States and internationally. A nursing faculty at a university in Thailand reported that regular exercise cuts in half the levels of stress that 102 Thai women reported prior to engaging in a regular exercise routine (Sunsern, 2002).

• **Prayer.** Prayer is the most commonly used form of complementary and alternative medicine in the world (Hales, 2007). However, only in recent years has science launched rigorous investigations of the effect that prayer has on health outcomes.

Praying directly to a higher power affects both the quality and quantity of life, claims Dr. Harold Koenig, director of Duke University's Center for the Study of Religion/Spirituality and Health. It boosts morale; lowers agitation, loneliness, and life dissatisfaction; and enhances ability to cope in men, women, the elderly, the young, the healthy, and the sick (Koenig, 2007). Furthermore, Koenig found that in one study almost half of the patients cited religion (and often prayer, as an expression of religion) as the most significant factor in helping them cope with the stress associated with illness (Koenig, Kvale, & Ferrel, 1988).

In a national survey, 35 percent of Americans prayed for health concerns. Of that 35 percent, 75 percent were praying for personal wellness and 22 percent were praying for alleviation of specific medical conditions. Among those who prayed because of a medical condition, 69 percent found prayer very helpful (McCaffrey, 2004).

• **Humor.** Dr. Richard Blonna, Professor of Community Health at William Paterson University says, "It is physiologically impossible to be stressed when you are laughing. Laughter creates a physiological state that is incompatible with stress" (Blonna, 2005, p. 166). Mounting evidence from the scientific community confirms Solomon was right when he said "a cheerful heart is good medicine" (Proverbs 17:22). For more than two

decades Norman Cousins, editor of the *Saturday Review of Literature*, wrote about how humor not only helped him fight off life-threatening illness but helped hundreds of others as well. Professor Keith Karren and colleagues argue in their book *Mind/Body Health* that, similar to the "runner's high" caused by a release in endorphins by running, a "laughter high" likewise exists (Karren, Hafen, & Smith, 2002). Three of the most important humor skills are to

• see the absurdity in difficult situations,
• take yourself lightly while taking your work seriously, and
• have a disciplined sense of joy (Metcalf & Felible, 1992).

Becoming Stress Hardy: Serious Stress Management

Everyone wants to be an overcomer, but they'd prefer not to encounter obstacles along the way. Instead of trying to limit and manage stressful situations, maybe it would be beneficial to spend some time discovering how to increase the capacity to withstand and even thrive in stressful situations. To borrow from agriculture, how can a person become more **stress hardy**? Used of plants, *hardy* means capable of surviving unfavorable conditions. Used of people, stress hardy means capable of keeping cool under pressure (Kobasa, 1979).

During the late 1970s and early 1980s, United States federal deregulation caused a great upheaval in the telecommunications industry, and thousands of people lost their jobs. Dr. Susan Kobasa from the University of Chicago was studying managerial and employee behavior at AT&T during this time. She reported that most employees acted like hunted animals, frantically trying any means they could think of—company politics, verbal harassment, threats of litigation, and so on—to avoid getting laid off. A few, however, remained calm and optimistic. They kept their job performance consistent and even encouraged and organized focus groups with their colleagues to brainstorm for positive solutions. Kobasa coined the term *stress hardy* to describe the latter group of employees.

Even more incredible and heroic examples of stress hardiness come from people who have been persecuted for their faith. In 168 AD, the Roman authorities arrested the well-known bishop Polycarp of Smyrna, who had studied under the apostle John:

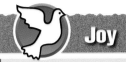

I climbed a mountain and the view from the top was gorgeous. I finished an exhilarating game of squash. I finished a lengthy cycle ride. These were victories of health, friendship, and personal goals. God again blessed me!

True joy is a gift (Psalm 4:7). **Joy** is the ability to respond to God's triumphs: seeing, feeling, and expressing celebration in God's victories. It is a response often shared in a festive manner with others. It is not a simple add-on in the Christian life but is listed significantly as the second fruit of the spirit. Does experiencing joy have that kind of priority in your life?

Joy is a response to the awesomeness of God's having revealed himself and offering salvation (Isaiah 9:3; 12:2–3; Matthew 13:44; 1 Thessalonians 1:6). This life-changing event causes "rejoicing in heaven" (Luke 15:7, 10) and should transform mourning into dancing (Psalm 30:11; Jeremiah 31:13). Do you realize how great a gift salvation is? Is that joy evident in your life experience?

Jesus brought joy to the world before his birth (Luke 1:44) and after he rose from the dead (Matthew 28:8). Jesus' followers lived in "joy and amazement" (Luke 24:40–41) and worshipped him with great joy (Luke 24:52–53). They recognized his victories and allowed joy to overtake them.

Joy is also a response to God's blessing. When the Israelites returned from captivity they were filled with gladness. The psalmist wrote that the Israelites were "like men who dreamed. Our mouths were filled with laughter, our tongues with songs of joy" (Psalm 126:1–2). Those people were so happy they were drunk with laughter! Proverbs reminds us that "a happy heart makes the face cheerful" (Proverbs 15:13; see also Proverbs 10:28; 12:20; 15:13) and a cheerful heart is "good medicine" (17:22) and "has a continual feast" (15:15). Can you allow gladness and joy to overtake you (Isaiah 35:10; 51:3,11; 52:8)? Remember how David danced for joy when the ark returned, and how his wife, Michal, remained barren because she was a kill-joy (2 Samuel 6:17–23)?

For those too crushed by circumstances to experience joy, think of David. In his confession about the sin with Bathsheba, he asked God, "Let me hear joy and gladness; let the bones you have crushed rejoice. . . . Restore to me the joy of your salvation" (Psalm 51:8, 12). David was also able to confess that God's "consolation brought joy to my soul" (Psalm 94:19). Isaiah later asked God: "Strengthen the feeble hands, steady the knees that give way; say to those with fearful hearts, 'Be strong, do not fear. . . .' Then will the lame leap like a deer, and the mute tongue shout for joy" (Isaiah 35:3–4, 6; see also Romans 15:13; Acts 8:8). God will provide victory and joy even in the painful times of life.

Paul says, "Rejoice in the Lord always, I will say it again: Rejoice" (Philippians 4:4)! Sometimes people need to be told to rejoice as a reminder to get off the track of "Go, go, go! Produce, produce, produce!" Then they can openly receive the gift of joy and celebrate God's triumphs.

Count God's blessings to you and give thanks for each of them. Take a moment to relax and enjoy God's goodness to you. Can you feel the healing? Do you remember how good it felt to receive a genuine smile, to give one, and to laugh your head off with friends? The Holy Spirit offers joy to those who open their hearts to him.

Joy: Take some time and write out the blessings and victories God has given in your life (from your learning to ride a bike to God's claiming you as his child). Sit back and chuckle and experience God's joy.

_____

_____

_____

_____

_____

"Swear by Caesar," demanded the hostile Roman proconsul. "Take the oath and I will release you. Curse Christ!" The bishop stood firm. "Eighty-six years have I served the Lord Jesus Christ, and He has never once wronged me," he said. "How can I blaspheme the King who has saved me?"

"I have wild beasts ready to tear you to pieces if you do not change your mind," said the proconsul. "Let them come, for my purpose is unchangeable," the old man replied. Unmoved by any threats, and unwilling to renounce his Savior, Polycarp was sentenced to be burned alive. As the Roman guards were about to nail him to the stake, he told them, "Leave me as I am. He who gives me the strength to endure the fire will enable me to remain still within it." Dumbfounded, the guards agreed and simply tied his hands with a rope. And as the flames consumed his flesh, only the bishop's lips moved. They were uttering praise to God. (DC Talk, 1999, p. 136)

The type of hardiness described in that story is something every follower of Christ wants. But how do we get it? Kobasa reported that there are three particular traits characteristic of stress hardy individuals: commitment, control, and challenge (Kobasa, 1979). These variables have deep spiritual roots.

Commitment

What is the most stressful situation you can imagine? How about having everything you own taken away, being separated from your family, and being imprisoned in a concentration camp? That's what happened to Victor Frankl, an Austrian psychiatrist imprisoned in a Nazi concentration camp during World War II (Frankl, 1984). The Germans made the existence of the prisoners as unbearable as possible: too little food, rags for clothing, beds full of lice, and continuous forced labor. One of Frankl's primary observations during this bleak experience involved human perseverance under pressure. He noticed how some prisoners just gave up. They experienced what he called "passive death," by surrendering their will to live. In stark contrast, some of the prisoners refused to be broken. Instead of giving up, they fought to survive.

The primary characteristic between the two groups, Frankl noted, was having a reason to live. Prisoners who survived this living hell had something left to do with their lives; there was a commitment that they wanted to fulfill. They felt a need to see their families one more time, to say "I love you" to a spouse, or to exact revenge on those who mistreated them. In short, prisoners who had a well-defined purpose survived. After being freed from prison, Frankl wrote the book, aptly titled *Man's Search for Meaning*, in which he stated, "Nothing is more likely to help a person overcome or endure troubles than the consciousness of having a task in life" (Frankl, 1984, p. 28).

Since then, Frankl's observations have been verified further. Oncology researchers reported that having a commitment to overcome can dramatically affect an individual's survival rate from cancer. In a longitudinal study published in the prestigious journal *Lancet*, researchers divided 57 women who were diagnosed with early breast cancer into one of three categories according to how the patients approached their illness: "stoic accepter," "hopeless/helpless," and a "fighting spirit." After 10 years, 25 percent of the stoic accepters were alive, 20 percent of the hopeless/helpless patients were alive, and 70 percent of the people in the fighting spirit group were alive (Pettingale et al., 1985)!

Control

People in control aren't objects acted on; instead, they act. Having control is being in charge of one's decisions and life. Perhaps one of the most common emotions students verbalize is being overwhelmed or out of control. The last century has seen unprecedented change. Those changes have dramatically affected day-to-day lifestyles. young women living 100 years ago in colonial America may have had one primary task to complete on a given day, like to do the laundry. Today, students read assignments, catch up with friends, answer the phone, watch TV, and gulp down a meal in 20 minutes or less.

We live in a new world. Some commercials present modern couples relaxing by the pool and sipping a drink while modern technological conveniences do all the work. In reality many of these devices make it possible to transport work virtually anywhere, and people are never out of contact with those who want to reach them. Perhaps a more accurate image of modern conveniences would be a ball and chain.

Effective time management can provide a sense of calm and control because it increases productivity. Productivity for students usually results in increased grade point averages. In one study that examined several predictors of college academic success, researchers discovered that the most consistent and powerful forecaster of college academic achievement was not high school grades or even SAT (Scholastic Aptitude Test) scores, but rather time-management practices (Crespian & Becker, 1999). The primary investigators of this study subdivided a college student's time-management strategies into three categories according to how well each predicted academic success:

1. **Daily planning.** The most effective strategies were to make a daily to-do list, to establish a clear idea of what to accomplish each day.

2. **Attitude toward time.** The second category to predict success was a student's attitudes toward time, which included feeling in charge of his or her own time, not worrying about lack of time, and a general awareness of time.

3. **Long-range planning.** The final category was long-range planning, which included setting semester or term objectives and planning ahead.

Isn't it interesting that creating a daily to-do list, a common strategy, ranked among the highest predictors of academic success? If you don't have a daily to-do list already, start one today; it may just help you ace this class. You can find help for putting together an effective to-do list in the Application Activities section at the end of this chapter.

T. S. Eliot said, "Learning to live a simple life is one of life's supreme complexities" (Draper, 1992). This section on time management is far from being exhaustive and is meant only to be a primer to get you thinking about how to make better use of your time. If you're looking for some additional suggestions, pick up Elaine St. James' thoughtful little book titled *Simplify Your Life: 100 Ways To Slow Down And Enjoy the Things That Really Matter* (1994). It's a quick and easy read that is loaded with recommendations.

Challenge

The third attribute associated with hardiness is challenge. Kobasa defined challenge as how people perceive a change. Hardy individuals view change as an inevitable part of life and recognize the need for flexibility to meet the demands of an ever-changing world. Less hardy individuals see change as threatening, destructive, and, in some cases, evil. They are comfortable with the status quo, how things have always been, and "the way it's done around here." They fight against even minor, inconsequential changes with the tenacity of a world-class boxer.

The book *Who Moved My Cheese?*, by Spencer Johnson, speaks poignantly about how to either benefit or suffer from attitudes about change (Johnson, 1993). Since its first printing in 1998, *Who Moved My Cheese?* remained on the *New York Times'* business bestseller list for a remarkable five years (*New York Times* Business, 2003). For more than 200 weeks it was on the *Publishers Weekly* hardcover bestsellers list (Publishers Weekly, 2004). What is so remarkable about this book? Its allegorical tale describes two mice, Sniff and Scurry, and two little people, Hem and Haw, living in a maze, which represents life. "The cheese" in this story is meant to be a metaphor for how businesses, organizations and families achieve success. In order to thrive, continual change and adaptation must occur. On the other hand, stagnation and refusing to change will only end in extinction. Some sobering words to consider. The bottom line messages of this book are outlined as follows (Johnson, 1993, p. 74):

- Change Happens: They Keep Moving the Cheese.
- Anticipate Change: Get Ready For the Cheese to Move.
- Monitor Change: Smell the Cheese Often So You Know When It Is Getting Old.
- Adapt to Change Quickly: The Quicker You Let Go of Old Cheese, the Sooner You Can Enjoy New Cheese.
- Enjoy Change! Savor the Adventure and Enjoy the Taste of New Cheese!

Depression

Everyone experiences sadness at times, but some people have something far more serious: **clinical depression**—long periods of despondency that cripple them physically, cognitively, socially, and spiritually. **Depression** is a mental illness, not a character flaw or a sign of weakness. The National Institute of Mental Health estimates that approximately 19 million Americans endure depression each year (National Institute of Mental Health, 2006). Of those, a growing number are college

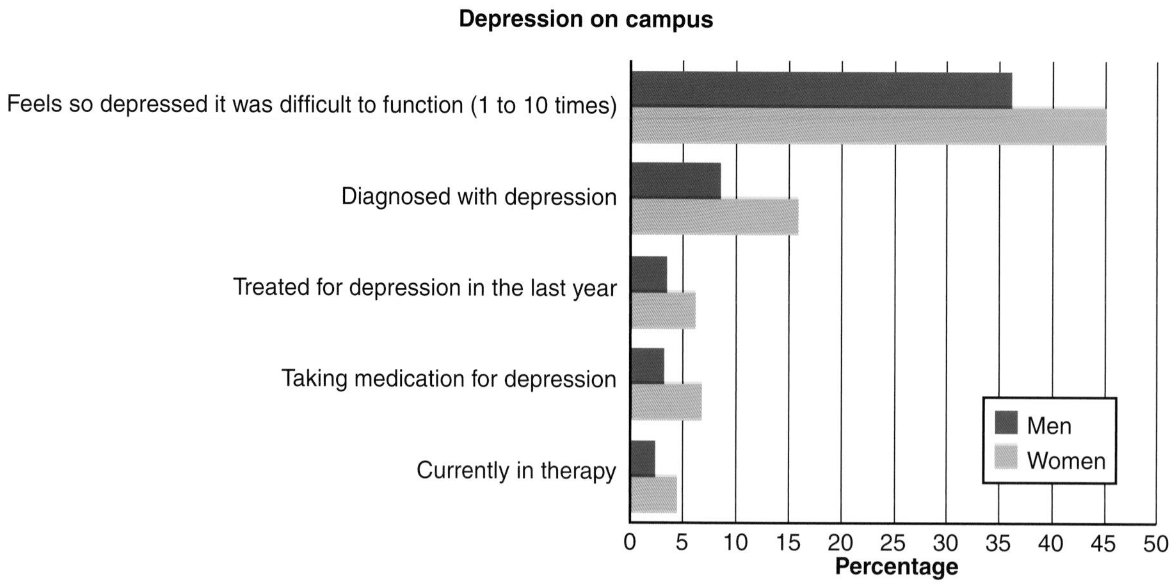

Depression on campus

FIGURE 9.7   Results from American College Health Association-National College Health Assessment (ACHA-NCHA) Web Summary. Updated April 2006. Available at www.acha-ncha.org/data_highlights.html.

students (see figure 9.7) (American College Health Association, 2006).

Symptoms

According to the American Psychiatric Association (2000), a person is clinically depressed if he or she exhibits one of the following symptoms for at least two weeks:

1. Sadness or hopelessness
2. A loss of interest in activities that were once enjoyed

In addition, four or more of these symptoms must be present:

1. A change in appetite that causes weight gain or weight loss
2. Too much sleep or not enough sleep
3. Restlessness and an inability to sit still or the feeling that moving takes too much effort
4. Persistent fatigue
5. Feelings of unworthiness or guilt without any reason
6. Significant problems with memory, concentration, or decision making
7. Frequent thoughts about death or suicide

Bad moods ordinarily disappear after a day or two, and normal grief after a loved one dies may last for more than a year. These usually do not *significantly* interfere with day-to-day activities. Clinical depression, however, impairs spiritual life, social life, and academic and vocational life. Young people with this condition see their grades drop, neglect their duties and obligations, and become isolated (Birmaher et al., 1996). Depressed teenagers are more likely than depressed children to have trouble eating and sleeping and to entertain suicidal thoughts, and more likely than depressed adults to be irritable (American Academy of Child and Adolescent Psychiatry, 1998).

The trajectory and the severity of depression vary from person to person. Sometimes mild symptoms last for a long time without going away, and at other times severe symptoms last for a short time but recur. The condition often returns, and people who have one episode of depression are more likely to have another.

Causes

Most experts believe that depression results from a combination of biological, psychological, and social factors, such as these:

- Sin
- Genetics

- Chemical imbalances
- Stress or trauma
- Inadequate social support
- Negative and irrational thoughts

Sin

Although you won't find this acknowledged in secular sources, all human suffering, including depression and other forms of mental illness, exists because of sin. Not all suffering, however, exists because of the sin of the sufferer.

> As he went along, [Jesus] saw a man blind from birth. His disciples asked him, "Rabbi, who sinned, this man or his parents, that he was born blind?"

> "Neither this man nor his parents sinned," said Jesus, "but this happened so that the work of God might be displayed in his life." (John 9: 1–3).

It's true that sinful attitudes and sinful choices can result in depression, but don't automatically conclude that a depressed person is to blame for his or her condition. Respond instead with compassion and understanding. If diseases that afflict the body are a result of the general distortion of God's creation by the fall, then so are diseases that afflict the mind. Also, many times the problem is caused by the sin of others. For example, victims of rape and sexual molestation and children of distant, divorced, or abusive parents often experience depression.

Genetics

Depression runs in families. One in fifteen (six to eight percent) of the general U.S. population will develop depression, but the rate is three times higher among people who have a parent or sibling that is clinically depressed. Keep in mind, though, that genetic factors increase the risk of, but do not cause, depression. People with a higher risk are more sensitive to potential triggers, such as the effects of negative or stressful environments (Birmaher et al., 1996).

Chemical Imbalances

The neurotransmitters relevant to depression are serotonin, norepinephrine, and dopamine (Garrett, 2003). Their exact role in depression is unclear, but many different types of imbalances in these brain chemicals are associated with depression (Kalat, 2001).

Some medications, such as those that regulate blood pressure, can cause depression. After a person stops taking the medication, the symptoms usually disappear.

Stress or Trauma

Significant life changes that cause stress can also lead to depression. Such stressors might be social, such as the death of a loved one or the end of a valued relationship, or stressors of other kinds, such as poverty or long-term illness. The more numerous the stressors a person experiences in a short time, the greater the risk of his or her becoming depressed.

Teenagers and young adults experience a lot of separation and loss. They leave home, family, and their old neighborhood to go to college. They begin and end friendships and romantic relationships. Some psychologists believe that separation and loss can lead to hostile feelings toward the lost person—for example, an ex-boyfriend or ex-girlfriend—and that this hostility, turned inward, causes depression. Feelings of loneliness, alienation, and rejection, all common during adolescence, are potential causes as well (Brage & Meredith, 1994).

Inadequate Social Support

It's a vicious cycle. People who lack the social skills to have fun times, make good friends, land top jobs, and attract the opposite sex can become disappointed, then depressed (Lewinsohn, 1974). Unfortunately, depressed people are depressing. Their irritability and pessimism cause other people to avoid them, and their increasing lack of social support can intensify their condition, particularly in women. Counselors often train these people in social skills to help break the cycle.

Negative and Irrational Thoughts

- "I'm a total failure unless I am liked by every significant person in my life."
- "It's horrible when things don't turn out the way I want them to."
- "If I'm not sure about an upcoming event, I must worry about it."
- "Unless I'm competent at everything, I'm worthless."

Brain Communication

The control center of human thinking and function is the brain. Brains are primarily made up of billions of nerve cells (or neurons). It is the ability or lack of ability of these nerve cells to communicate effectively with one another that lies at the heart of many physiological problems. Figure 9.8 provides a closer look at exactly what is occurring at the neurological level.

Like snowflakes, no two neurons are exactly the same, yet each one has a similar structure. A neuron consists of a cell body containing the nucleus; a long fiber, called the axon, which can range from less than an inch (a few centimeters) to several feet (more than a meter) in length; an axon terminal, or ending; and multiple branching fibers called dendrites. For communication to occur between

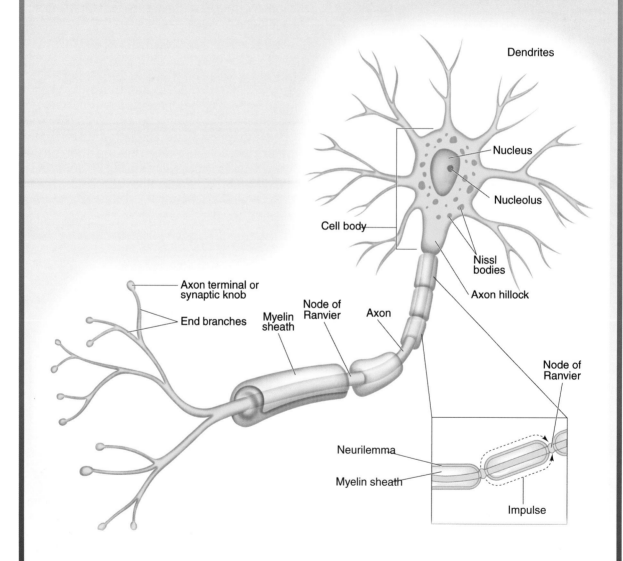

FIGURE 9.8 The anatomy of neurons.

Reprinted, by permission, from J. Wilmore and D. Costill, 2004, *Physiology of sport and exercise,* 3rd ed. (Champaign, IL: Human Kinetics), 62.

(continued)

(continued)

neurons an electrical signal travels along the axon terminal where chemical messengers called neurotransmitters are stored. These neurotransmitters flow out of the axon terminal and cross a synapse to receptors on an adjoining dendrite. Receptors are protein molecules designed to bind with neurotransmitters. Although this process sounds lengthy, it takes about 1/10,000 second for a neurotransmitter and a receptor to come together.

This process can become compromised through either a failure to excite and release neurotransmitters (sending) or in the receptors' failure to effectively take up neurotransmissions (receiving). When these neurological and chemical communications fail, abnormalities in thinking, feeling, or behaving may result. Some of the most promising and exciting research in neuropsychiatry (a subspecialty of psychiatry that deals with mental disorders attributable to diseases of the nervous system) is focusing on correcting such malfunctions. One example is the neurotransmitter serotonin. Serotonin and its receptors have been shown to affect mood, sleep, behavior, appetite, memory, learning, sexuality, and aggression; thus it plays a role in several mental disorders (Hales, 2005). Although this branch of science is relatively new, it holds promise to thousands of people who have neurological and chemical imbalances.

Irrational, pessimistic, and self-defeating thoughts like these can cause depression and keep it going once it starts. Depression makes people likely to think negatively about themselves ("I am unattractive and unlovable"), their world ("Nobody cares about me") and their future ("I'll never find a spouse or a job, and I'll never be happy") (Beck, 1970; Sacco & Beck, 1995). Depressed people will assume the worst possible outcome in any situation (catastrophizing), assume that because one event turned out badly others will too (overgeneralizing), and believe that they are to blame for anything bad that happens around them, even when they aren't responsible (personalizing) (Beck, 1967). They think, irrationally, that they can do nothing to improve a bad situation, so they shouldn't even bother trying. This attitude is called *learned helplessness* (Seligman, 1974).

When you receive a low grade on a test, do you attribute it to your own stupidity, to insufficient study time, to an incompetent teacher, to unfair test questions, or to something else? What determines your response, other than the simple facts of the matter, is **attribution**, or the meaning we ascribe to the events and circumstances that occur in our lives (McFarland & Miller, 1994). A person prone to depression will tend to attribute a poor grade to his own ineptitude and believe that he will continue to fail for a long time and in many other areas. A person not prone to depression might take a more optimistic view of the event and consider it an isolated incident, the result of a bad day (Abramson, Seligman, & Teasdale, 1978; Jacobson et al., 1996). Events themselves are not depressing; what is important is how you handle them. Perfectionism, the habit of tying your self-worth to unachievable goals, can easily make you depressed.

Where do such thoughts come from? Some sources might includes examples set by parents and other authority figures, early-in-life experiences of rejection, and a lack of understanding of God's truth.

Treatment

Only 30 percent of clinically depressed people seek professional help. The rest are either too embarrassed to go to "a shrink" or think that the symptoms will disappear on their own. Sometimes the symptoms do go away. If you have them for more than two weeks, however, it's best to seek professional help. Even if your condition is mild, without treatment you run the risk of sinking into a deeper state. Other people's efforts to cheer you up can improve a bad mood, but they can't cure clinical depression. The sooner you get help, the better your chances for a quick and complete recovery. If you are having suicidal thoughts, seek *immediate* professional help. Most colleges have staff members who are trained to deal with these issues.

The goals of any treatment program for depression are

- to improve your mood;
- to improve your ability to function normally at home, at school, and at work;
- to improve your overall quality of life; and
- to prevent a relapse.

Before you undergo a treatment program, have your symptoms evaluated by a professional to make sure they are genuinely the result of clinical depression, not just a bad mood, grief, or another condition. The most effective therapy combines medication and counseling, though either one alone can sometimes be enough. Psychiatrists and physicians can prescribe medication; psychiatrists, clinical psychologists, licensed professional counselors, and social workers can perform counseling. Christians may feel most comfortable with Christian counselors who incorporate scripture and prayer into the process.

Medication

Antidepressants are designed to correct imbalances in the neurotransmitters implicated in depression (Geddes & Butler, 2002). They restore functioning to predepression levels; they do not alter your personality. The newer ones, such as Prozac, Paxil, and Celexa, work for most adults. Though they are equally effective, their side effects vary widely (Geddes & Butler, 2002), so discuss with a professional which one is best for you. Don't start or stop taking medication without supervision, because the consequences may be very unpleasant.

Medications that decrease psychiatric symptoms have brought relief to millions of people. About half of all Americans will take a psychiatric drug at some point in their lives (Hales, 2007). This statistic includes people suffering from depression, anxiety, sleeping difficulties, eating disorders, alcohol or drug dependence, impaired memory, or other disorders that disrupts the intricate chemistry of the brain. Psychiatric drugs are now among the most widely prescribed drugs in the United States (Hales, 2007).

The vast majority of antidepressants are designed to correct chemical imbalances in the body (Geddes & Butler, 2002). A new generation of more precise and effective psychiatric drugs has increased the success rate of treating mental disorders significantly. How significantly? About 70 percent of people treated with antidepressants report feeling better within 6 to 10 weeks (Hales, 2007).

Although pharmacological advances have been made, it is important to keep in mind that every individual is unique and that pharmacology is not an exact science. Therefore, it may take several trials to determine the appropriate drug and dosage to treat a specific person's depression. Furthermore, humans are in a constant state of change. This means that any pharmaceutical drug needs to be monitored and in many cases adjusted to meet the ever-changing biology of the body.

Counseling

The most effective form of counseling for depression, with a success of rate of 65 to 85 percent, is called **cognitive-behavioral therapy** (Marcotte, 1997; Clarke et al., 2003; Cuijpers, 1998). Based on the theory that irrational or pessimistic thoughts and actions cause and subsequently intensify depression, it aims to replace those bad habits with good ones. For instance, instead of saying to himself, "I failed this test, so I will fail all my tests," a client will be taught to say, "I failed this test, so I'll study harder and do better on the next one." If he lacks supportive relationships, he may be trained in social skills. If he is anxious, he may be taught relaxation techniques.

In **rational-emotive therapy**, the counselor directly and often confrontationally challenges the client's negative thoughts in an attempt to convince her that they should be rejected because they do not make sense (Ellis, 1962). A less confrontational means to the same end is to lead the client to discover that her thoughts are unjustified and to reformulate them in a healthier way.

Many Christian counselors prefer those techniques because they view a person's beliefs, either negative or positive, as an integral part of spiritual life (Backus & Chapian, 1980; Crabb, 1977). Spiritual directors or counselors often refer to these beliefs as *faith*. Regardless of terminology, the ideas help provide answers to these big questions of life: Who created the universe? Why am I here? Where am I going? Faith also helps explain the smaller, more personal questions about identity, success, and failure. Inevitably, at the root of human actions and attitudes, a set a beliefs exists that people embrace to be true. Spiritual mentors see the need to root out illogical, untrue, and harmful beliefs about others and self as an essential part of personal growth.

What To Do if You Are Depressed

Medication and counseling take a few weeks to take effect. While you wait, these steps may help you manage. They may also help prevent a relapse after your treatment ends.

1. **Keep God central.** Pray and ask God for help. You will always need him to strengthen you, but you will especially need him when you are depressed. Trust that no matter how badly you feel, he has not abandoned you. He has promised, "Never will I leave you; never will I forsake you" (Hebrews 13:5). Try to understand your depression as an opportunity for spiritual growth. If it is a result of guilt, remember God's unconditional love and forgiveness. If it is a result of perfectionism, learn to find your self-worth in who you are in God. Pray for the people who are standing with you during this hard time; they will need strength, patience, wisdom, and understanding.

2. **Maintain a positive attitude.** First, as hard as it is, try to be optimistic. When negative thoughts occur, fight them. "Positive thinking is . . . grounded in the conviction that life is embraced by God's unconditional grace" (Ellens, 1999, p. 885). Never give up hope that your condition will improve. Trust that the Lord has better things in store for you.

Second, focus on what you *can* still do and don't worry about what you can't. Don't let yourself sink into self-pity or feelings of worthlessness. Accept the fact that your energy and productivity are lower than normal, and work within your limits. If you can, cut back on your course load at school or on your hours at work. Don't define the meaning of your life or your worth as a human being in terms of how much you can accomplish. Remember that God doesn't expect more of you than you can do, and he doesn't love you for your achievements.

3. **Don't make any major life changes.** Major life changes are difficult and stressful to cope with when you are well; when you are depressed, they can be overwhelming and aggravate your condition.

4. **Get support from friends and family.** Don't be ashamed that you are depressed, and don't be embarrassed to ask for help. Jesus commands that Christians bear one another's burdens. Doing so is a blessing and a privilege.

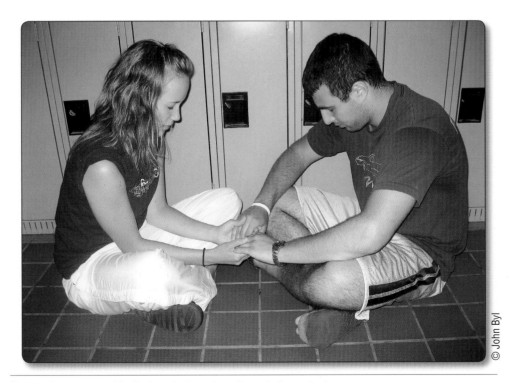

Supportive prayer with God and others is extremely important.

If someone you know is depressed, pray. Be available. Spend some quiet time with him or her. Respond with kindness and understanding, not with blame or condemnation. Don't offer too much advice, but encourage your friend to get professional help—*especially* if he or she is contemplating suicide (see sidebar on this page).

Suicide

According to official records, about 30,000 Americans commit **suicide** every year (Center for Disease Control and Prevention, 2004). Experts believe, however, that the actual number is higher, because many suicides are misreported as accidents. Furthermore, this figure does not include unsuccessful suicide attempts.

Suicide is the eighth leading cause of death among Americans as a whole, and the third leading cause of death among Americans aged 15 to 24. Between 7 and 8 percent of high school students attempt it, and about 10 percent of high school and college students seriously consider it (Mazza, 1997).

Depression, more than any other factor, increases a person's likelihood of attempting suicide (Angst, Angst, & Stassan, 1999). Between 50 and 70 percent of people who commit suicide clearly satisfy the criteria for clinical depression. More than 90 percent of adolescents who commit suicide have a known psychological disorder at the time of their deaths, and more than half of them have had it for more than two years (American Academy of Child and Adolescent Psychiatry, 1998). Half of the teenagers who take their own lives have depression (Hales, 2007).

Warning Signs of Suicide

The circumstances surrounding each suicide are different, but there are several common warning signs. People who talk about suicide are more likely to attempt it (Marttunen et al., 1998). People who end up taking their own lives drop hints of this during conversation; so if you hear someone threatening suicide, take the threat seriously. The biggest warning sign, however, is a previous suicide attempt. About 40 percent of people who successfully commit suicide have tried it in the past (Zametkin, Alter,

& Yemini, 2001). The statistic is between 50 and 80 percent in the case of adolescents (Shafii et al., 1985). If the circumstances that pushed a person to attempt suicide have not been dealt with, it is likely that the person will try to attempt suicide again (Blumenthal & Kupfer, 1988; Stevens, 2001). Other warning signs include preparing a will, giving away treasured items, and showing a morbid interest in death or the afterlife. Suicides are often preceded by seriously stressful or traumatic experiences, such as loss of something or someone important, rejection by others, the end of a romantic relationship, humiliation, arrest, or dismissal from work or school. Sometimes few or no warning signs are present, as is the case with most adolescent males who have been publicly humiliated (Marttunen et al., 1998). People are more likely to commit suicide if they lack the social support and personal resources to help them cope (Blumenthal & Kupfer, 1988; Stevens, 2001).

What To Do if Someone You Know Is Suicidal

After a loved one takes his or her life, family and friends are often plagued with questions like these:

- Where did things go wrong?
- Why didn't I pick up on this sooner?
- What should I have done differently?

There are no easy answers to those questions. However, there are a couple of practical suggestions for when you are in the company of others you care about:

1. **Take suicidal talk seriously.** Don't minimize pain or glibly assure the person that "everything will work out," because that com-

(continued)

(continued)

municates you don't understand or appreciate her pain. If you are unsure whether the person is serious about ending it all, ask directly.

2. **Someone who is suicidal may think that no one cares; you must show him you do.** Genuine listening and concern from others make people less likely to commit suicide; but indifferent, angry, or shaming responses can increase the possibility.

3. **Determine why the person is considering taking her life.** Often she will have many problems, but one that is especially significant. Encourage her to identify and clarify that key issue. Then suggest rational solutions to it. Help her to see that suicide is an irrational solution—and not the only possible one (review the discussion of cognitive therapy). Capitalize on any doubts, fears, or hesitations she may have about it.

4. **Strongly urge the individual to seek professional help.** Your loving concern is no substitute for professional help. Just because you talk the person out of suicide once doesn't mean the problem is over. Anything that has driven a person to consider suicide is a deep and serious issue that cannot be solved overnight.

5. **As you work through these steps, remember to incorporate your faith.** As a Christian, you maintain deep convictions about the sanctity of life, a source of abiding and sustaining hope, and a God who listens to prayer and is able to comfort and heal people.

Christians throughout the ages have consistently believed that deliberately taking one's own life is wrong; life is a gift from God, and only he has the right to end it. Though Job suffered and longed for death, he never considered suicide. (He did wish that he had never been born). As Robert Scott Peck says in the first line of his book, *The Road Less Traveled*, "Life is difficult" (Peck, 1976, p. 1). Although this truth is inescapable, God promises that, in the midst of the pain, he is present (Psalm 23).

Happiness and Life Satisfaction

Historically, mental health professionals have primarily focused on what is wrong. The goal has been to help anxious, depressed, and paranoid people reach a state of normalcy. As Dr. Martin Seligman, past president of the American Psychological Association, said, "We wanted to help people move from a minus five to a zero" (Wallis, 2005, p. A2). Now, a new breed of mental health practitioners and scientists are examining the conditions that contribute to **happiness** and well-being. New questions are being asked: "How do we get people from a zero to a plus five?" (Wallis, 2005, p. A2). Here are some of the findings.

World Happiness

Dr. Edward Diener, psychologist at the University of Illinois, was chief investigator for one of the largest global studies on the issue of happiness that has ever been conducted (Diener, Diener, & Diener, 1995). More than 100,000 surveys were conducted in 55 different countries representing a combined population of 4.1 billion people. A large subset of this data, 18,032 responses, came from college students. Figure 9.9 identifies countries with the highest measures of subjective well-being, and figure 9.10 lists the lowest.

Prescription for Happiness: Fact or Fiction?

Before we identify the traits that characterize people reporting the highest levels of happiness, we'll spend a little time busting some myths about what brings happiness.

Myth 1: Money

There is a positive relationship between income and happiness, but rich people on average are only slightly happier than individuals with a more average income. According to research by Diener and others, money contributes most substantially to personal happiness when people move from poverty to having adequate funds (Diener, Diener, & Diener, 1995). At the point basic needs are met, additional income does little to increase a sense of satisfaction. Since the end of World War II, income has almost tripled in the United States

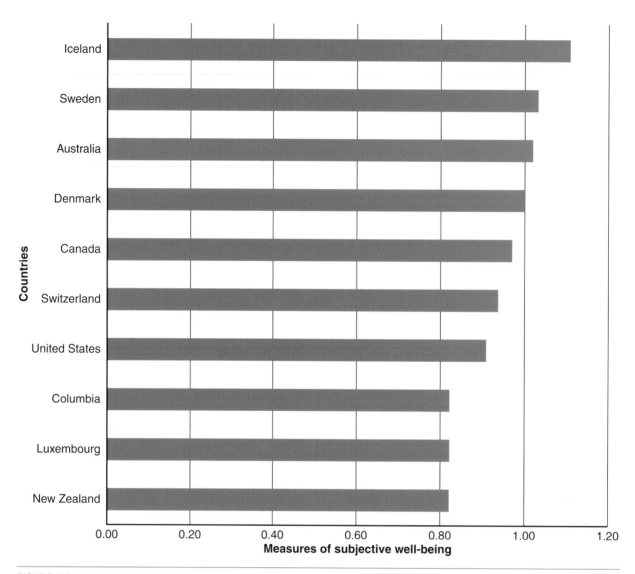

FIGURE 9.9   Top 10 countries for measures of subjective well-being.

Data from Diener, Diener, & Diener, 1995.

(after controlling for inflation), and house size has more than doubled. Americans currently have the most buying power of anyone in the world. Yet, if you were to chart the number of Americans who report being "very happy" during the same time, the line would be as flat as a table top (Easterbrook, 2007).

Myth 2: Education

Neither a good education nor high IQ paves the road to happiness. Two researchers at the University of Amsterdam tested their hypothesis that schooling and IQ positively affect health and happiness. Individuals in their study that had a

higher intelligence and increased education had a greater than average propensity for health, although it did not affect happiness (Hartog & Oosterbeek, 1997). It was Ernest Hemingway who said, "Happiness in intelligent people is the rarest thing I know" (The Quotations Page, 2007).

Myth 3: Youth

If you were to find the "fountain of youth," you may be forever young but this does not guarantee happiness. As a matter of fact, older people consistently rate their satisfaction with life higher than young adults do (Wallis, 2005). Older adults are

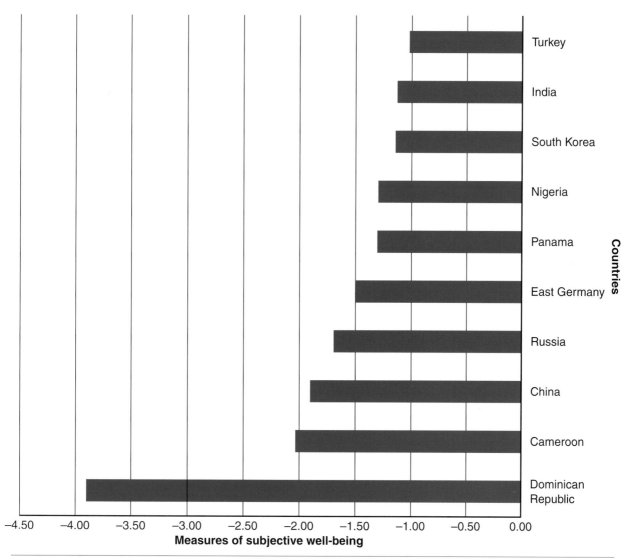

FIGURE 9.10 Bottom 10 countries for measures of subjective well-being.

Data from Diener, Diener, & Diener, 1995.

less prone to dark moods. According to a survey by the Center for Disease Control and Prevention, young adults aged 20 to 24 are sad on an average of 3.4 days per month, compared to 2.3 days for people aged 65 to 74 (Center for Disease Control and Prevention, 2005).

Myth 4: Weather

Studies show warm, sunny days can enhance one's mood, but there is no evidence that weather has a more permanent effect on happiness (Sanders & Brizzolara, 1982). People who live in southern California may think they are happier than those living in the American Midwest—but when con-

trolling for age, gender, income, education, and social connectedness, this is simply not true (Wallis, 2005).

Reality: What Is the Source of Happiness?

What factors do predict life satisfaction? What characteristics do individuals with the highest levels of happiness have in common? An argument could be presented for a number of different variables; but, by virtue of the quantity and quality of the evidence, love and faith should be on everyone's short list.

Strong Social Relationships

The degree to which relationships affect happiness is evident in the answers to some probing questions. *Time* magazine asked three such questions in a poll of 1,000 American adults (Wallis, 2005). Figures 9.11 and 9.12 and table 9.3 show the responses.

In a survey of 222 college students, psychologists found the "happiest" 10 percent, as determined by six different rating scales, shared one distinctive characteristic: a rich and fulfilling social life. Almost all were involved in rewarding relationships with family and friends and were committed to spending time with them. Although many were involved in romantic relationships, that was not a prerequisite for fulfillment. The happiest students spent the least time alone, and their friends rated them highest on good relationships (Diener & Seligman, 2002).

Spiritual Faith

Recently, interest in spirituality and well-being has exploded. Prior to 1982, approximately 100 scholarly articles on the relationship between religion and health were published in academic journals. Twenty years later, from 2000 to 2002, more than 1,000 scholarly articles were published on those topics (Paul, 2005). Clearly defined patterns are emerging from the rapidly expanding research that strongly suggest religion is not just beneficial for the soul. Religious people are less depressed, less anxious, and less suicidal than the nonreligious.

They are better able to cope with crises like illness, divorce, and bereavement. Additionally, faith seems to boost a person's overall feelings of fulfillment. Michael McCullough, associate professor of psychology and religious studies at the University of Miami, said that in a comparison of individuals with equivalent levels of depression, "the more religious person will be a little less sad" (Paul, 2005, p. 46). Studies show that the more a person attends church services, reads scripture, and prays, the better he or she will score on measures of happiness—specifically, frequency of positive emotions and overall sense of satisfaction with life (Paul, 2005). When Jesus said, "I have come that they may have life, and have it to the fullest," he meant it (John 10:10)!

Next Steps

You have read about a broad range of emotional territory in this chapter. Beginning with the exposed cliff edges of anxiety, you moved into the dark caverns of depression. Finally, you scaled the mountain to catch a glimpse of happiness. As is true of most journeys, you've caught only a glimpse of what each of these emotions can teach us. As you continue, you no doubt will return to each of these three places in a deeper and more intensive manner. Until then, perhaps you can consider some of the "travel suggestions" outlined in this chapter that will make your return visit less confusing and more insightful.

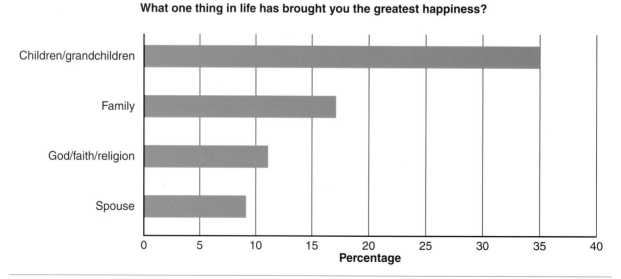

What one thing in life has brought you the greatest happiness?

FIGURE 9.11   The top four responses reflect two values: family and faith.

Adapted from Wallis, 2005.

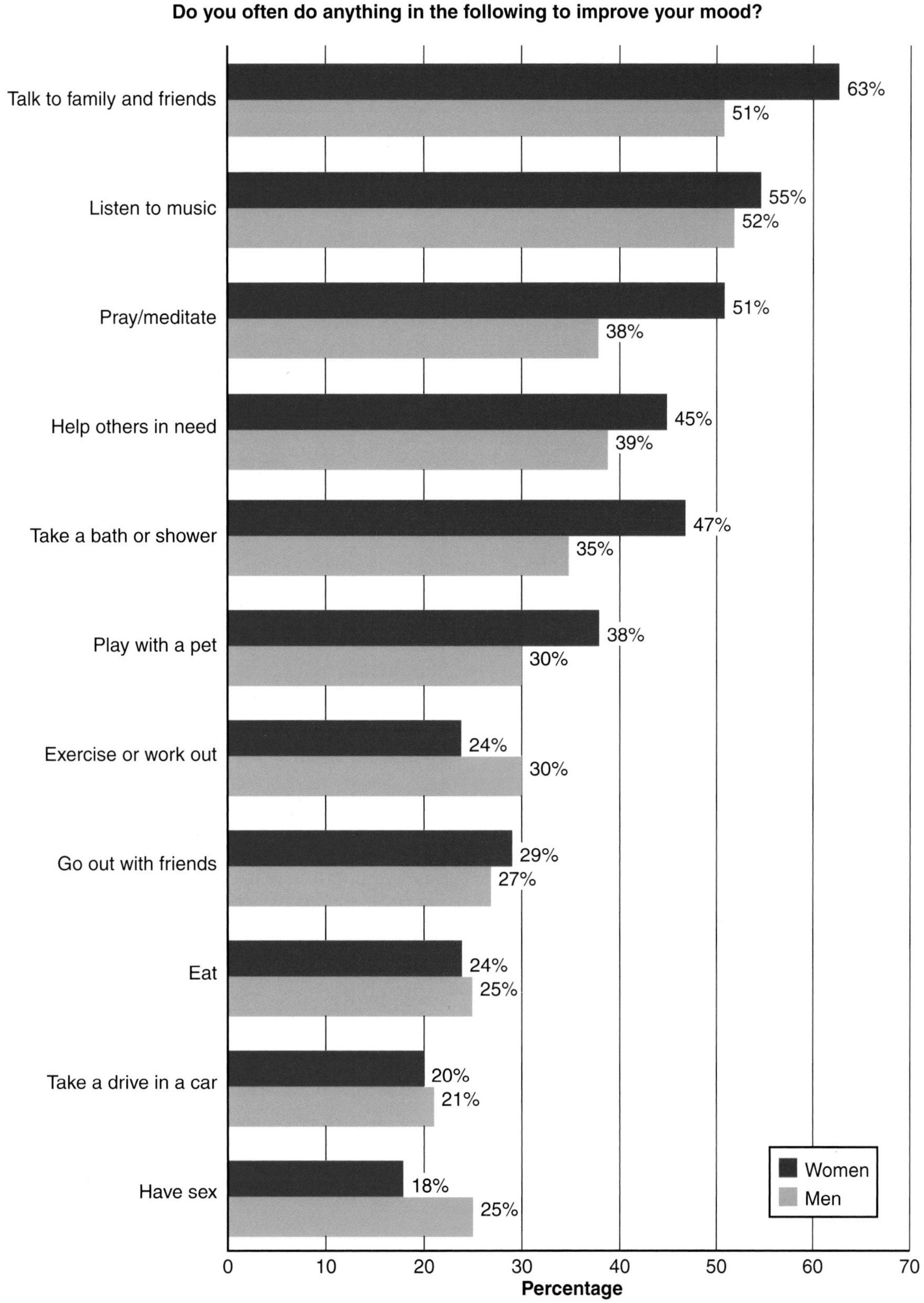

Do you often do anything in the following to improve your mood?

FIGURE 9.12   When people want to feel better temporarily they turn to friends, family, and faith.

Adapted from Wallis, 2005.

Table 9.3 What Are Your Major Sources of Happiness?

Responses	Percentage of those surveyed selecting this response
Relationships with my children	77%
Friends	76%
Contributing to the lives of others	75%
Relationship with spouse/partner	73%
Degree of control over life and destiny	66%
Things I do during leisure activity	64%
Relationship with parents	63%
Spiritual life	62%
Holidays	50%

Adapted from Wallis, 2005.

Key Terms

activating event, or stressor
all-or-nothing thinking
arousal
attribution
clinical depression
cognitive-behavioral therapy
cognitive restructuring, or reframing
deep breathing
depression
drive theory
emotional reasoning
fight-or-flight response
general adaptation syndrome (GAS)

happiness
individualized zones of optimal functioning
    (IZOF)
inverted-U theory
joy
labeling
mental filtering
post-traumatic stress disorder (PTSD)
psychoneuroimmunology (PNI)
rational-emotive therapy
stress
stress hardy
suicide

Review Questions

1. Identify the primary branch of science investigating the mind–body connection.
2. Describe the ABCs of stress.
3. Diagram three current models of how stress affects performance.
4. Identify three primary types of stressors.
5. Describe three traits of a stress-hardy person.
6. List six potential factors that may fuel depression.
7. Identify four action steps for treating depression.
8. List three warning signs of suicide.
9. List the two strongest predictors of happiness.

Application Activities

1. **Stress test**

   The assessment on page 224 was designed by Dr. Archibald Hart, author of *Adrenaline and Stress* (Hart, 1998). It can quickly help you identify your stress load.

2. **Building an effective to-do list**

   Creating a to-do list fundamentally involves two activities: listing and prioritizing. The first step is to think about everything that you would like to or must accomplish in a week. Despite your best intentions, you won't be able to make this list exhaustive; simply do the best you can. As other items come to mind you can add them to your list later.

   After listing each item, the next step is to prioritize them. One tried and true method for doing that involves letters and numbers.

First, go through your list and place an A beside the items you absolutely *must* get done during the week. Place a B next to items that *need* to get done, but not necessarily during the week. Finally, Cs go beside items you would *like* to get done at some time.

Now go back to all your As and prioritize them (with numbers) according to how important and urgent each is. Whatever item on your list that gets the A1 priority is, by definition, the most important and urgent item you have to accomplish. Begin working here before going on to the next item, A2. You may find yourself at the end of the day being able to mark only one or two items off your list. Don't be discouraged by this because you have accomplished the most important and time-sensitive task.

Stress Assessment

Write a number next to each question, according to the following scale. When you are finished, add up all the numbers and look at the key below.

0 – I seldom or never feel this way.

1 – I sometimes (once a month or so) feel this way.

2 – I often (more than once a month) feel this way.

3 – I almost always feel this way.

1. Do you feel moody and have difficulty getting up in the morning? ____

2. Do you experience slight fevers, signs of the flu, a sore throat, or tender lymph nodes? ____

3. Are mornings the worst times of your day, with evenings being better? ____

4. Do you fall asleep easily but wake early without being able to fall asleep again? ____

5. Have you ever found yourself staring at a computer monitor, keyboard, or book, barely able to keep your head from dropping? ____

6. Do you feel mentally sluggish, confused, and unresponsive? ____

7. Has your short-term memory worsened, and do you have trouble concentrating? ____

8. Has your daily activity dropped to below half of what it was before? ____

9. Are your emotions relatively blunted, and do you often feel apathetic? ____

10. Does your body ache all over, as if it is weaker than it used to be? ____

11. When you exercise, do you feel debilitated for more than 12 hours afterwards? ____

12. Does your work stress you out to the point that you want to escape from it? ____

13. Do you get headaches? ____

14. Do you find yourself desperately wanting to avoid being with other people? ____

15. Are you more impatient, irritable, nervous, angry, or anxious than you used to be? ____

Total score: ____

If your score is . . .

Below 12: Your fatigue is within normal limits. Cut back on unnecessary stress wherever you can and improve your sleeping habits (see chapter 10).

12 to 22: You have type 1 fatigue, which is temporary and not serious. You can reverse it by lowering your stress level, taking a vacation or sabbatical, or increasing your rest and sleep time. If these things don't help, consult a professional.

23 to 32: You have type 2 fatigue, which is longstanding and serious. A simple short break will not relieve it. You are suffering from chronic stress, depletion of adrenaline, and most likely a compromised immune system. You probably need to make a major lifestyle change and get professional help.

Above 33: You have type 3 fatigue, which is a "disease state." You are at risk for serious depression, hormonal imbalances, and physical illnesses such as chronic fatigue syndrome. You *must* get professional help.

From P. Walters and J. Byl, 2008, *Christian paths to health and wellness* (Champaign, IL: Human Kinetics). Adapted, by permission, from A.D. Hart, 1998, *Adrenaline and stress* (Waco, TX: Word).

References

Abramson, S.Y., Seligman, M.E.P., & Teasdale, J.D. (1978). Learned helplessness in humans: A critique. *Journal of Abnormal Psychology, 87*: 49-74.

American Academy of Child and Adolescent Psychiatry. (1998). Summary of the practice parameters for the adolescent and treatment of children and adolescents with depressive disorders. *Journal of the American Academy of Child and Adolescent Psychiatry, 37*: 1223-1239.

American College Health Association. (2006). National College Health Assessment. Retrieved November 6, 2006, from www.acha-ncha.org/data_highlights. html.

American Institute of Stress. (2002). American's #1 health problem. Retrieved May 29, 2002, from www. stress.org.

American Psychiatric Association. (2000). *American Psychiatric Association: Diagnostic and statistical manual of mental disorders* (4th ed.). Washington, DC: American Psychiatric Association.

Anderson, G.E. (1972). *College schedule of recent experience.* Fargo, ND: North Dakota State University.

Angst, J., Angst, F., & Stassen, H.H. (1999). Suicide risk in patients with major depressive disorder. *Journal of Clinical Psychiatry, 60*: 57-62.

Backus, W., & Chapian, M. (1980). *Telling yourself the truth.* Minneapolis: Bethany Fellowship.

Beck, A.T. (1967). *Depression: Clinical, experimental, and theoretical aspects.* New York: Harper & Row.

Beck, A.T. (1970). *Depression: Causes and treatment.* Philadelphia: University of Pennsylvania Press.

Benton, S.A., Robertson, J.M., Tsent, W.C., Newton, F.B., & Benton, S.L. (2003). Changes in counseling center client problems across 13 years. *Professional Psychology, Research and Practice, 34*(1): 66-74.

Birmaher, B., Ryan, N.C., Williamson, D.E., Brent, D.A., Kaufman, J., & Dahl, R.E. (1996). Childhood and adolescent depression: A review of the past 10 years. *Journal of the American Academy of Child and Adolescent Psychiatry, 35*: 1427-1440.

Blonna, R. (2005). *Coping with stress in a changing world.* Boston: McGraw-Hill.

Blumenthal, S.J., & Kupfer, D.J. (1988). Overview of early detection and treatment strategies for suicidal behavior in young people. *Journal of Youth and Adolescence, 17*: 1-23.

Bradberry, T.G.J. (2003). *The emotional intelligence quickbook: Everything you need to know.* San Diego, CA: Talentsmart.

Brage, D., & Meredith, W. (1994). A causal model of adolescent depression. *The Journal of Psychology, 128*: 455-468.

Brain Mind Bulletin. (1989). Princeton study: Student stress lowers immunity. *Brain Mind Bulletin, 14*: 1,7.

Burns, D. (1989). *The feeling good handbook.* New York: Penguin.

Canadian Mental Health Association. (2006). Stress at work. Retrieved November 4, 2006, from www.cmha. ca/bins/index.asp.

Cannon, W. (1932). *The wisdom of the body.* New York: Norton.

Center for Disease Control and Prevention. (2004). Suicide: Fact sheet. Retrieved August 18, 2007, from ww.cdc.gov/ncipc/factsheets/suifacts.htm.

Center for Disease Control and Prevention. (2005). National center for injury prevention and control. Retrieved June 4, 2007, from www.cdc.gov/ncipc/ wisqars.

Cialdini, R. (2000). *Influence: Science and practice.* Boston: Allyn & Bacon.

Clarke, G.N., DeBar, L.L., Lewinsohn, P.M., Kazdin, A.E., & Weisz, J.R. (2003). Cognitive-behavioral group treatment for adolescent depression. In A.E. Kazdin & J.R. Weisz (Eds.), *Evidence-based psychotherapies for children and adolescents* (pp. 120-134). New York: Guilford Press.

Crabb, L. (1977). *Effective biblical counseling.* Grand Rapids, MI: Zondervan.

Crespian, T., & Becker, J. (1999). Effects of time management practices on college grades. *Journal of Educational Psychology, 83*: 405-410.

Cuijpers, P. (1998). A psychoeducational approach to the treatment of depression: A meta-analysis of Lewinsohn's coping with depression course. *Behavior Therapy, 29*: 52-65.

DC Talk. (1999). *Jesus freaks.* Tulsa: Albury.

Diener, E., Diener, M., & Diener, C. (1995). Factors predicting the subjective well-being of nations. *American Psychological Association, 69*(5): 851-864.

Diener, E., & Seligman, M.E.P. (2002). Very happy people. *Psychological Science, 13*(1): 81-84.

Draper, E. (1992). *Draper's book of quotations for the Christian world.* Wheaton, IL: Tyndale House.

Easterbrook, G. (2007). The real truth about money. *Newsweek*: A32.

Ellens, J.H. (1999). Positive thinking. In D.G. Benner & P.C. Hill (Eds.), *Baker encyclopedia of psychology and counseling* (2nd ed.) (pp. 885-886). Grand Rapids, MI: Baker.

Ellis, A. (1962). *Reason and emotion in psychotherapy.* Secaucus, NJ: Prentice-Hall.

Ellis, A., Gordon, J., Neenan, M., & Palmer, S. (1997). *Stress counseling.* New York: Springer.

Ellison, C. (2002). *From stress to well-being.* Nashville, TN: Nelson Reference & Electronic Publishing.

Frankl, V. (1984). *Man's search for meaning.* New York: Touchstone.

Garrett, B. (2003). *Brain and behavior.* Belmont, CA: Wadsworth.

Geddes, J., & Butler, R. (2002). Depressive disorders. *Clinical Evidence, 7*: 867-882.

Goleman, D. (1995). *Emotional intelligence.* New York: Bantam.

Goleman, D., Boyatzis, R.E., & McKee, A. (2002). *Primal leadership: Realizing the power of emotional intelligence.* Boston: Harvard Business School Press.

Gould, D., & Tuffey, S. (1996). Zones of optimal functioning research: A review and critique. *Anxiety, Stress and Coping, 9*: 53-68.

Greenberg, J. (2002). *Comprehensive stress management* (7th ed.). Boston: McGraw-Hill.

Hales, D. (2005). *An invitation to health* (11th ed.). Belmont, CA: Wadsworth.

Hales, D. (2007). *An invitation to health* (12th ed.). Belmont, CA: Wadsworth.

Hanin, Y.L., Spielberger, C.D., & Diaz-Guerrero, R., (1986). State-trait anxiety research on sports in the USSR. In C.D. Spielberger & R. Diaz-Guerrero (Eds.), *Cross-cultural anxiety* (vol. 3) (pp. 45-64). New York: Hemisphere Publishing Corporation/Harper & Row Publishers.

Hart, A.D. (1998). *Adrenaline and stress.* Waco, TX: Word.

Hartog, J., & Oosterbeek, H. (1997). *Health, wealth, and happiness: Why pursue a higher education?* Amsterdam: Unpublished manuscript.

Health Canada. (2006). Impact of work-life conflict. Retrieved November 4, 2006, from www.hc-sc.gc.ca/index_e.html.

Hill, W.F. (1957). Comments on Taylor's drive theory and manifest anxiety. *Psychological Bulletin, 54*(6): 490-493.

Holmes, T., & Rahe, R. (1967). The social readjustment rating scale. *Journal of Psychosomatic Research, 11*: 213-218.

Jacobson, N.S., Dobson, K.S., Truax, P.A., Addis, M.E., Koerner, K., & Gollan, J.K. (1996). A component analysis of cognitive-behavioral treatment for depression. *Journal of Consulting and Clinical Psychology, 64*: 295-304.

Johnson, S. (1993). *Who moved my cheese?* New York: Penguin Putnam.

Kalat, J.W. (2001). *Biological psychology* (7th ed.). Belmont, CA: Wadsworth.

Karren, K.J., Hafen, B.Q., & Smith, N. (2002). *Mind/body health: The effects of attitudes, emotions, and relationships* (2nd ed.). San Francisco: Benjamin Cummings.

Kessler, R.C. (2000). Posttraumatic stress disorder: The burden to the individual and to society. *Journal of Clinical Psychiatry, 6*: 4-12.

Kobasa, S. (1979). Stressful life events, personality, and health: An inquiry into hardiness. *Journal of Personality and Social Psychology, 37*: 1-11.

Koenig, H. (2007). Personal interview with Diane Hales. In D. Hales, *An invitation to health* (pp. 53). Belmont, CA: Thomson.

Koenig, H., Kvale, J., & Ferrel, C. (1988). Religion and well-being in later life. *The Gerontologist, 28*(1): 18-27.

Lazarus, R., & Susan, F. (1984). *Stress, appraisal, and coping.* New York: Springer Publishing Company.

Lewinsohn, P.B. (1974). A behavioral approach to depression. In R.J. Friedman & M.M. Katz (Eds.), *The psychology of depression: Contemporary theory and research* (pp. 157-178). Washington, DC: Winston-Wiley.

Marcotte, D. (1997). Treating depression in adolescence: A review of the effectiveness of cognitive-behavioral treatments. *Journal of Youth and Adolescence, 26*: 273-284.

Marttunen, M.J., Henriksson, M.M., Isometsa, E.T., Helkkinene, M.E., Aro, H.M., & Lonnquist, J.K. (1998). Completed suicides among adolescents with no diagnosable psychiatric disorders. *Adolescence, 26*: 669-681.

Matthews, G., Zeidner, M., & Roberts, R. (2002). *Emotional intelligence: Science and myth.* Cambridge, MA: MIT Press.

Mazza, J.J. (1997). School-based suicide prevention programs: Are they effective? *School Psychology Review, 26*: 382-397.

McCaffrey, A.M. (2004). Prayer for health concerns: Results of a national survey on prevalence and patterns of use. *Archives of Internal Medicine, 164*(8): 858-862.

McFarland, C., & Miller, D.T. (1994). The framing of relative performance feedback: Seeing the glass as half empty or half full. *Journal of Personality and Social Psychology, 66*: 1061-1073.

Merriam-Webster. (2007). Worry. Retrieved June 8, 2007, from www.merriam-webster.com/dictionary/worry.

Metcalf, C.W., & Felible, R. (1992). *Lighten up: Survival skills for people under pressure.* New York: Perseus.

Miner, M., & Rawson, H. (1997). *American heritage dictionary of American quotations.* New York: Penguin.

National College Health Association. (2006). National College Health Assessment. Retrieved October 11, 2006, from www.acha-ncha.org/data_highlights.html.

National Institute of Mental Health. (2006). Depression. Retrieved November 6, 2006, from www.nimh.nih.gov/publicat/depwomenknows.cfm#intro.

New York Times Business. (2003). Bestseller list. Retrieved June 11, 2003, from www.nytimes.com/pages/business/index.html.

Ornstein, R., & Sobel, D. (1989). *Healthy pleasures.* Reading, MA: Addison-Wesley.

Paul, P. (2005). The power to uplift. *Newsweek*: A46-48.

Peck, M.S. (1976). *The road less traveled.* New York: Simon & Schuster.

Pettingale, K.W., Morris, T., Greer, S., & Haybittle, J.L. (1985). Mental attitudes to cancer: An additional and prognostic factor. *The Lancet* (March 30): 750.

Publishers Weekly. (2004). Publishers Weekly bestsellers. Retrieved May 15, 2006, from www.publishersweekly.com/bestsellerslist/1.html?channel=bestsellers.

Rein, G., Atkinson, M., & McCraty, R. (1995). The physiological and psychological effects of compassion and anger. *Journal of Advancement in Medicine, 8*: 87-105.

Riga, A. (2006). Business awakes to the cost of stress. *The Gazette* (February 27): 16.

Sacco, W.P., & Beck, A.T. (1995). Cognitive theory and therapy. In E.E. Beckham & W.R. Leber (Eds.), *Handbook of depression* (2nd ed.) (pp. 95-104). New York: Wiley.

Sanders, J.L., & Brizzolara, M.S. (1982). Relationships between weather and mood. *Journal of General Psychology, 107*(1): 155.

Sapolsky, R. (2004). *Why zebras don't get ulcers* (3rd ed.). New York: Henry Holt & Company, Inc.

Sax, L. (1999). *The American freshman.* Los Angeles: Cooperative Institutional Education Research Institute.

Seligman, M.E.P. (1974). Depression and learned helplessness. In R.J. Friedman & M.M. Katz (Eds.), *The psychology of depression: Contemporary theory and research.* Washington, DC: Winston-Wiley.

Shafii, M., Carrigan, S., Whittinghill, J.R., & Derrick, A. (1985). Psychological autopsy of completed suicide in children and adolescents. *American Journal of Psychiatry, 142*: 1061-1064.

Spence, J.T., & Spence, K.W. (1996). The motivational components of manifest anxiety: Drive and drive stimuli. In C.D. Spielberger (Ed.), *Anxiety and behavior.* New York: Academic Press.

St. James, E. (1994). *Simplify your life.* New York: Hyperion.

Stevens, L.M. (2001). Adolescent suicide. *Journal of the American Medical Association, 286*: 31-94.

Sunsern, R. (2002). Effects of exercise on stress in Thai postmenopausal women. *Health Care for Women International, 23*(8): 924-932.

The Quotations Page. (2007). Quotes from Ernest Hemingway. Retrieved November 11, 2006, from www.quotationspage.com.

U.S. Department of Education. (2006). Average undergraduate college costs 2002-03. Retrieved November 4, 2006, from www.ed.gov/students/prep/college/thinkcollege/early/students/edlite-college-costs.html.

Wallis, C. (2005). The new science of happiness. *Newsweek*: A4-9.

Walters, P., Gustafson, J., Williams, B., & Carlson, K. (2006). What your students are really thinking. Paper presented at the Christian Society of Kinesiology, Sport, and Leisure. Boston.

Weinberg, R., & Gould, D. (2003). *Foundations of sport and exercise psychology* (3rd ed.). Champaign, IL: Human Kinetics.

Yerkes, R.M., & Dodson, J.D. (1908). The relation of strength of stimulus to rapidity of habit-formation. *Journal of Comparative and Neurological Psychology, 18*: 459-482.

Zametkin, A.J., Alter, M.R., & Yemini, T. (2001). Suicide in teenagers. *Journal of American Medical Association, 286*: 3120-3125.

Suggested Readings

Burns, D. (1989). *The feeling good handbook.* **New York: Penguin.**

This best-selling book describes common mental distortions that can destroy our sense of well-being. Methods for combating these distortions are outlined.

Frankl, V. (1984). *Man's search for meaning.* **New York: Touchstone.**

Frankl, imprisoned in a Nazi concentration camp, describes the concept that man's deepest driving force is to search for meaning and purpose in life.

Goleman, D. (1995). *Emotional intelligence.* **New York: Bantam.**

This book describes the five crucial skills of emotional intelligence and shows how they determine our success in relationships, work, and even our physical well-being.

Johnson, S. (1993). *Who moved my cheese?* **New York: Penguin Putnam.**

An analogy of mice and mankind, this book describes how we must "move with the cheese" in our ever-changing environment.

Mackenzie, A. (1997). *The time trap: The classic book on time management.* **New York: American Management Association.**

This classic book has time-tested methods and principles for effectively managing your time.

Peck, M.S. (1976). *The road less traveled.* **New York: Simon & Schuster.**

The author discusses how discipline and love make up the essential emotional framework for spiritual and psychological health.

Suggested Web Sites

www.nimh.nih.gov

A resource provided by the National Institute of Mental Health for information on all aspects of mental health, including stress and depression.

www.save.org

SAVE: Suicide Awareness Voices of Education is an organization dedicated to increasing public awareness of depression and suicide.

www.nmha.org

Mental Health America, formerly known as National Mental Health Association, is one of the largest nonprofit organizations dedicated to improving mental health.

www.apa.org

The American Psychological Association is the largest psychological association in the world. It is primarily dedicated to assisting mental health care professionals, yet it has a multitude of helpful resources for the general public.

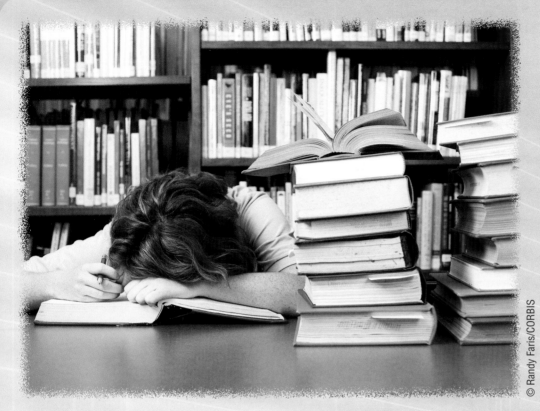

© Randy Faris/CORBIS

CHAPTER

10

Sleep Habits and Wellness

Peter Walters

After reading this chapter, you should be able to do the following:

❶ Understand the scope of sleep deprivation.

❷ List the reasons for sleep deprivation.

❸ Understand the effects of sleep deprivation.

❹ Identify sleep stages and sleep cycles.

❺ Examine how much sleep you need.

❻ Learn how to improve your quality of sleep.

❼ Explore a biblical view of rest and sleep.

Creation is filled with rhythms and cycles. The earth joins a multitude of celestial beings in predictable lunar cycles. The daily cycle of photosynthesis allows plants to flourish. Every water droplet is part of a hydrologic cycle. Conception is made possible during a menstrual cycle. Three weeks after conception, the heart begins a cardiac cycle. Upon exiting the womb, a baby's respiratory cycle begins. These cycles often become so automatic their presence is hardly noticed. Yet, human existence is maintained by these subtle rhythms.

The most basic movements of many cycles can be broadly defined as the expansion and contraction of motion. Ocean waves advance toward the shore and then retreat back into the ocean. The sun rises, then sets. While breathing, our lungs expand and then contract.

Some cycles happen so quickly and with such frequency that it is tempting to overlook the small undulating patterns. For example, it is easy to see only forward motion when watching an Olympic track sprinter run 100 meters in less than 10 seconds. The forward motion is created only through a cycle of the legs reaching out (expansion) and pushing back (contraction).

Several years ago I was struck by the title of one popular book by Christian author Charles Swindoll, *Three Steps Forward, Two Steps Back* (Swindoll, 1997). That pattern was familiar to me, and I thought about how wasteful it is to move in a direction contrary to the one intended. My preference is for advancement, progress, and production. Yet after more careful refection, I began to understand that human movement is only made possible through both extension and flexion.

Contraction without relaxation equals immobilization. The retreats are what allow movement to continue. Some have commented about how amazing the human heart is because it never rests. Yet in truth, one-half of the cardiac cycle is devoted to relaxation or retreat.

The photograph on this page shows what occurs when the nervous system involuntarily sustains muscular contraction. This person is suffering from an advanced case of tetanus, which is sometimes referred to as lockjaw. Tetanus is caused by a bacterial infection that usually begins with a dysfunction of the trigeminal nerve's causing the face and neck muscles to spasm. This paralysis continues to expand throughout the body until the respiratory system is affected, leading to oxygen deprivation and eventually suffocation. If

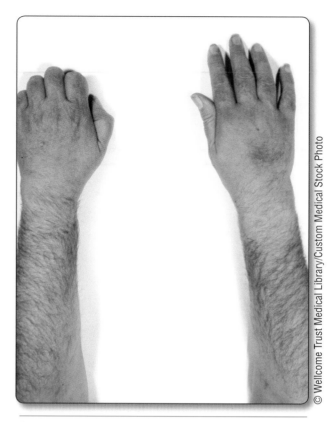

Tetanus causes severe muscular contractions that do not subside (see left hand).

left untreated, tetanus kills 3 out of 10 individuals who are infected (Health Square, 2007).

Many rhythms, such as the cardiac and respiratory cycles, work involuntarily. One discussed in this chapter (sleep) is under voluntary control. Although a person may feel tired, the ultimate decisions about when to go to bed and what time to get up is up to the individual. For many college students who are living away from home for the first time, this new freedom is exciting. They are able to determine how late to stay out, when to pull an all-nighter, and how late to sleep.

Consequences are firmly attached to most of our choices. The most critical factor in getting up early before an 8:00 class is not remembering to set the alarm or even having the will power to get out of bed when the alarm goes off, but bedtime the night before. Like a row of dominos, each decision affects subsequent ones. Just as night follows day, the level of emotional stability, mental alertness, and physical stamina are affected by many of the choices we make.

200 Hours Without Sleep

New York City, January 1959—Peter Tripp, the flamboyant and fame-seeking disc jockey (DJ) for the Big Apple's WMGM radio, was determined to shatter the world record for sleeplessness and garner national attention in the process. His goal: a 200-hour "wakeathon" to raise money for the March of Dimes (Coren, 1996; Bullman & Milne, 1998). A creative and energetic entrepreneur as well as a smooth talker, Tripp had invented the Top 40 playlist and the radio talk show, both of which would become staples of radio programming in his time. He was arguably the most popular DJ alive. He knew better than to rest on his laurels. He hoped that this stunt would make him the topic of cocktail conversations and dinner table discussions from coast to coast.

Because no one could predict the effects of more than eight days without sleep, Tripp's concerned coworkers urged him not to undertake this challenge without expert supervision. Tripp casually agreed to allow Dr. Floyd Cornelison, from Jefferson Medical College in Philadelphia, and Dr. Louis West, from the University of California, to monitor his health.

Dr. West had seen firsthand what sleep deprivation could do to a person. As a young psychiatrist working at an Air Force base in Texas, he examined American pilots who had been captured by the Chinese during the Korean War and who were tortured by being forced to stay awake for days at a time. Several of these men believed they were not the same after this ordeal. After extensive testing, West agreed. He found that their experiences in prison had caused permanent cognitive damage and altered their personalities. Knowing the danger, he tried to discourage the DJ from his foolhardy feat. But for Tripp, national celebrity and a place in the record books were worth the risk. He told both doctors that he was going ahead, with or without them.

The purpose of this chapter is to help you learn how your choices pertaining to sleep affect many aspects of your well-being and to make good decisions about sleep. I hope that you'll discover the benefits of synchronizing your sleep to the rhythm of your individual sleep cycle.

Chronic Sleep Deprivation

Not many people take **sleep deprivation** to the extreme that Peter Tripp did (see sidebar on this page). But studies show that *the majority of Americans today are consistently sleep deprived* (Murphy & Delanty, 2007). One sleep expert claims, "If we operated machinery the way we are now operating the human body, we would be accused of reckless endangerment" (Moore-Ede, 1993, p. 36). According to another, "The fact that nearly everyone is chronically sleep deprived has led to an acceptance of less than ideal daytime alertness as normal" (Dement & Vaughan, 1999, p. 231). This hasn't always been the case, as you can see from figure 10.1.

Sleep Thieves

While it may surprise you that your ancestors got 10 hours of sleep each night, most people in unindustrialized countries still sleep that much. What really needs explaining is the three-hour drop, one hour of which has happened in the last three decades. What vandals have pilfered so much sleep? The answer is complex and personal, but this section will deal with some of the more common sleep thieves.

Academic Workload

Japan, as you may know, is a competitive place. This is especially true in the academic arena, where the selection process for higher education has been called "hellish" and "warlike" (Wikipedia, 2005). One major source of stress and anxiety is the series of national college entrance exams. To prepare for these tests, high school students often attend special "cram schools," called *juku,* in the evenings, then study into the wee hours of

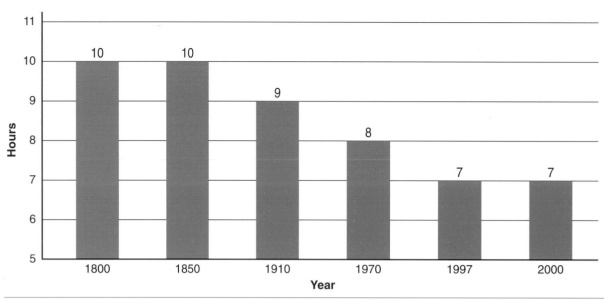

FIGURE 10.1   Average hours of sleep Americans get per night by year.

Based on National Sleep Foundation Web site, 2005.

Sunday Spent in the Library

Do you feel like you just can't get everything done that needs to be accomplished? If so, you're not alone. In a recent survey, more than one-quarter of Americans 18 years of age and older said they could not be successful vocationally while getting the sleep they need (Walters, 2005).

The phrase "24/7" has not been in the vernacular that long, but students know what it means from experience. Ask the college student who eats lunch in less than 18 minutes while pecking away at a laptop computer and talking with a friend on a cell phone, "How is it going?" Most likely, you will hear one of these common refrains: "Wiped out!" "Exhausted!" "Whipped!"

It is interesting to observe some of the more common ways college students respond to this apparently universal problem. Drowning underneath an ocean of papers, class assignments, and projects, many students say they just need to "work harder." Maybe that reflexive response is what led a large group of students at one Christian college to petition college administrators to open the college library on Sundays. This petition gained momentum from irate community members who were upset over the fact that their public library was being overtaken on Sundays by students from the Christian college.

What does this kind of behavior say about the way that Christian college students live their lives? Maybe it says that they are very serious about academic rigor and intellectual excellence. On the other hand, it may mean that they have jumped aboard the 21st-century treadmill, leaving little time for solitude, reflection, and spiritual renewal.

the morning. A commonly quoted proverb among Japanese students is, "Pass with four, fail with five" (Coren, 1996, p. 128). They are referring to hours of sleep per night.

Colleges and universities in the United States that emphasize academic rigor make no apologies for burdening their undergraduates with workloads that leave them with little time for rest or leisure. When golf champion Tiger Woods decided to drop out of Stanford to turn professional, a reporter asked him what he was looking forward to. His reply? "More sleep." Graduate schools, too, especially in medicine, law, and business, make it clear that students can't both sleep and excel.

Books, however, are not the only things that come between students and their pillows. Most students spend a lot of time and energy

- defining their social identities,
- dealing with the inevitable ups and downs of human relationships, and
- beginning the painstaking and often painful process of picking a life partner.

In a survey of young adults aged 18 to 29, more than half of the respondents said they often stayed up later than they should to watch TV or surf the Internet (Maas, 1998).

Together, these factors make students some of the most sleep-deprived people in the land. Studies at Cornell University (Maas, 1998) and five different Christian colleges (Walters, 2005) found that the average student sleeps only 6.1 hours per night (see figure 10.2). Compare this with the U.S. population as a whole (see figure 10.3).

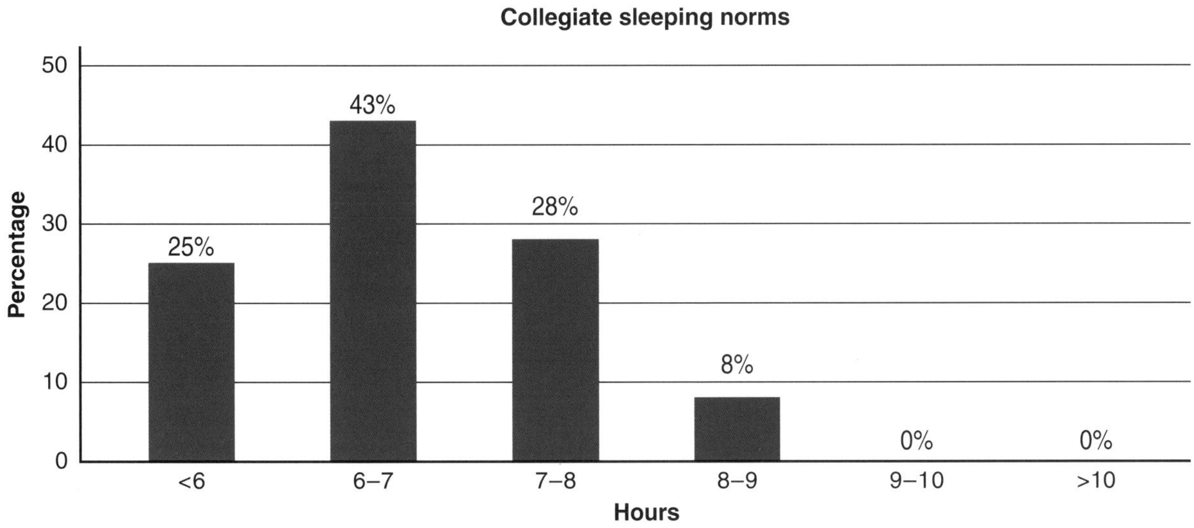

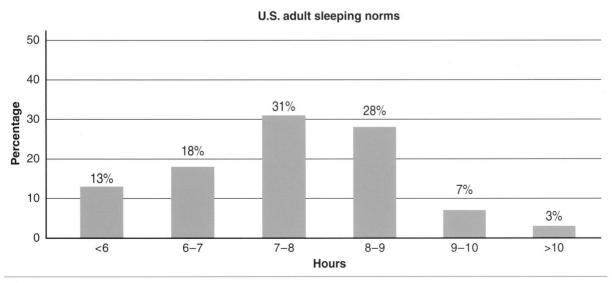

FIGURE 10.2   Only eight percent of college students report sleeping eight or more hours per night.

Adapted from Walters, 2005.

FIGURE 10.3   In contrast to college students, 38 percent of American adults receive an average of eight or more hours of sleep per night.

National Sleep Foundation, 2005.

Work

Evidence suggests that people take the hectic lifestyle they learn at school into the workplace. A sociologist estimated that in 1969, a typical two-parent, middle-class American family with two children worked for 5,420 hours per year. The wife worked for 2,465 hours as a homemaker and the husband worked both inside and outside the home for 2,965 hours. Today, however, a similar family works for 6,488 hours, in great part because women now work outside the home as well (Schor, 1993). This additional 1,058 hours is equivalent to another half-time job (see figure 10.4).

Data from the National Sleep Foundation (NSF) reveal a strong correlation between the number of hours a person works and the number of hours he or she sleeps. Forty-five percent of adults polled

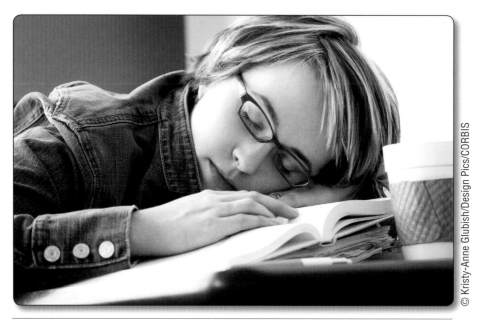

Students cite academic pressure as the leading cause of less sleep.

© Kristy-Anne Glubish/Design Pics/CORBIS

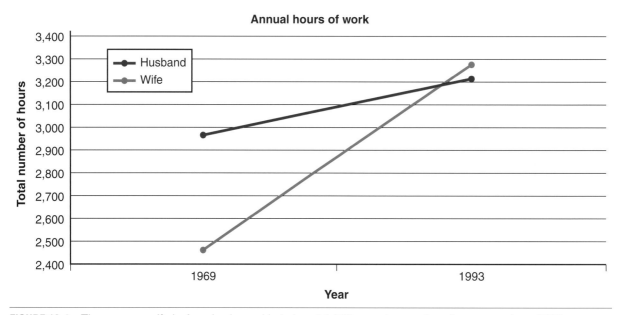

FIGURE 10.4   The average wife in America has added almost 1,000 more hours of work per year since 1969.

Adapted from Schor, 1993.

in 2001 said they were sleeping less in order to be more productive (National Sleep Foundation, 2001) (see figure 10.5).

Pain of Humanity

Respected pastor and teacher A.W. Tozer said, "In an effort to get the work of the Lord done we often lose contact with the Lord of the work, and quite literally wear our people out" (Draper, 1992, p. 115). It is hard not to be completely engulfed by the suffering sea of humanity, especially today when global needs are so evident. About one-sixth of the world's population goes to bed hungry every night, more than half of the world's citizens earns less than a dollar per day, and the AIDS epidemic is expanding (World Health Organization, 2006). Resting amid crises like those seems not only selfish but also ruthless, callous, and unmerciful. It's like taking a coffee break when people are drowning.

Yet to a group of young Christian activists vigorously battling societal ills that the Trappist monk, Thomas Merton, said this:

There is a pervasive form of contemporary violence among us, which is activism and overwork. The rush and pressures of modern-day life are the most innate forms of this violence. To allow oneself to be carried away with a multitude of conflicting concerns, to surrender to too many demands, to commit oneself to too many projects, to want to help everyone and everything, is to succumb to violence. The frenzy of our activism neutralizes our work for peace because it kills the root of inner wisdom that makes our work fruitful. (Muller, 2000, p. 36)

Judas accused Jesus of allowing careless waste when Mary anointed his feet with a bottle of perfume worth one year's wages (see John 12:1–7). Jesus replied with a sharp retort, "Leave her alone." Then he added that poverty and pain will always be a part of human existence. Since the fall of Adam, toil and suffering have been part of the human drama. In the midst of this hard reality, Christ willingly accepted a lavish display of love, and so should his followers.

Ignorance

Any recipe for a healthy lifestyle must include at least these three ingredients: exercise, diet, and rest. Much has been written about the first two. More than 3,000 books, not to mention magazine articles, are in print on diet alone. Yet very little has been written about rest, recovery, or sleep. For instance, I reviewed 10 different health and wellness textbooks targeted for distribution in

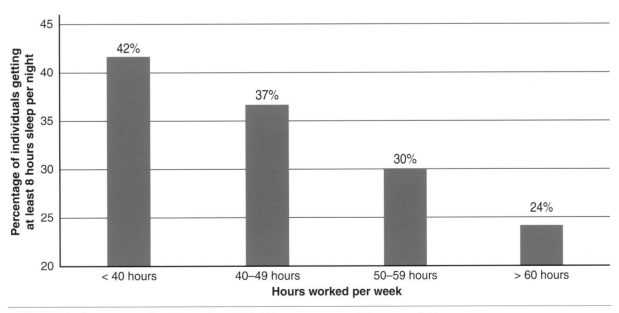

FIGURE 10.5 Percentage of workers who get eight hours or more of sleep per night.
Adapted from Schor, 1993.

North America and found that they devoted less than two percent of their space to the topic (Walters, 2000). As a result, Americans and Canadians know very little about sleep: what it is, why they need it, when to do it, how to do it, or how much is required. In fact, a lot of them are sleep deprived and don't even know it! This ignorance is anything but bliss; it keeps many people miserable.

Test Your Sleep IQ

In a 1999 survey by the National Sleep Foundation, 83 percent of American adults failed the following sleep quiz (National Sleep Foundation, 1999). Take it and see how you do. You may be surprised.

Sleep I.Q.

True or false?

1. During sleep, your brain rests. _____
2. You cannot learn to function normally with one or two fewer hours of sleep a night than you need. _____
3. Boredom makes you feel tired, even if you have had enough sleep. _____
4. Resting in bed with your eyes closed cannot satisfy your body's need for sleep. _____
5. Snoring is not harmful as long as it doesn't disturb others or wake you up. _____
6. Everyone dreams every night. _____
7. The older you get, the fewer hours of sleep you need. _____
8. Most people don't know when they are sleepy. _____
9. Raising the volume of your radio will help you stay awake while driving. _____
10. Sleep disorders are due mainly to worry or psychological problems. _____
11. The human body never adjusts to a night shift. _____
12. Most sleep disorders go away even without treatment. _____

From P. Walters and J. Byl, 2008, *Christian paths to health and wellness* (Champaign, IL: Human Kinetics). Reprinted, by permission, from National Sleep Foundation, 1999, *The sleep quiz* (Washington, DC: National Sleep Foundation).

Answers to Sleep Quiz

1. *False.* Though your body rests, your brain doesn't. While you sleep, your brain prepares you for mental alertness and peak functioning the next day, especially during the REM (rapid eye movement) phase.

2. *True.* The need for sleep is biologically encoded. Although children need more sleep than adults, how much sleep any individual needs is genetically determined. Most adults need around eight hours of sleep to function at their best. You can teach yourself to sleep less, but not to need less sleep.

3. *False.* People usually don't feel tired when they are active, but when they take a break from activity or feel bored, they may notice that they are sleepy. The main cause of sleepiness is sleep deprivation. Boredom doesn't cause sleepiness; it merely reveals it.

(continued)

4. *True.* Sleep is as necessary to your health as food and water are, and rest is no substitute for it. When you don't get the sleep you need, your body builds up a **sleep debt** that can only be paid with sleep.

5. *False.* Snoring may indicate the presence of a life-threatening sleep disorder called **sleep apnea**. People with sleep apnea snore loudly and awaken repeatedly during the night gasping for breath. These repeated awakenings lead to severe daytime sleepiness, which increases risk of accidents and heart problems. Ninety-five percent of people with sleep apnea remain unaware that they have a serious disorder.

6. *True.* Most people don't remember their dreams, but everyone does dream every night. Dreams are most vivid during REM sleep.

7. *False.* Sleep needs remain constant throughout adulthood. Older people often awaken more frequently and sleep less during the night, but they tend to make up for that during the day. Sleep difficulties are *not* a normal or inevitable part of aging, although they are too common. If poor sleeping habits, pain, or other health conditions make sleeping difficult, a physician can help.

8. *True.* Researchers have seen thousands of people answer "no" to the question "Are you sleepy?" only to fall asleep as soon as they are given the opportunity!

9. *False.* If you're having trouble staying awake while driving, the only short-term solution is to pull over to a safe place and take a short nap or have a caffeinated drink. Doing both—for example, drinking coffee and then napping before the caffeine kicks in—may be even better. Studies show that loud music, gum chewing, and open windows all fail to keep sleepy drivers alert. The only long-term solution is to start out well-rested after a good night's sleep.

10. *False.* Most people who report **insomnia** (difficulty falling asleep or staying asleep) give stress as the reason. But stress only accounts for a fraction of sleep disorders, which have a variety of causes. Sleep apnea, for instance, is caused by the obstruction of the airway during sleep. Narcolepsy, whose symptoms are severe daytime sleepiness and sudden sleep attacks, appears to be genetic. No one knows what causes restless legs syndrome, in which uncomfortable sensations in the legs occur and are relieved temporarily by motion.

11. *True.* Human beings, like all other living things, have **circadian rhythms** that affect when they feel alert and when they feel sleepy ("circadian" means "around the day," that is, at 24-hour intervals). The rhythms are set by the cycle of daylight. During travel across time zones, your body quickly adjusts because the cycle changes; but when you work a night shift, your body never adjusts because this cycle does not change. No matter what shift you work, even if you have been working it for years, you will feel sleepy between midnight and 6:00 a.m. and will have trouble sleeping during the day. If you have to work nights, however, avoid caffeine during the last half of your shift, stay away from alcohol and stimulating activities before you go to bed, and block out as much light and noise as you can when going to sleep.

12. *False.* Sleep disorders must be treated. Unfortunately, many people who have them don't realize they are problems that *can* be treated. The cure may be surgical, pharmacological, behavioral (for example, going to sleep and waking up at the same time every day, scheduling naps, or losing weight), or a combination of these. Untreated sleep disorders can ruin your quality of life, your performance at work, and your relationships with other people.

Are You Sleep Deprived?

The test on this page, devised by the Stanford University Center for the Diagnosis and Treatment of Sleep Disorders, is simple and reliable (Maas, 1999).

Sleep Deprivation Quiz

Answer Yes or No to the following five questions *based on your behavior over the last six months.*

1. Do you frequently fall asleep if given a sleep opportunity? (A *sleep opportunity* is defined as at least 10 minutes in a cool, dark, and quiet environment.)
2. Do you frequently need an alarm clock to wake up?
3. Do you frequently catch up on sleep during weekends?
4. Do you frequently take naps during the day?
5. When you wake up, do you feel tired most mornings?

From P. Walters and J. Byl, 2008, *Christian paths to health and wellness* (Champaign, IL: Human Kinetics).

Notes on These Questions on Sleep Deprivation

1. This question may be hard for you to answer, especially if your day is so busy that you rarely have sleep opportunities. But if the mere thought of 10 minutes in a cool, dark, and quiet room seems very appealing to you, chances are you may need them!

2. Forty-six percent of American adults answer yes to this question (National Sleep Foundation, 1995). Figure 10.6 identifies the frequency with which adults, 18 years of age and older, reported needing an alarm clock to wake up. An alarm clock is an artificial way to wake up and disturbs natural sleep rhythms. After a restful night of sleep, your sleep will become progressively lighter until you wake up automatically—a healthier and more pleasant way to get yourself out of bed.

3. According to the National Sleep Foundation, more than half of adults sleep for longer

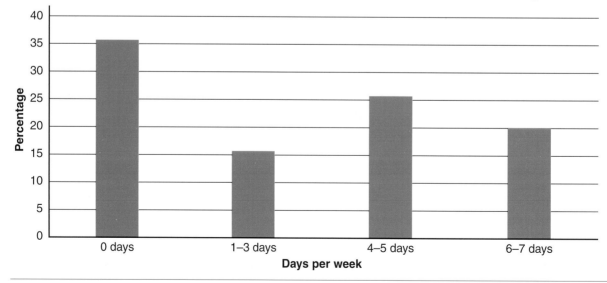

Percentage of adults who report needing an alarm clock to wake up in the morning

FIGURE 10.6   Approximately 65 percent of adults use an alarm clock to wake up.

Adapted from National Sleep Foundation, 2001.

on weekends than on weekdays (National Sleep Foundation, 2001).

4. More than half of surveyed college students report napping during the day (National Sleep Foundation, 2001). Adults take fewer naps than children do for the simple reason that sleeping on the job is generally frowned upon.

5. That is, do you wake up feeling refreshed, or do you need a tow truck to drag you out of bed? This has nothing to do with whether you're a "morning person" or not. By *refreshed*, I don't mean eager to do jumping jacks or to solve complex academic problems, but rather having a sense of being rested and regenerated by your night's sleep. More than half of younger adults answer yes to this question—that is, they don't feel refreshed in the mornings.

If you answered yes to two or more of the questions, you need more sleep. This puts you in a category with two-thirds of the U.S. population (National Sleep Foundation, 2001).

World Record for Sleeplessness

Realizing they could not talk Tripp out of his objective, Cornelison and West decided to take advantage of this rare research opportunity and agreed to observe him. On January 20, 1959, Tripp began. Confidently broadcasting from a glass booth in the middle of Times Square, he announced his plan to break the world record. He told listeners that he was in the best physical condition of his life and that a team of medical professionals would be with him around the clock, monitoring his health and making sure he didn't fall asleep.

Tripp's first symptom, predictably, was drowsiness. During his regular broadcasts he felt as good as ever, but the hours between seemed to stretch on endlessly. The EEGs, blood and urine analyses, and psychological tests that he took each day helped keep him from nodding off, but the medical staff constantly had to prod him to keep him awake.

After 48 hours, Tripp's mood changed dramatically. The usually good-natured and easygoing disc jockey became irritable and easily angered. Getting a haircut from his favorite barber, whom he had known for years, Tripp began to ridicule the man and finally swore at him so harshly that he brought the barber to tears.

By the third day, Tripp's mental abilities began to decline. Instead of his famous fast-paced chatter, he spoke in slow and cumbersome sentences and often seemed to be at a loss for words. He could no longer concentrate on anything, and he began to have difficulty remembering things. Even worse, he began to experience mental delusions. Changing his shoes, he noticed a cobweb in one of them that wasn't there. Specks on the table seemed to be scurrying about like insects. He became convinced that a rabbit was running loose in the broadcasting booth.

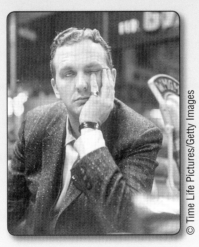
Tripp struggling to stay awake.

© Time Life Pictures/Getty Images

After five days, the hallucinations became more vivid and more frequent. A doctor's tie was jumping out of place. Furry worms swarmed about on another doctor's coat. When Tripp opened a drawer, flames spurted out. He heard voices. Tripp was certain that the staff was playing practical jokes on him, but he was actually dreaming while he was awake. By the seventh day, the sleepless DJ often could no longer remember who or where he was.

(continued)

(continued)

On the morning of the eighth day, the situation reached a crisis. For days Tripp had been imagining, with increasing intensity, a terrible conspiracy against him. Now, as a well-known neurologist, dressed in black, had him undress and lie down on the examining table, Tripp had a sudden "realization." He thought the man was an undertaker who had come to bury him alive! Screaming in terror, Tripp fled the examination room and ran naked down the corridor. Cornelison had to tackle him to keep him from running out of the building. Everyone on the observation team was very concerned but, less than 24 hours away from his goal, they decided to continue. Somehow Tripp managed to finish the day, and after his evening broadcast and a final battery of tests, he went to bed and slept for 24 straight hours. He held the world record for consecutive hours awake: an amazing 201.

Tripp awoke calm and refreshed, his terrors and hallucinations gone. It appeared that the effects of more than eight days of sleep deprivation had been completely cured by one day of sleep. But his wife was the first to perceive that something had changed inside him. His happy-go-lucky demeanor had soured into a pessimistic and argumentative one. They began to fight, and eventually divorced. On the air, too, people noticed a difference, and his ratings began to drop. For the rest of his life, Tripp wandered from town to town and from job to job, unable to establish roots. Those 201 sleepless hours were the defining moments of his career—but not in the way he had expected.

In 1964, a 17-year-old high school student broke Tripp's 1959 record (Veasey et al., 2002). Randy Gardner stayed awake for 264 hours with the help of friends, TV, reporters, and pinball. Despite the fact that Gardner reported no detrimental effects, Lt. Commander John Ross of the U.S. Naval Medical Neuropsychiatric Research Unit said that on the fourth day Gardner had a delusion that he was a famous football player. He later mistook a street sign for a person. On the eleventh day he was asked to count down from 100 by sevens. He stopped at 65 because he forgot what he was doing (Veasey et al., 2002). Several sleep experts agree that long-term sleep deprivation has the potential for serious consequences (Coren, 1996; Dement & Vaughan, 1999; Veasey, et al., 2002).

One clear message from these two experiments is that extreme sleep deprivation is dangerous and should not be attempted by anyone without close medical supervision.

Bullman & Milne, 1998; Coren, 1996.

The Effects of Sleep Deprivation

Peter Tripp's experiences are a fairly accurate case study of the consequences of sleep deprivation (see sidebars on pages 231 and 239-240). The following is a more formal list of the six effects of sleeplessness, in the order in which they usually occur:

1. General fatigue
2. Emotional irritability
3. Cognitive impairment
4. Physical impairment
5. Psychosis
6. Death

General Fatigue

The first symptom is a general feeling of drowsiness and lack of energy. According to some experts, fatigue is the fastest-growing health problem reported by adults in developed nations. According to one study, in less than a century there has been almost a 60 percent growth in the number of individuals who report being tired in the morning and sluggish throughout the day (Pasztor, 1996).

Fatigue doesn't feel good, but the real danger is that it dramatically increases the chances of getting in an accident.

- The U.S. National Highway Safety Administration estimates that approximately 100,000 accidents, 71,000 injuries, 15,000 deaths, and $12.5 billion in monetary losses per year are directly attributable to drowsy drivers (National Sleep Foundation, 2007a).

- According to the National Transportation Safety Board, fatigue is the number one factor that detrimentally impacts the ability of pilots (Pasztor, 1996).

- Sixty-two percent of adults (72 percent of men and 54 percent of women) reported driving while feeling drowsy; 27 percent (36 percent of men and 20 percent of women) said they dozed off while driving in the past year (National Sleep Foundation, 2007a).

- In a report submitted to Congress by the National Commission on Sleep Disorders, 56 percent of shift workers reported falling asleep at least once a week while on the job (National Commission on Sleep Disorders Research, 1993).

- Sleep-related crashes are most common in young people, who tend to stay up late, sleep too little, and drive at night. A study by the state of North Carolina found that 55 percent of such crashes involved people aged 25 or younger (National Sleep Foundation, 2007a).

The good news is that fatigue is easily dealt with. One study indicated that alertness increased by approximately 25 percent with just one additional hour of sleep (Leung & Becker, 1992).

Emotional Irritability

People with sleep deprivation are more prone to depression, irritability, anger, frustration, and anxiety (Stickgold, Winkelman, & Wehrwein, 2004). Furthermore, good emotional memories are reinforced and bad ones dampened during certain phases of sleep. One scientist speculates that if someone sleeps well following a distressing experience, he or she may be less likely to have post-traumatic stress syndrome. In the most recent poll conducted by the National Sleep Foundation, a new group of questions was added to investigate the relationships between sleep and the emotional health of teenagers (National Sleep Foundation, 2005). Some of the results included the following:

- 73 percent of students who reported being the most unhappy, tense, and nervous said they consistently did not get enough sleep.

- 55 percent of the students with the best mood compared to 20 percent of the students with the worst mood reported getting the sleep they needed most nights.

- 59 percent of students with the worst mood said they "often feel too tired," compared to 19 percent of the students with the best mood.

- 51 of the students with the worst mood compared to 18 percent of students with the best mood said they had trouble falling asleep.

Christians have a tendency to overspiritualize things. But moods and emotions have a physical component, and sometimes the best remedy for a short fuse or a bad attitude is not more prayer or Bible study but simply more sleep. Any mother will tell you how greatly sleep affects her child's temper. Needing sleep is one thing people don't grow out of.

Cognitive Impairment

An old joke: "Q. How do you get to Carnegie Hall? A. Practice, practice, practice." A new finding: Sleep between practice sessions may be just as crucial to success. According to a recent Harvard experiment, people's scores on memory tests improve when they sleep soundly for at least six hours the night after they learn something. But if they are deprived of sleep the night after they learn it, their memory of it will never improve, even if they sleep normally on subsequent nights (Moore-Ede, 1993).

Students don't have to choose between bed and books. Better grades come with more, not less, sleep. Researchers who compared academic records to sleep questionnaires for both high school students and medical students found that the ones with the best grades consistently reported sleeping longer. The moral of this story is that the way to get more As is to get more Zs (Moore-Ede, 1993).

Physical Impairment

It's true that Peter Tripp did not show any signs of physical impairment during his wakeathon except for a drop in core body temperature. Keep in mind, though, that his job didn't require much fitness and that he didn't do any physical activity except a

Gentleness

I recall an elder in a church who valued men wearing a tie and suit for a church service. The elder met a man at church who was dressed neatly but who was not wearing a suit and tie. The elder gruffly spoke to the other man, "Why aren't you dressed!?" The other man felt his heart sink, and with tears in his eyes he left the worship service before it ever began. Harshness in our words and actions can severely wound others.

Gentleness is a gift from the Holy Spirit (2 Corinthians 10:1). Christ's kingly mission on earth was exemplified in gentleness (Matthew 21:5; Zechariah 9:9). Jesus invites people: "Come to me, all you who are weary and burdened, and I will give you rest. Take my yoke upon you and learn from me, for I am gentle and humble in heart, and you will find rest for your souls" (Matthew 11:28–29). "Like a lamb to the slaughter" (Isaiah 53:7), Jesus died on the cross to bring peace and rest, or wellness.

The Bible teaches that gentleness must especially be evident in those in leadership positions (1 Timothy 3:3), because people grow when nurtured by gentleness. Perhaps more importantly, gentleness is a sign of "God's chosen people" (Colossians 3:12). This gift must be put to use. For example, scripture encourages restoring with gentleness a person caught in sin (Galatians 6:1; 1 Peter 3:15). Gentleness does not produce anxiety precipitated by fear, but recovery nurtured by love. Healing takes place through gentle restoration.

There is a happy ending to the story of the gruff elder. The elder and offended person later met for coffee to reconcile their differences. As the elder apologized, he confided that he was having difficulties in his own life, and that his gruffness and cutting humor were inappropriate ways of coping with those difficulties. The elder's gruffness put a barrier between the two people before worship; gentleness and forgiveness over coffee brought healing. Lack of gentleness brings pain; gentleness brings healing and wellness.

Gentleness: If you lacked gentleness in a recent situation, apologize to that person and experience the Spirit's powerful healing. Describe.

_____

_____

_____

_____

_____

_____

little bit of walking. We now know that sleep deprivation decelerates reaction time (see figure 10.7) (Kribbs & Dinges, 1994; National Sleep Foundation, 2007c), diminishes muscular strength (Reilly & Piercy, 1994), and decreases cardiorespiratory endurance by as much as 11 percent (Martin, 1981; National Sleep Foundation, 2007c).

Psychosis

Political, military, and religious groups have long used sleep deprivation as a means of brainwashing and torture. Sleep deprivation causes people to become emotionally unstable and lose their grip on reality. Although the thought of seeing space aliens or singing frogs may seem funny, the consequences can be quite serious. For obvious reasons, few experiments have been done in which subjects are extensively sleep deprived, so many questions about these later stages remain unanswered. Case studies such as Tripp's, however, indicate that permanent damage may occur (Bullman & Milne, 1998; Coren, 1996).

Death

Any animal will eventually die if not permitted to sleep. Rats will die after about two weeks (Wikipedia, 2005). It's very difficult to kill people this way because they will begin to experience several-second intervals of "microsleep;" but a rare, incurable hereditary disease called *fatal familial insomnia* completely eliminates the ability to sleep, with deadly results (Wikipedia, 2005).

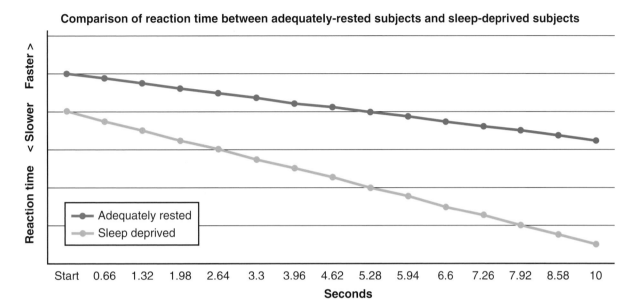

Comparison of reaction time between adequately-rested subjects and sleep-deprived subjects

Seconds: Start, 0.66, 1.32, 1.98, 2.64, 3.3, 3.96, 4.62, 5.28, 5.94, 6.6, 7.26, 7.92, 8.58, 10

— Adequately rested
— Sleep deprived

FIGURE 10.7   Reaction time decreases with sleeplessness.

Data from Kribbs and Dinges, 1994.

Keeping the Sabbath?

From ancient civilizations to modern society, people from every part of the globe have set aside one day of the week for physical and spiritual renewal. In fact, each of the seven days of the week has been designated as a Sabbath at one time.

Sabbath Around the World

Monday	Greek
Tuesday	Persian
Wednesday	Assyrian
Thursday	Egyptian
Friday	Turkish
Saturday	Jewish
Sunday	Christian

Tan, 1982.

Jews and Christians have debated the rules of the Sabbath for more than 2,000 years. The Talmud, which contains a vast array of ancient Jewish laws, has 24 chapters and 38 subcategories dedicated to Sabbath regulations.

In this point/counterpoint discussion, I am going to limit the focus to one simple question. Should 21st-century Christians set aside one day of the week for renewal? For sake of continuity, I'll call this unique day a Sabbath. I won't discuss particulars, such as what day of the week Sabbath should be, spiritual practices that should be included, or behaviors that should be prohibited.

Proponents of setting aside one day of the week for rest are quick to point out God's example in the creation narrative in Genesis. After six days of work, the creator God rested.

(continued)

Thus the heavens and the earth were completed in all their vast array. By the seventh day God had finished the work he had been doing; so on the seventh day he rested from all his work. And God blessed the seventh day and made it holy, because on it he rested from all the work of creating that he had done. (Genesis 2:1–3)

Not only did God rest, but he also blessed this day and made it holy. When God gave Moses what we now know as the Ten Commandments, he referred back to his creation example and commanded the Israelites to do likewise.

Remember the Sabbath day by keeping it holy. Six days you shall labor and do all your work, but the seventh day is a Sabbath to the Lord your God. On it you shall not do any work, neither you, nor your son or daughter, nor your manservant or maidservant, nor your animals, nor the alien within your gates. For in six days the Lord made the heavens and the earth, the sea, and all that is in them, but he rested on the seventh day. Therefore, the Lord blessed the Sabbath day and made it holy. (Exodus 20:8–11)

Many noteworthy Christians have chosen to abide by God's command to keep the Sabbath, in some cases to their personal detriment.

Perhaps one of the most notable examples in the 20th century was Eric Liddell, a Scottish track star whose story became popular through the movie *Chariots of Fire* (Hudson, 1981). Liddell refused to run in an Olympic qualifying race because it was being held on Sunday, despite the threat of his not being able to participate in the 1924 Olympic Games.

Like Liddlell, many Christians in the 19th and 20th centuries were quite serious about not working on the Sabbath. The first man of flight, Wilbur Wright, refused an appeal of the King of Spain who requested an aerial display on Sunday (Tan, 1982). And former president Ulysses S. Grant refused an invitation of the president of France to join his entourage for a day at the races:

It is not in accord with the custom of my country, or with the spirit of my religion to spend Sunday in that way. I will go to the house of God. (Tan, 1982, p. 1,389)

History is filled with individuals who advised others of the merits of Sabbath renewal:

"Sunday is the golden clasp that binds together the volume of the week."

—Henry Wadsworth Longfellow (1807–1882) (Draper, 1992, p. 956)

"If your soul has no Sunday, it becomes an orphan."

—Physician and missionary, Albert Schweitzer (Gibbs, 2004, p. 90)

"Jesus spoke about the ox in the ditch on the Sabbath. But if your ox gets in the ditch every Sabbath, you should either get rid of the ox or fill up the ditch."

—Billy Graham (Draper, 1992, p. 109)

There are some spiritually minded Christians, however, who believe that the practice of keeping a Sabbath is not a model for Christians today.

Although God rested on the Sabbath, Jesus seemed to disobey many of the Jewish Sabbath laws right in front of religious officials.

- Matthew 12:1–7 Picks grain for consumption on the Sabbath
- Matthew 12:9-14 Heals a man with a shriveled hand on the Sabbath
- Luke 13:10–17 Heals a woman who had been crippled for 18 years on the Sabbath
- Luke 14:1–6 Heals a man suffering from dropsy on the Sabbath
- John 5:1–18 Heals an invalid by the pool of Bethesda, then orders him to unlawfully pick up and carry his mat on the Sabbath
- John 9:13–16 Heals a blind man with cakes of mud on the Sabbath

(continued)

Each time Jesus was questioned by the religious leaders about his disrespect for the Sabbath, he responded by showing he cared more about loving people than properly keeping the Sabbath: "The Sabbath was made for man, not man for the Sabbath" (Mark 2:27).

In addition to Christ's behavior, additional support for not keeping the Sabbath is the fact that the commandment to keep the Sabbath is the only one of the Ten Commandments not repeated in the New Testament (Lawrence, 1990).

Other passages add to the scriptural evidence that keeping the Sabbath was a command relevant to Old Testament believers but not required for New Testament disciples. Note what Paul says concerning the Sabbath in his letter to the Colossians:

> When you were dead in your sins and in the uncircumcision of your sinful nature, God made you alive with Christ. He forgave us all our sins, having canceled the written code, with its regulations, that was against us and that stood opposed to us; he took it away, nailing it to the cross. And having disarmed the powers and authorities, he made a public spectacle of them, triumphing over them by the cross. Therefore do not let anyone judge you by what you eat or drink, or with regard to a religious festival, a New Moon celebration or a Sabbath day. These are a shadow of the things that were to come; the reality, however, is found in Christ. (Colossians 2:13–17)

In his letter to the Galatians, Paul urges followers of Christ not to be enslaved by the old system of keeping the law, which seems to include having particular days be "special."

> Formerly, when you did not know God, you were slaves to those who by nature are not gods. But now that you know God—or rather are known by God—how is it that you are turning back to those weak and miserable principles? Do you wish to be enslaved by them all over again? You are observing special days and months and seasons and years! I fear for you, that somehow I have wasted my efforts on you. (Galatians 4:8–11)

Finally, some scholars believe that New Testament believers should strive for perpetual rest in Christ instead of rest only one day each week.

> There remains, then, a Sabbath-rest for the people of God; for anyone who enters God's rest also rests from his own work, just as God did from his. Let us, therefore, make every effort to enter that rest, so that no one will fall by following their example of disobedience. (Hebrews 4:9–11)

As you can see from these opposing positions, scripture passages seem to support conflicting viewpoints. Which view do you believe God desires for his disciples today?

Most people will never experience the more severe and dangerous symptoms of sleeplessness. Still, many will go through their lives tired and cranky. Without the energy to remember birthdays or write letters or return phone calls, or the spirit to make jokes or take risks or have adventures, they will find it hard to build meaningful relationships. Instead of being a "fountain of joy," people become a drain. Worst of all, these people may be so exhausted that they don't even care. Those who say, "I'll sleep when I'm dead," may miss out on a lot while they're alive.

The Architecture of Sleep

Sleep stages fall into two broad categories: **rapid eye movement (REM)** and **non-rapid eye movement (NREM)**. NREM is the deeper type of sleep, and most physical restoration happens during NREM. **Electroencephalography (EEG)**, which measures **brain waves,** shows that each of the four stages of NREM has its own distinctive brain wave pattern, as you can see in figure 10.8. These are the four stages of NREM:

Stage 1. **Theta brain waves**

Stage 2. Theta brain waves with sleep spindles and K complexes

Stage 3. Theta and **delta brain waves**

Stage 4. Delta brain waves

Stages 1 and 2 of NREM

In the first stage of NREM sleep, which lasts between 10 seconds and 10 minutes, your heart rate, breathing rate, and metabolic rate all decrease, and your muscles begin to relax. You begin to disengage from the world around you. Most people in stage 1 sleep, however, can be awakened by a gentle nudge or a soft whisper and will claim that they weren't asleep yet. The second stage is where theta brain waves are mixed with **sleep spindles** and K complexes. Stage 2 lasts between 5 and 20 minutes and is a transition between light sleep and deep sleep. People awakened at this point typically acknowledge that they were, indeed, asleep.

Stages 3 and 4 of NREM

Moving into deeper stages, the third and fourth stage of sleep in amplitude and low in frequency is characterized by high delta brain waves. That is why these stages are also called *slow wave sleep*. The third stage is another transitional phase, and lasts between 5 and 20 minutes. Stage 4 sleep is the deepest stage of sleep. Blood supply to the brain drops, and all but the essential bodily functions shut down. Stage 4 lasts between 5 and 40

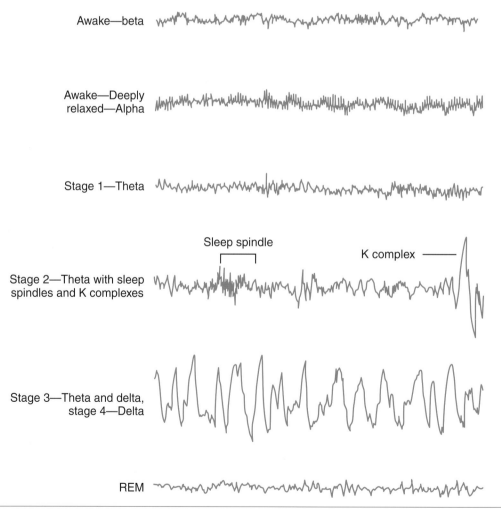

FIGURE 10.8   Electroencephalograph images of various stages of wakefulness and sleep.

Adapted from Encarta, 2004.

minutes. Stage 3 and 4 sleep is where the majority of physical restoration occurs. During these stages, 80 percent of our daily amount of growth hormone is released. This places the body in a super compensation mode. Our skin cells multiply at twice the normal rate, the body defends itself against pathogens, and the immune system rejuvenates. Deep sleep is like getting a major "tune-up" for the body. So just how important is sleep for physical growth and development? Animal and human studies have both demonstrated that prolonged failure to get deep sleep can permanently stunt growth (Obal et al., 2003; Bonuck, Parikh, & Bassila, 2006).

REM Sleep

At this point, approximately an hour after you fell asleep, blood flow to your brain increases, your body temperature rises, and your pulse, respiration, and blood pressure all begin to quicken. Under your closed eyelids, your eyes begin to rapidly dart back and forth. It is from this strange phenomenon that REM sleep gets its name. Most dreams occur during the REM phase, which lasts between 1 and 20 minutes; when awakened from REM sleep, more than half of sleepers report that they were dreaming. While your eyes race, your body is paralyzed because all motor signals are blocked at the brainstem. Experts believe that this is to keep you from acting out your dreams. In rare cases this protective mechanism fails, as it did for the unfortunate young man who dreamed he was an NFL player and tried to tackle the wall beside his bed (Moore-Ede & LeVert, 1998)! REM sleep is essential for mental renewal; like a librarian that reshelves books and magazines, the brain organizes mental material during REM sleep.

You have now completed one **sleep cycle**. This entire sequence will be repeated several times a night, depending on how much you sleep. In subsequent cycles, however, deep sleep is shorter and REM sleep is longer. Each cycle takes about 90 minutes.

How Much Sleep Do You Need?

It depends. If you are a. . .

Giant sloth, koala	20 hours per 24-hour period
Opossum	19
Cat	16
Dog	15
Mouse	13
Jaguar	10
Chimpanzee	9
Human, rabbit, pig, rhinoceros	8
Gray seal, dolphin	6
Cow, goat, donkey, sheep	4
Horse, elephant	3

Becker, 2005; Bestfriendspetcare.com, 2007; Encarta, 2004.

The general recommendation for human beings is to get about eight hours of sleep a night. This figure comes from two sources: the statistical average for men and women who were allowed to sleep as much or as little as they wanted, and a study published in the *Journal of Sleep Research* that examined sleep and mortality rates (Wingard & Berkman, 1983). Keep in mind, though, that this is an average, and that individual sleep needs can vary significantly from it (Dement & Vaughan, 1999). Thomas Edison got by with four hours of sleep a night, and Bill Clinton with only five or six. On the other hand, Albert Einstein needed 10, and Calvin Coolidge 11 (Coren, 1996)! Sleep need is like shoe size: the average man wears a size 9-1/2 (8-1/2 UK; 42-1/2 Continental), but shoe stores still sell plenty of pairs of 8s (7s and 40-1/2s) and 13s (12s and 47s). Furthermore, sleep needs are dynamic before age 20, as you can see in table 10.1 (Condor, 2001).

Determining *your* personal sleep needs requires no special equipment or expert assistance, but it does take a little bit of discipline. First, set yourself a regular bedtime to stabilize your biological clock. Second, make sure you are not disturbed or awakened in the morning. A good time to do this experiment might be when you are on vacation and have no early morning demands. Third, simply let nature take its course. Students who do this usually report sleeping 10 to 12 hours the first night, 9 to 10 hours the next few nights, and then progressively shorter periods until their sleep becomes regular. During the first few nights they are paying back accrued sleep debt. Within two weeks, most people find that their sleep time stabilizes between seven and nine hours. I must emphasize again, though, that sleep needs are individual. Don't force yourself into a sleep pattern; relax and see what happens. You will be amazed at how your body develops a natural sleep rhythm, how you no longer need an alarm clock, and how great you feel. People say they feel lighter, charged with energy, able to focus like never before, and are less troubled by people and circumstances. They are experiencing sleep the way God designed it.

Table 10.1 The Changing Sleep Requirements of Children

Age	Hours of sleep needed
Newborn	16 – 18 hours broken up throughout the day
1 year	14 hours, including one or two naps
2 years	11 – 12 hours, including an afternoon nap
3 years	12 – 12.5 hours; some children stop taking naps by this age
4 years	11.5 – 12 hours; more children stop taking naps by this age
5 years	11 hours; most children stop taking naps by this age
6 years	10.75 – 11 hours
7 years	10.5 – 11 hours
8 years	10.25 – 10.75 hours
9 years	10 – 10.33 hours
10 years to puberty	9.75 – 10 hours
Adolescent	9.25 hours

Adapted from Condor, 2001.

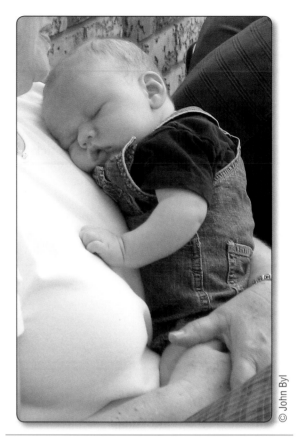

© John Byl

Many people wish they **could** sleep this soundly.

How to Sleep Like a Log

The expression "sleep like a log" is somewhat inaccurate, first because of how much goes on inside the brain while you sleep (as you have just learned), and second because most people shift posture about 20 times during the night (Maas, 1998). "Sleep like a baby" is probably a worse comparison, however. Do you really want to sleep irregularly for 17 hours a day, frequently waking up and crying? Here are some suggestions for having good **sleep hygiene**—a term recently coined to describe quality sleeping habits.

1. **Establish a consistent sleep schedule.** Go to bed and wake up at the same time 365 days a year. Many experts believe that after getting enough sleep, this is the most important thing you can do to wake up feeling refreshed (Dement & Vaughan, 1999). As evidence, they cite the fact that 80 percent of shift workers report problems sleeping (Moore-Ede, 1993). Constantly changing your bedtime keeps your circadian rhythm from being established. You will be constantly off balance, as if someone were holding onto your arm while you are jogging. Fortunately, you don't need to go to bed and get up at *exactly* the same time every day. Changes of less than 30 minutes earlier or later will not adversely affect your biological clock (National Sleep Foundation, 2002). Benjamin Franklin popularized the proverb, "Early to bed, early to rise makes a man healthy, wealthy and wise." More accurately, the statement would be, "Consistently to bed, consistently to rise . . . ."

2. **Get regular exercise.** Some of the most troubled sleepers are elderly people. On average, they tend to sleep intermittently and get less deep sleep. Trying to discover how to improve this situation, researchers studied the effect of exercise on the sleeping behavior of older people. Sixty-seven adults aged 50 to 76 were divided into two groups. One group did 30 to 40 minutes of aerobic exercise at 60 to 70 percent of maximum heart rate, four times a week. The other group did not. After 16 weeks, the subjects in the exercise group took 50 percent less time to fall asleep and increased their quality sleep time by one hour (Dement &

Vaughan, 1999). This is not an isolated study, and its results are not only true for the aged. A careful analysis of 44 different studies shows that people who exercise consistently go to sleep faster, have longer bouts of deep sleep, and sleep longer than people who don't (Kubitz et al., 1996). One caveat: For some people, exercising too late in the day acts as a stimulant. They find that exercising in the evening makes it harder to go to sleep (Stickgold, Winkelman, & Wehrwein, 2004). If you are one of those people, do your exercise at least four hours before you go to bed.

3. **Establish a bedtime ritual.** This is one of the most common recommendations made by sleep experts (Coren, 1996; Dement & Vaughan, 1999; National Sleep Foundation, 2007b; Zammit, 1997). Many people say they nod off effortlessly after following a simple routine. Some popular rituals are drinking a glass of milk, reading a book, turning down the covers a certain way, taking a warm bath, or brushing and flossing their teeth. The routine must be regular and consistent to be effective. Many proponents of these rituals also recommend using your bed only for sleep. They believe that doing work, talking on the phone, or watching TV while in bed sends conflicting messages about what should happen there.

4. **Create a quality sleeping environment.** Three words: quiet, dark, and cool. Getting quiet can be difficult, especially if you live in a college dorm. Fortunately, earplugs can reduce noise, and there are other devices that produce "white noise," or soothing sounds like rain, waterfalls, or ocean waves, to mask disturbing noises. Many people find that they sleep better with the fan on.

You can make your room dark by getting opaque blinds for your windows, turning off your computer screen and other electronic devices, turning digital clocks away from you, and stuffing a towel under the door to eliminate light from the hallway. If those measures are not enough, you can purchase eye masks that block out light.

What's true of porridge is true of temperature for sleeping as well: Some like it hot; some like it cold. Couples who sleep together often squabble about it. Preferences about covers and bed temperature vary by individual, but the majority of people like the room they're sleeping in to be about 65 degrees Fahrenheit (18 degrees Celsius) (Maas, 1999).

5. **Invest in a quality bed and sleeping accessories.** Most people will spend almost a third of their lives (an average of 23.4 years) in bed, so making it comfortable is worth the investment.

- Generally, bigger is better. Make sure your bed is at least six inches (15.24 centimeters) longer than you are tall (Maas, 1999). If you sleep with someone else, don't settle for anything smaller than a queen-size mattress.

- When it comes to sheets, a well-recognized independent consumer group reported cotton as the winner (Consumer Reports, 2006b). In their investigation, the variables evaluated were comfort, ease of care, and durability. Cotton performed well in each of the three categories. Although there are a number of personal preferences in bedding, cotton is a good place to begin looking.

- Fold your pillow in half and squeeze out the air. A pillow with proper support will return to its original shape, but a broken one will stay folded. Down or feather pillows seem to be the most popular (Maas, 1999).

Consumer Watch: Mattresses and Sheets

Egyptian cotton, jersey knit, flax linen, cellulose modal, pima cotton, synthetic polyester, or smooth satin—what type of sheets are best? Will the quality of your sleep improve on a mattress made of space-age memory foam or one with adjustable air pressure? These are some of the questions facing consumers who are making choices about where and on what type of material they will spend one-third of their lives. An estimated 70 million Americans complain about sleeplessness, so there is plenty of need for wise advice (National Sleep Foundation, 2005). One popular consumer magazine receives more inquiries about mattresses than about any other product except cars (Consumer Reports, 2006a). Following are some sound suggestions that will make you a savvy shopper.

(continued)

(continued)

1. A comfortable mattress is a matter of personal opinion. There are no clear winners when it comes to mattress preferences (Consumer Reports, 2006a). The optimal surface is purely subjective, says Dr. Clete Kushida, director of the Stanford University Center for Human Sleep Research (Kushida, 2006). Because preferences for firmness, materials, and size vary so widely, it is critical to try before you buy. Do not be embarrassed—try lots of different mattresses before making a purchase. A good sales person should encourage you to take your shoes off and spend some time on your back, stomach, and side to find the mattress that feels best to you.

2. Contrary to popular opinion, if you have lower-back pain, a firm mattress is not always better. One study published in *The Lancet* suggested that people who have lower-back pain would benefit from a medium-firm sleeping surface (Kovacs, 2003). If a mattress is too firm, it won't support all body parts evenly and may cause discomfort at the heaviest points (hips and shoulders). If it's too soft, the person could sink into the surface and have a hard time moving. Dr. Alan Hedge, professor of ergonomics at Cornell University, noted that the best mattress supports the spine at all points while allowing it to maintain its natural curve (Consumer Reports, 2006a).

3. Thread count of sheets matters up to a point. Thread count is determined by counting the number of vertical and horizontal threads in one square inch (2.5 square centimeters) of fabric. Many manufacturers suggest higher thread counts are better. Yet a recent report examining the softness, durability, and comfort of sheets concluded that sheets between 200 and 400 threads per square inch rated highest overall. Thread counts exceeding 400 usually did not have increased benefits, only increased price.

4. When it comes to fabric, cotton is still king. In tests examining easy care, comfort, and durability, traditional cotton was the clear winner (Consumer Reports, 2006b). After 20 washings, many of the sheets made of luxury materials lost color, shrank so much they would no longer fit, or simply began to unravel.

5. Finally, you do not have to shop at specialty bedding stores to find high-quality cotton sheets with thread counts between 200 and 400. The highest rated sheet in one consumer magazine was a cotton sheet with thread count of 300 from the retail store Target (Consumer Reports, 2006b).

Only One Who Never Sleeps

I lift up my eyes to the hills—where does my help come from? My help comes from the Lord, the Maker of heaven and earth. He will not let your foot slip—he who watches over you will not slumber; indeed, he who watches over Israel will neither slumber nor sleep. (Psalm 121:1–4)

Next Steps

Robert Murray McCheyne (1813–1843) of Edinburgh, Scotland, was a young man ablaze with passion for Christ and His Kingdom. An ordained pastor of St. Peter's Church in Dundee when he was 23, McCheyne made such an impact that one listener said of him, "He preached with eternity stamped upon his brow. I trembled, and never felt God so near" (Rice, 2005). For the next six years McCheyne zealously and tirelessly presented the gospel of Jesus Christ to all who would listen. In 1839, he made a trip to the Holy Land to evangelize the Jews, and upon his return contributed to a great revival that swept across Scotland and northern England. Soon afterward, however, his health began to fail. Ignoring the urging of his concerned friends, he refused to rest and continued to push himself to the limit. Finally, as the young preacher lay on his deathbed at only 29 years of age, he whispered to a friend at his side, "God gave me a message to deliver and a horse to carry it.

Alas, I killed the horse, and now I cannot deliver the message" (Sanders, 1997, p. 136).

McCheyne's story dramatically and tragically shows that even a passion for the glory of God must be balanced with an understanding of physical limitations. God has infused rhythms everywhere in creation, from the rising and the setting of the sun; to the ebb and flow of the ocean's tides; to the waxing and waning of the moon; to the succession of the seasons; to the birth, growth, decay, and death of organic creatures; and to the repeating stages of the sleep cycle. It's important to respect and live by these rhythms rather than fight them, because the Lord has pronounced them "very good." Although the creator God does not sleep, He certainly does not begrudge his children their slumber. Verses in scripture that warn against sloth are balanced by others like Psalm 127:2, which says, "In vain you rise early and stay up late, toiling for food to eat—for he grants sleep to those he loves." Jesus urged his followers, "If anyone would come after me, he must deny himself and take up his cross and follow me" (Matthew 16:24). He also said, "Come to me, all you who are weary and burdened, and I will give you rest" (Matthew 11:28).

It is really a matter of balancing labor and leisure. Mother Teresa, who worked with the Sisters of Charity in Calcutta, India, acknowledged that a person's gifts and abilities are to be used up so she can be filled by God:

Our intellect and other gifts have been given to be used for God's greater glory, but sometimes they become the very god for us. That is the saddest part: We are losing our balance when this happens. We must free ourselves to be filled by God. (Draper, 1992, p. 109)

Key Terms

brain waves

circadian rhythm

delta brain waves

electroencephalography (EEG)

gentleness

insomnia

non-rapid eye movement (NREM)

rapid eye movement (REM)

sleep apnea

sleep cycle

sleep debt

sleep deprivation

sleep hygiene

sleep spindles

sleep stages

theta brain waves

Review Questions

1. To what degree is sleep deprivation a problem?

2. What societal changes have encouraged individuals to sleep less?

3. Identify the effects of sleep deprivation in the order in which they occur.

4. Diagram the stages and cycles of sleep.

5. Identify the process for determining how much sleep you need.

6. List several reasons for improving the quality of sleep.

Application Activities

1. Complete a more comprehensive sleep test to evaluate potential sleep problems at the Sleepnet Web site: www.sleepnet.com.

2. Keep a seven-day sleep/alertness log to evaluate your individual sleep, nap, and alertness levels. This can be especially helpful to students who want to study during periods of maximum alertness.

Sleep/Alertness Log

Degree of Alertness

5: Feeling active, vital, alert, or wide awake

4: Functioning at a high level but not at my peak

3: Awake, relaxed; responsive but not fully alert

2: Lethargic, sluggish, slow

1: Foggy, losing interest in remaining awake

0: Fighting sleep

| Fill out this section when you rise in the morning. | | | | | | | Fill out during waking hours. |
Date	Bedtime	Time until sleep onset	Number of awakenings, total length	Rise time	Number of naps, total length (yesterday)	Sleep time	See above (degree of alertness 0-5)
							1A 2A 3A 4A 5A 6A 7A 8A 9A 10A 11A 12N 1P 2P 3P 4P 5P 6P 7P 8P 9P 10P 11P 12MN
							1A 2A 3A 4A 5A 6A 7A 8A 9A 10A 11A 12N 1P 2P 3P 4P 5P 6P 7P 8P 9P 10P 11P 12MN
							1A 2A 3A 4A 5A 6A 7A 8A 9A 10A 11A 12N 1P 2P 3P 4P 5P 6P 7P 8P 9P 10P 11P 12MN
							1A 2A 3A 4A 5A 6A 7A 8A 9A 10A 11A 12N 1P 2P 3P 4P 5P 6P 7P 8P 9P 10P 11P 12MN
							1A 2A 3A 4A 5A 6A 7A 8A 9A 10A 11A 12N 1P 2P 3P 4P 5P 6P 7P 8P 9P 10P 11P 12MN
							1A 2A 3A 4A 5A 6A 7A 8A 9A 10A 11A 12N 1P 2P 3P 4P 5P 6P 7P 8P 9P 10P 11P 12MN
							1A 2A 3A 4A 5A 6A 7A 8A 9A 10A 11A 12N 1P 2P 3P 4P 5P 6P 7P 8P 9P 10P 11P 12MN
							1A 2A 3A 4A 5A 6A 7A 8A 9A 10A 11A 12N 1P 2P 3P 4P 5P 6P 7P 8P 9P 10P 11P 12MN
7-day average (total of weekly averages)							1A 2A 3A 4A 5A 6A 7A 8A 9A 10A 11A 12N 1P 2P 3P 4P 5P 6P 7P 8P 9P 10P 11P 12MN

From P. Walters and J. Byl, 2008, *Christian paths to health and wellness* (Champaign, IL: Human Kinetics).

References

Becker, M. (2005). How much do dogs sleep? *The Daily Item* (August 10).

Bestfriendspetcare.com. (2007). How long do cats sleep? Retrieved June 27, 2007, from www.bestfriendspetcare.com/Pet_FAQs/cats-sleep.cfm.

Bonuck, K., Parikh, S., & Bassila, M. (2006). Growth failure and sleep disordered breathing: A review of the literature. *International Journal of Pediatric Otorhinolaryngology, 70*(5): 769-778.

Bullman, J., & Milne, C. (1998). *The sleep files* [3 videocassettes (ca. 156 min.)]. New York: Ambrose Video.

Condor, B. (2001). Early to bed. *Chicago Tribune*: 1, 6.

Consumer Reports. (2006a). How to buy a mattress without losing sleep. *Consumer Reports* (June).

Consumer Reports. (2006b). Sheets: Wake-up call. *Consumer Reports* (June).

Coren, S. (1996). *Sleep thieves: An eye-opening exploration into the science and mysteries of sleep.* New York: The Free Press.

Dement, W., & Vaughan, C. (1999). *The promise of sleep.* New York: Delacorte Press.

Draper, E. (1992). *Draper's book of quotations for the Christian world.* Wheaton: Tyndale House.

Encarta. (2004). Dictionary/encyclopedia. Retrieved June 24, 2004, from http://encarta.msn.com/Default.aspx.

Gibbs, N. (2004). And on the seventh day we rested. *Time, 164*(5):90-91.

Health Square. (2007). Lockjaw: What you should know. Retrieved August 9, 2006, from www.healthsquare.com/mc/fgmc9036.htm.

Hudson, H. (1981). *Chariots of fire.* United Kingdom: Ladd Company & Warner brothers.

Kovacs, F.M. (2003). Effect of firmness of mattress on chronic non-specific low-back pain. *The Lancet, 362* (November 15): 1594-1595.

Kribbs, N.D., & Dinges, D. (1994). Vigilance decrement and sleepiness. In J.O.R. Harsh (Ed.), *Sleep onset mechanisms* (pp. 113-125). Washington, DC: American Psychological Association.

Kubitz, K.A., Landers, D.M., Petruzzello, S.J., & Han, M. (1996). The effects of acute and chronic exercise on sleep: A meta-analytic review. *Sports Medicine, 21*: 277-291.

Kushida, C. (2006). *Sleep deprivation: Basic science, physiology, and behavior.* Philadelphia, PA: Taylor & Francis.

Lawrence, R. (1990). *365 devotional commentary.* Colorado Springs, CO: Cook Communications Ministries.

Leung, L., & Becker, C.E. (1992). Sleep deprivation and house staff performance. *Journal of Occupational Medicine, 34*: 1153-1160.

Maas, J.B. (1998). *Asleep in the fast lane: Our 24-hour society.* Ithaca, NY: Cornell University Psychology Film Unit.

Maas, J.B. (1999). *Power sleep* (1st ed.). New York: Harper Perennial.

Martin, B.J. (1981). Effects of sleep deprivation on tolerance of prolonged exercise. *European Journal of Applied Physiology and Occupational Physiology, 47*: 345-354.

Moore-Ede, M. (1993). *The twenty-four-hour society: Understanding human limits in a world that never stops.* Boston: Addison-Wesley Publishing Company.

Moore-Ede, M., & LeVert, S. (1998). *The complete idiot's guide to getting a good night's sleep.* New York: Alpha.

Muller, W. (2000). *Sabbath: Restoring the sacred rhythm of rest.* New York: Bantam Doubleday Dell.

Murphy, K., & Delanty, N. (2007). Review article: Sleep deprivation: A clinical perspecitve. *Sleep and Biological Rhythms, 5*(1): 2-14.

National Commission on Sleep Disorders Research. (1993). *Report on the National Commission on Sleep Disorders research.* Washington, DC: National Commission on Sleep Disorders Research.

National Sleep Foundation. (1995). *Sleep in America.* Princeton: Gallop Organization.

National Sleep Foundation. (1999). *The sleep quiz.* Washington, DC: National Sleep Foundation.

National Sleep Foundation. (2001). *Sleep in America.* Washington, DC: National Sleep Foundation.

National Sleep Foundation. (2002). *Sleep in America.* Washington, DC: National Sleep Foundation, 1-28.

National Sleep Foundation. (2005). *Sleep in America.* Washington, DC: National Sleep Foundation.

National Sleep Foundation. (2007a). Facts and stats. Retrieved June 5, 2007, from www.sleepfoundation.org/site/c.hulXKjM0IxF/b.2495307/k.8A0F/Facts_and_Stats.htm.

National Sleep Foundation. (2007b). Healthy sleep tips. Retrieved June 5, 2007, from www.sleepfoundation.org/site/c.hulXKjM0IxF/b.2417321/k.BAF0/Healthy_Sleep_Tips.htm.

National Sleep Foundation. (2007c). Sleep and sports: Getting the winning edge. Retrieved June 5, 2007, from www.sleepfoundation.org/site/c.hulXKjM0IxF/b.2419139/k.AE9B/Sleep_and_Sports_Get_the_Winning_Edge.htm.

Obal, F., Alt, J., Taishi, P., Gardi, J., & Krueger, J. (2003). Sleep in mice with nonfunctional growth hormone-releasing hormone receptors. *American Journal of Physiology: Regulatory, Integrative & Comparative Physiology, 53*(1): R131.

Pasztor, A. (1996). An air-safety battle brews over the issue of pilots' rest time. *The Wall Street Journal* (July 1): A1.

Reilly, T., & Piercy, M. (1994). The effect of partial sleep deprivation on weight-lifting performance. *Ergonomics 37,* 107-115.

Rice, J.R. (2005). Preacher bibliographies. Retrieved July 20, 2005, from www.swordofthelord.com/biographies/MccheyneRobertMurray.htm.

Sanders, O. (1997). Don't kill the horse. *Leadership, 7*(3): 136.

Schor, J. (1993). *The overworked American: The unexpected decline of leisure.* New York: Basic Books.

Stickgold, R., Winkelman, J., & Wehrwein, P. (2004). You will start to feel very sleepy. *Newsweek* (January 19): 58-60.

Swindoll, C. (1997). *Three steps forward, two steps back.* Nashville, TN: Word.

Tan, P.L. (1982). *Encyclopedia of 7,700 illustrations.* Rockville, MD: Assurance.

Veasey, S., Rosen, R., Barzansky, B., Rosen, I., & Owens, J. (2002). Sleep loss and fatigue in residency training. *Journal of the American Medical Association, 288*(9): 1116-1124.

Walters, P. (2000). Sleep: The forgotten factor. Paper presented at the annual National Wellness Conference, Stevens Point, WI.

Walters, P. (2005). Sleep: The forgotten factor: Part II. Paper presented at the annual National Wellness Conference, Stevens Point, WI.

Wikipedia. (2005). Sleep deprivation. Retrieved June 7, 2007, from http://en.wikipedia.org/wiki/Sleep_deprivation.

Wingard, D.L., & Berkman, L.F. (1983). Mortality risk associated with sleeping patterns among adults. *Journal of Sleep Research, 6*(2): 102-107.

World Health Organization. (2006). Millennium development goals. Retrieved October 20, 2006, from www.who.int/mdg/goals/goal1/en.

Zammit, G. (1997). *Good nights.* Kansas City, MO: Andrews and McMeel.

Suggested Readings

Bass, D. (1997). Rediscovering the Sabbath. *Christianity Today, 41*(10): 38-43.

This journal article describes the process for learning "anew" the benefits of Sabbath rest.

Coren, S. (1996). *Sleep thieves: An eye opening exploration into the science and mysteries of sleep.* **New York: The Free Press.**

This book provides an eye-opening exploration into the science and mysteries of sleep.

Dement, W., & Vaughan, C. (1999). *The promise of sleep.* **New York: Delacorte.**

This may be the best single book on sleep that exists for the layman.

Maas, J. B. (1999). *Power sleep.* **New York: Harper Perennial.**

This is a good place to begin educating yourself about the importance of proper sleep hygiene.

Muller, W. (2000). *Sabbath: Restoring the sacred rhythm of rest.* **New York: Bantam Doubleday Dell.**

This journal article emphasizes the importance of sacred rhythms for emotional, physical, and spiritual renewal.

Peterson, E. (1994). The good-for-nothing Sabbath. *Christianity Today, 38*(4): 34.

Peterson describes the joy of following the Creator's example of Sabbath rest.

Suggested Web Sites

www.sleepnet.com

Sleepnet: "Everything you wanted to know about sleep but were too tired to ask."

http://med.stanford.edu/school/psychiatry/coe

Stanford University Medical School is one of the leading sleep research institutions in the world. You will find a wealth of information related to sleep disorders.

www.sleepfoundation.org

National Sleep Foundation: Organization dedicated to surveying sleep behavior and potential solutions for millions of Americans who have sleep-related problems.

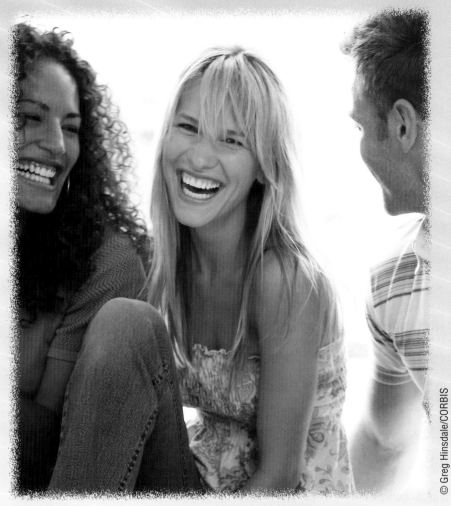

© Greg Hinsdale/CORBIS

Personal Relationships and Wellness

Peter Walters

After reading this chapter, you should be able to do the following:

1. Discover the value of human relationships.
2. Explore your personality, values, and spiritual gifts.
3. Appreciate the connection between relational and physical well-being.
4. Identify cultural shifts that make intimacy more difficulty in modern times.
5. Examine four principles for pursuing deeper relationships.

Stunning! Spectacular! Exhilarating! Irresistible! An eye-popping, action-packed thriller! You'd be a fool to miss it!

Open your newspaper to the movie listings any day of the year, and you'll see wildly enthusiastic endorsements like those splashed in an enormous font across the pages. Most people who've seen a few movies, however, learn to take those mad ravings with a grain of salt. Everyone knows that no mere human could possibly live up to the hype.

God, on the other hand, is a master of understatement. To jaded ears, scripture sounds minimalist and muted. After Jesus had fasted for 40 days in the harsh Judean wilderness he was probably hallucinating with hunger, his reserves were depleted, and his organs and muscles were in a catabolic state. The Bible says only, "He was hungry" (Luke 4:2). Christ's excruciating death, graphically reenacted in the movie *The Passion of the Christ*, is sickening to watch. It was described by the Gospel writer Luke with four simple words: "There they crucified him" (Luke 22:33).

God's modesty is even more remarkable in the Genesis creation account. He created amazing things: the sun, a fiery ball of fusion reactions 1.3 million times larger than the earth; microscopic single-celled organisms, each more complex than a jet-engine factory; 400 billion stars that make up the Milky Way galaxy alone; and 2 million known species of animals and 260,000 known species of plants on this planet. All that sprang solely from the mind and will of one mighty being, and the creator calls them, simply, "good" (Genesis 1:10, 12, 18, 21, 25).

When God, then, does choose to emphasize something, it's important to stop and listen. Only one event in the Genesis creation narrative is highlighted and pronounced "*very* good": the creation of people. One of the Bible's most profound and most quoted, but least understood, passages says, "So God created man in his own image, in the image of God he created him; male and female he created them" (Genesis 1:27).

Value of Relationships

Relationships are, without question, one of the most important things humans have. Nearly everyone, when it comes down to it, would rather give up careers, plans and ambitions, time and money, comfort and security, and even health than lose someone he or she loves. It would be rare

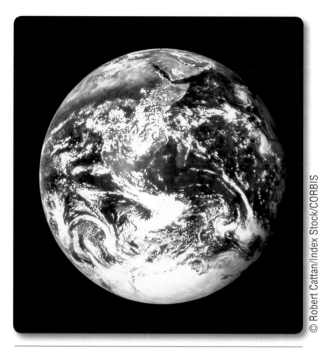

God created Adam from a fistful of earth.

for a mother to run into a burning house to save her china instead of her children. A man in love wouldn't trade his fiancée for a new automobile. Relationships are treasures, and they're delicate. With skill, care, and continual nurturing, they'll grow and blossom, but they'll wither and die if they're neglected.

I'll take the analogy a little further: The best gardeners are those who know most about the soil and climate conditions they have to work with, about each plant's unique features and growing patterns, and about the needs of and potential dangers for each plant. In this chapter I hope you'll learn to cultivate and care for your relational "gardens."

The first step in this process is to develop a careful understanding of your own personality, values, and gifts. More than half of this chapter is devoted to exercises in self-understanding. While this may seem strange in a chapter about relationships, this approach is based on the assumption that as you develop a keener awareness of self you will be able to see others more clearly. Anne Morrow Lindbergh, in her book *Gift by the Sea* (1992, p. 38), said the following:

When one is a stranger to one's self then one is estranged from others too. If one is not in touch with one's self then they can not touch others. . . . Only when one is connected to one's core can one be connected to others.

Sigmund Freud, perhaps one of the best-known psychologists of all time, argued that self-insight is one of the most critical steps in personal growth and that it is virtually impossible to know others intimately before knowing oneself (Freud, 1953). Therefore, the first aim in the chapter is to help you carefully examine your inner world so you can reach deeply into another's.

One model that visually illustrates this initial step is called the **Johari Window.** The two originators of this model, Joseph Luft and Harry Ingham (their first names combine to name the window), identified four areas of self-knowledge. Each quadrant of knowledge is illustrated in figure 11.1 (Luft, 1955).

> The top-left box represents what you and others know about you.
>
> The bottom-left quadrant represents what you know about yourself but others do not.
>
> The top-right quadrant represents what others know about you but you do not.
>
> The bottom-right quadrant is unknown to self and others.

The exercises in the beginning sections of this chapter are targeted at reducing the size of the "unknown" and "blind spot" quadrants and expanding what you know about yourself. As the knowledge about yourself grows, you have a choice about what you will reveal to others.

Digging Deeper

As you move into this self-exploration, not everything you find will please you. If you are honest with yourself, you will see weaknesses, flaws, failings, and outright evil. God's most precious creation becomes dreadful when it's warped by sin. In Dante's *Divine Comedy*, the pilgrim narrator must first descend to the pit of hell before he can begin his journey outward and upward (Alighieri, 1998). It's a difficult challenge to stand naked before God asking him to expose the dark corners of the heart. As you do it, remember the words of Jean Nicholas Grou:

> God in his wisdom only gives the grace of self-knowledge gradually; if he were to show us our true selves suddenly, we should despair and lose all courage. But as we perceive and conquer the more glaring faults, his gracious lights shows us the subtler, more hidden imperfections; and this spiritual process lasts all throughout life. (Draper, 1992, p. 236)

Be honest, but don't be discouraged; remember that God loves you as you are, and he has the power and the will to help you change.

	Known to self	Not known to self
Known to others	Common	Blind spot
Not known to others	Façade	Unknown

FIGURE 11.1 Four areas of self-knowledge.

Adapted from Luft, 1955.

Filled Up but Still Empty

This is an excerpt from an interview with Brad Pitt published in *Rolling Stone* magazine:

Pitt: Man, I know all these things are supposed to seem important to us—the car, the condo, our version of success—but if that's the case, why is the general feeling out there reflecting more impotence and isolation and desperation and loneliness? If you ask me, I say toss all this—we gotta find something else. Because all I know is that at this point in time, we are heading for a dead end, a numbing of the soul, a complete atrophy of the spiritual being. And I don't want that.

Rolling Stone: So if we're heading toward this kind of existential dead end in society, what do you think should happen?

Pitt: Hey, man, I don't have those answers yet. The emphasis now is on success and personal gain. I'm sitting in it, and I'm telling you, that's not it. I'm the guy who's got everything. I know. But I'm telling you, once you've got everything, then you're just left with yourself. I've said it before and I'll say it again: It doesn't help you sleep any better, and you don't wake up any better because of it. (Heath, 1999)

Personality

Have you ever wondered why two people who seem to have nothing in common at all just "click," or why others who seem to share a great deal never hit it off? The answer probably has to do with their personalities. If it's not the most important factor, **personality** is at least the most immediate factor that affects how individuals relate to each other. Consider what you notice when you meet new people. Right after you become aware of physical appearance, you begin picking up clues about personality. Personality comes before any deeper qualities like gifts, interests, values, and life goals.

The Odd Couple

Many personal clashes are personality clashes. Nothing illustrates this point better than Neil Simon's 1968 television comedy *The Odd Couple* (Simon, 1968). If you haven't watched it, do. After his wife Frances kicks him out of the house, Felix Ungar (played by Jack Lemmon) can't bring himself to jump out of the 12th-story window, and he decides instead to move in with his recently divorced friend, Oscar Madison (played by Walter Matthau). Unfortunately, despite their similar life situations, their personalities couldn't be more poorly suited for each other. Though his name means "happy," Felix is sensitive and emotional, always teary-eyed over his wife and kids. He complains about his back, his shoulder, his stomach, and his sinuses. He's polite, punctilious, and demanding, a stickler for rules and deadlines. He spends his days at Oscar's place preparing meatloaf and coleslaw, wrapping the leftovers in plastic, washing the dishes, installing a dehumidifier, spraying clouds of air freshener, vacuuming the carpet, fluffing the towels in the bathroom, and sterilizing the poker deck.

Oscar, on the other hand, is somewhat of a grouch. Unlike Felix, he's often fuming and snarling. He has a cavalier attitude toward his poker game, his apartment, his child-support payments, and the rest of his life, too. He leaves half-eaten plates of food around the apartment, drops cigarette butts on the floor, and throws dishes against the wall when he's angry. He talks loudly, makes lewd jokes, and flirts with waitresses. Predictably, then, after less than a week of living together, Felix and Oscar can't stand each other. Their relationship nearly comes to blows.

Simply put, personality is the unique way a person thinks, feels, and behaves. This definition is vague and nebulous, to be sure, but so is the common use of the term. *Personality* is a term that attempts to capture what makes people different, other than age, race, gender, appearance, culture, background, intelligence, and other abilities. It's at the heart of a question like, "What kind of person is Xavier?" or "What would Yolanda do in that situation?" It means roughly the same as *temperament* or *disposition*. The increasing popularity of personality tests, one of which you will take later in this chapter, has helped to narrow and sharpen the concept; and by the end of the chapter's discussion of the results, you should have a pretty good idea of what it means.

Psychologists believe that personality is established early in human development, usually by age eight, and remains fairly consistent throughout life. Like concrete, or like the human skeleton, once it is set it is difficult to alter. Premarital counselors often advise, "If you don't like his basic personality, don't marry him—you'll be stuck with it!"

Of course, Felix and Oscar's troubles had at least as much to do with major character flaws as with incompatible personalities, and I'm not saying that *those* can't be changed. With God's grace and with hard work, any two people can get along. Neither am I suggesting that personality differences are always a source of conflict. They can be a source of interest, even delight. Still, they must be seriously taken into account.

Your Personality Type

Isabel Myers and Kathryn Briggs developed a **personality type** model based on Carl Jung's writings (Keirsey & Bates, 1984). Their model is more sophisticated than the medieval theory of the humors (which classified people as sanguine, melancholic, choleric, or phlegmatic personalities according to the bodily fluid they believed was dominant), or the popular but simplistic Type-A versus Type-B distinction. The Myers-Briggs model classifies personalities into 16 types, based on four variables:

1. How are you energized?
2. How do you prefer to receive information?
3. On what basis do you make decisions?
4. How do you structure your life?

Each variable can have one of two values, depending on preference in the four variables:

Source of energy	(E) Extroversion or	(I) Introversion
Receiving information	(S) Sensing	or (N) Intuition
Decision making	(T) Thinking	or (F) Feeling
Orientation	(J) Judging	or (P) Perceiving

You'll read about each of those terms in the next paragraphs. Then you will be asked to identify which characteristic best describes your preference. As you make your judgments, remember that rarely is anyone exclusively an introvert or exclusively an extrovert, exclusively a thinking type or exclusively a feeling type, and so on. Imagine each variable as a seesaw, or a balance scale. Different people have different "tilts" in one direction or the other. Also, most people can behave in both ways when necessary but prefer one of them. It's a lot like hand dominance: You can use both your hands, but you prefer to hold pens, eat soup, and throw baseballs with one hand rather than the other.

It is also important to keep in mind the following information about personality types:

1. **All classifications, even this one, are artificial.** They are useful and have a lot of explanatory power, but ultimately they are human creations. They are, at some level, arbitrary. It's not as if God made people out of 16 different molds, or that "ESFJ" (substitute your type here) is written into your DNA code.

2. **All classifications are fallible.** They are only as accurate as your answers to the questions.

3. **All classifications are personality *types*, not personalities.** Everyone's personality is different, including the personalities of people with the same test results. You may even find that none of the labels really fits.

4. **Your four-letter sequence does not define you.** Treat it as a description of, not a prescription for, how you think, feel, and behave. Don't let it put you in a box.

5. **The classifications are not value judgments.** There are no "bad" or "good" personality types.

With those limitations in mind it's time to get started identifying your preferences. As you read the following descriptions, identify which letter best describes you (Kise, Stark, & Hirsh, 1996).

How Are You Energized?

Extroverts (about 75 percent of the population) tend to be energized by being around people, working in groups or teams with tangible results. They process their thoughts by sharing them with others, getting their input, and modifying their views based on those interactions. Introverts, by contrast, are energized by the inner world of their ideas and imaginations. They prefer to work alone or to interact one on one. They would rather process their thoughts silently and share them only when they are finalized. For more information on these variables, see table 11.1.

How Do You Prefer to Receive Information?

Sensing types (about 75 percent of the population) are focused on what they receive through their five senses: sight, hearing, touch, taste, and smell. They value hard facts; they pay attention to details; they are concerned with what is. Intuitive types listen to their hunches. They think in analogies, and they love to draw connections between different areas of knowledge. They rely less than

sensing types do on their five senses and more on what you might call a "sixth sense." Other people may say that they live in their own worlds. They are concerned with what could be and with new developments and new possibilities. For more information on these variables, see table 11.2.

On What Basis Do You Make Decisions?

Thinking types (about 75 percent of men, 25 percent of women) try to make decisions according to the canons of logic, consistency, and fairness. When they have objectively analyzed the situation, they are ready to proceed. Right or wrong, they are often perceived as being more committed to ideas, goals, and tasks than to people. Feeling types, however, rely heavily on their gut instincts as they make decisions. They usually consider

Table 11.1   Extrovert Type and Introvert Type

Extrovert types (E)	Introvert types (I)
Find interruptions stimulating	Find interruptions distracting
Are outgoing	Are reserved
Invite others in	Wait to be invited
Say what they're thinking	Keep their thoughts to themselves
Are energized from without	Are energized from within
Want to live it first	Want to understand it first
Focus on the outside	Focus on the inside
Take over	Step aside

Table 11.2   Sensing Type and Intuitive Type

Sensing types (S) prefer	Intuitive types (N) prefer
The useful	The innovative
Common sense	Insight
Accuracy	Creativity
Methodical approaches	Novel approaches
What is actual	What is possible
Practice	Theory
Identifying pieces	Identifying connections
The visible	The invisible

relationships more important than the work they are doing, so they seriously consider how their decisions will affect those relationships. They feel most at home where they can focus on people's needs and live according to their own personal values. For more information on these variables, see table 11.3.

How Do You Structure Your Life?

The terms *perceiving* and *judging* are not very helpful but, like the QWERTY keyboard, they have been so firmly established that they've stuck. Judging, in this context, has nothing to do with being judgmental, and perceiving has nothing to do with being perceptive. Judging types (about 50 percent of the population) like to plan their work, then work their plan. They like closure. Wherever they go, they leave organization and structure in their wake. They feel frustrated when things are out of place, and they must create some sense of order before they can work effectively. They believe that work should always come before play. On the other hand, perceiving types feel that planning gets in the way of living life to the fullest. They like things open-ended and spontaneous, and they tend to be adaptable and flexible. They want play to be part of work; they want work to be more fun. For more information on these variables, see table 11.4.

My guess is that Felix is an ISFJ and Oscar is an ENTP. What do you think? More important, what are your four personality preferences? List them below.

_____   _____   _____   _____

Table 11.3 Thinking Type and Feeling Type

Thinking types (T)	Feeling types (F)
Are logical and analytical	Are harmonious and personal
Are fair but firm, making few exceptions	Are empathetic, making many exceptions
Put business first	Put people first
Want recognition for exceeding requirements	Want recognition for personal effort
Decide with the head	Decide with the heart
Find flaws	Find strengths
Emphasize reasons	Emphasize values

Table 11.4 Judging Type and Perceiving Type

Judging types (J)	Perceiving types (P)
Are organized and efficient	Are flexible, juggling multiple tasks
Prefer planned events	Prefer serendipitous events
Want things settled and decided	Are open to late-breaking developments
Put work before play	Allow work and play to coexist
Accomplish tasks through consistent effort	Accomplish tasks through last-minute effort
Are systematic	Are spontaneous
Like things scheduled	Like things spur-of-the-moment
Enjoy finishing things	Enjoy starting things

Values

What are your highest **values**? Most Christians know the "right" answer to this question. It's something like, "God first, others second, me last." Christians know they're supposed to love God and love others, glorify God in all they do, and seek first the kingdom of God. They cut their spiritual baby teeth on these things. So when you're asked, as a Christian, what is most important to you or what you live by, the response is instinctive. It's as if you were asked what 9 times 5 equals. You don't have to think. You know what to say.

Don't misunderstand—teaching priorities is paramount for Christian discipleship. It's just that the point of this exercise is not to try to identify what your highest values *should be*, but what they *are*, and such automatic "church answers" have a tendency to get in the way of real, deep, honest thinking and introspection. Also, "values" in this context are broader than spiritual values alone. Values include everything that is important to you as a human being, from possessions to people to principles. Here are some questions meant to reveal your highest values:

- If you were going on a trip you wouldn't return from, what five things would you take with you? If the ship started to sink, which of them would you throw out first?

- If you knew you would die tomorrow, or next week, or next month, how would you spend your last days?

- What would you want said about you at your funeral? What would you want written on your tombstone?

Trying to answer questions like those can be useful, but it's hard to know what you would really do in those circumstances, and the exercise encourages the misperception that the deepest values emerge only under extreme pressure or in life-or-death situations. What really indicates your deepest values are the actions you have already performed. And the important actions to examine are the innumerable small and seemingly insignificant decisions you make day in and day out. The Grand Canyon was created by slow erosion over millions of years, not all at once in a single great catastrophe. In the same way, your character and values are formed gradually, almost imperceptibly,

What Do You Most Value in a Romantic Partner?

Dr. David Buss, a psychologist at the University of Michigan, sought to find out the characteristics people look for in a marriage partner. His study, published in the *American Scientist*, listed these common traits (Buss, 1985):

Adaptability

Kindness and understanding

Religious orientation

Creativity

Physical attractiveness

Good health

Desire for children

Good housekeeper

College graduate

Exciting personality

Intelligence

Good heredity

Good earning capacity

The list was given to a group of college students at a large secular institution, and they were asked to rank the items from most to least important, giving the trait deemed most important a numerical value of 1, the second most important trait a 2, and so on. Table 11.5 shows Buss' findings, which are grouped according to gender. Traits are listed in descending order, with the most valuable on top.

The same list was given to almost 1,000 college students enrolled in Christian colleges and universities (Walters et al., 2006). Table 11.6 represents how this group of students prioritized the same list of traits.

(continued)

(continued)

Table 11.5 Most Valuable Traits in a Romantic Partner: Secular University

Men	Women
1. Kindness and understanding	1. Kindness and understanding
2. Intelligence	2. Intelligence
3. Physical attractiveness	3. Exciting personality
4. Exciting personality	4. Good health
5. Good health	5. Adaptability
6. Adaptability	6. Physical attractiveness
7. Creativity	7. Creativity
8. Desire for children	8. Good earning capacity
9. College graduate	9. College graduate
10. Good heredity	10. Desire for children
11. Good earning capacity	11. Good heredity
12. Good housekeeper	12. Good housekeeper
13. Religious orientation	13. Religious orientation

Table 11.6 Most Valuable Traits in a Romantic Partner: Christian Colleges and Universities

Men	Women
1. Religious orientation	1. Religious orientation
2. Kindness and understanding	2. Kindness and understanding
3. Exciting personality	3. Exciting personality
4. Physical attractiveness	4. Intelligence
5. Intelligence	5. Physical attractiveness
6. Adaptability	6. Adaptability
7. Good health	7. Desire for children
8. Creativity	8. Good health
9. Desire for children	9. Creativity
10. College graduate	10. College graduate
11. Good housekeeper	11. Good earning capacity
12. Good heredity	12. Good housekeeper
13. Good earning capacity	13. Good heredity

Celibacy or Marriage?

Most evangelical churches are designed for married couples. Most evangelical leaders (clergy, elders, and deacons) are married. Pastors preach assuming their congregants are married, perhaps making an occasional reference to singles. Yet the number of singles either unmarried, widowed, or divorced has rapidly expanded in the last several years.

Consider the following statistics:

In 1940, fewer than eight percent of Americans lived alone. Today that proportion has more than tripled, reaching nearly 26 percent (U.S. Census Bureau, 2005a).

More than 45 percent of adult females and 40 percent of adult males in America are single (Duin, 2002).

Because the largest group of single adults in the United States has never been married (60 percent unmarried, 25 percent divorced, and 15 percent widowed [U.S. Census Bureau, 2005b]), it is time to consider the spiritual ramifications of this choice.

Celibacy has a long and distinguished history in the church. The apostle Paul says in 1 Corinthians 7:1, "It is good for a man not to marry." There is evidence that during the first century young widows were taking vows of celibacy (1 Timothy 5:9–12). By 110 AD, celibates could take vows that mirrored marital vows (Thomas, 2000). By the third century, lifelong vows of celibacy were not uncommon. By the fourth century, celibacy was commemorated by a full liturgical celebration (Oliver, 1994).

Within evangelical circles, views about people who practice celibacy range from "completely sold out to Jesus" to "second-class citizens who never fully realize the beauty of marriage." Is there a more Christ-like view to embrace? What are the unique challenges and benefits of singleness? How can singles be more effectively ministered to? And what unique ministry opportunities may single men and women be better suited for?

---

a little bit at a time. What you wear every day, whether you choose to spend your time studying or talking with friends, whether you go to class or habitually skip it to sleep in say at least as much about your values as what you think you would do if someone put a gun to your head.

For some help in values clarification, complete the application exercise at the end of this chapter titled "Your Highest Values." Take your time as you complete this assignment, resist the urge to identify what your values *should* be and hone in on the values you reflect in your day-to-day choices.

Spiritual Gifts

In addition to personalities and values, scripture says God gives **spiritual gifts.**

There are different kinds of gifts, but the same Spirit. There are different kinds of service, but the same Lord. There are different kinds of working, but the same God works

all of them in all men. Now to each one the manifestation of the Spirit is given for the common good. (1 Corinthians 12:4–8)

Eugene Peterson's (2003, p. 2083) New Testament paraphrase, *The Message*, puts the verse like this: "Each person is given something to do that shows who God is: Everyone gets in on it, everyone benefits. All kinds of things are handed out by the Spirit, and to all kinds of people."

The apostles and early church leaders frequently discussed and argued about the issue of spiritual giftedness, but today only about 25 percent of Christians say they know what their own spiritual gifts are (Barna, 2001). In this section I'll briefly describe the spiritual gifts mentioned in scripture, and then try to help you unwrap yours.

The New Testament mentions about 20 different spiritual gifts. Each of the several lists is different in content and terminology (but they overlap), and none is exhaustive. To avoid confusion and controversy, I have chosen to use the terms and descriptions from the book *Network: The Right People. . .In the Right Places. . .For the Right Reasons*, by Bugbee, Cousins, and Hybels (1994).

To gain insight into which of the spiritual gifts you possess, complete the second application activity at the end of the chapter. Because each person has traits that are visible to others but that he or she can't see—the spiritual equivalent of spinach stuck between the front teeth, if you like—it is necessary to seek others' input about spiritual giftedness. Get feedback from at least two people who know you well, one family member (because they probably know you the best) and one person not in your family (because they are less likely to be *too* familiar and, therefore, biased). Ask each to complete the application activity at the end of the chapter with you in mind. Where your results agree with theirs, treat it as confirmation. You may find, however, that you have hidden gifts that others do not recognize or that others affirm gifts in you that you didn't know you had. Either way, be open to what God wants to reveal to you about the special abilities he has divinely entrusted to you.

Your SHAPE

"Shape" refers to the way you are, in a broad sense. It can also serve as an acronym for the following:

Spiritual gifts

Heart (i.e., values)

Abilities (i.e., natural gifts)

Personality

Experience (Warren, 2002)

I haven't included a formal exercise in this chapter to help you identify your natural gifts or experience, but you might want to spend some time thinking about them. Your natural gifts—that is, your talents or aptitudes or abilities—are probably well known to you, but it would certainly be

---

 ## Freedom of Self-Acceptance

According to *Gramophone*, a leading magazine about classical music, Susan Graham is "America's favorite mezzo" (Graham, 2006). During Graham's rise to stardom, Jamie Fields, writer for *Texas Monthly* sought to compare Graham to one of opera's legendary mezzo-sopranos, Cecilia Bartoli (Fields, 1996). Fields asked Graham in an interview if Graham thought she could be the next Bartoli. Graham's response: "I'm not sure I want to be the next anyone. I'd rather be the first Susan Graham" (Fields, 1996, p. 36).

Graham's refusal to emulate other classical vocalists was perhaps one of the most important factors that resulted in her unique voice. Graham's response is similar to the message that the apostle Paul preached. Paul urged the Galatians in his letter to them to resist the temptation of comparing themselves to others:

Make a careful exploration of who you are and the work you have been given, and sink your teeth into that. Don't be impressed with yourselves. Don't compare yourselves with others. Each of you take responsibility for doing the creative best you can do with your life. (Galatians 6:4–5, *The Message*)

Those inspired words reflect the wisdom of how pride (being impressed with yourself) and comparison can kill the inner spirit. People who think other people are inferior swell with pride. Yet if they think everyone else is superior, they can easily sink into self-denigration. Neither mindset is what God wants for his people.

The first section in this chapter has been about discovering the unique way God wired you. As you begin to understand how the designer has uniquely crafted you, your aim should simply be to do the creative best you can. It doesn't matter how you stack up against others on academic assignments, within your chosen profession, or in society at large. If you do your best with your gifts, you can be free to become the person God masterfully created you to be. God won't ask you at the end of your life why you weren't more like Moses, Abraham, David, or Paul. He'll want to know instead how you used your unique service in Christ's kingdom.

worthwhile to reflect and write down what you believe they are. Think about the areas in life in which you've been successful (and don't limit yourself only to school or work). Think about the activities you really enjoy doing, because very few people find sustained pleasure in something for which they have no gift. In the long run, you will probably find the most fulfillment in life doing what you are good at. Many wise Christians believe that your specific gifts may indicate God's specific calling for you.

Be realistic with yourself about your weaknesses, too. Fooling yourself, or living in denial, typically leads to failure and frustration. You shouldn't neglect your shortcomings, but don't spend all your time trying to shore them up, either. You could spend a lifetime working on them and still be only average. But if you develop your gifts to the fullest, you can certainly make a positive impact on the world.

Keep in mind that everyone has a different combination of gifts, just as everyone has a different fingerprint. Maybe you feel dissatisfied with or discouraged by the shape you've been given. When you do the application activities at the end of the chapter, you might think that your personality is not as attractive as someone else's or that your true values aren't as solid or positive as you had hoped. You might see your gifts as "white elephants" that seem unremarkable. Read "Freedom of Self-Acceptance" on page 265 and reflect on what the apostle Paul says about who you are and the work you have been given to do.

Healthy Relationships and Healthy Bodies

At the beginning of the chapter, I discussed what the creator called "good" and "very good." There was one thing, however, that he called *not* good: "It is not good for man to be alone" (Genesis 2:18). God's divine pronouncement should be enough; nonetheless, a growing body of scientific literature indicates that isolation and loneliness have negative effects on health in unimaginable ways.

In one study (Ornish, 1990), 119 men and 40 women completed a psychological questionnaire and were tested for plaque build-up in their coronary arteries. After statistically controlling for other factors associated with heart disease, such as age, gender, hypertension, cholesterol, and smoking, the people who had fewer blockages were those who felt more loved and supported by other people. A second study (Berkman & Syme, 1979), this one encompassing 20,000 subjects in California and Finland, found similar results: Independent of all other relevant factors, the people who had the fewest social contacts were two to three times more at risk of death from heart disease than those who had the most social contacts.

The Abkhasians of Georgia (in central Asia, not in the United States) have caught the attention of health researchers. That group of people has the industrialized world's lowest mortality rate, and many of them live for more than 100 years. Scientists believe that one major reason for their longevity is their intricate web of social connections. The Abkhasians measure their worth and status in terms of the quality and quantity of family ties they have, and it is not uncommon for an Abkhasian to have more than 300 family members (Siegler, Longino, & Johnson, 1992)!

Read Dean Ornish's (1999) book *Love and Survival* for more on this subject. Dr. Ornish, a cardiovascular physician, was in search of a more effective treatment plan for his patients when he discovered what he calls "the healing power of love." His book reviews more than 100 studies on the relationship between physical and relational health, and concludes the following (1999, p. 30):

When I reviewed the scientific literature, I was amazed to find what a powerful difference love and relationships made upon the incidents of disease and premature death from virtually all causes.

Cultural Isolation and Loneliness

Most people would agree that the quality of human relationships has an impact that goes beyond social well-being. Novelist Jonathan Franzen wrote an editorial essay titled "Imperial Bedroom." In it he discussed how the social landscape has changed, describing a gradual decline in the number of personal, intimate relationships (Franzen, 1998, p. 48):

In 1890, an American typically lived in a small town. . . . Not only did his every purchase "register," but it registered in the eyes and the memory of shopkeepers who knew him, his parents, his wife, and his children. . . . Probably he grew up sleeping in the same bed with his siblings and possibly with his parents, too. Unless he was well off, his transportation—a train, a horse, his own two feet—either was communal or exposed him to the public eye.

Rejection— More Than Emotional

Social rejection is heartbreaking and gut-wrenching. According to a study published in the *Journal of Science*, social snubbings do affect more than just people's emotions. In fact, the feelings a person gets when ignored at a party or when not chosen for a team generate exactly the same brain wave patterns that he or she gets when experiencing real, physical pain. In the study, 13 volunteers were given a task and they didn't know it related to an experiment in social snubbing. During the experimental trials, each subject experienced social rejection. When that occurred, the EEG showed the same electrical patterns as when humans undergo visceral pain (Eisenberger, Lieberman, & Williams, 2003).

In the suburbs and exurbs where the typical American family lives today, tiny nuclear families inhabit enormous houses, in which each person has his or her own bedroom and, sometimes, bathroom. . . . It's no longer the rule that you know your neighbors. Communities increasingly tend to be virtual, the participants either faceless or firmly in control of the face they present. Transportation is largely private: The latest SUVs are the size of living rooms and come with onboard telephones, CD players, and TV screens; behind the tinted windows of one of these high-riding I-see-you-but-you-can't-see-me mobile PrivacyGuard units, a person can be wearing pajamas or a licorice bikini, for all anybody knows or cares.

One long-term study reported that almost one in four Americans do not have even one person to confide in (McPherson, Smith-Lovin, & Brashears, 2006). The study, conducted by researchers at Duke University and the University of Arizona, interviewed 1,467 subjects about their interpersonal relationships. The results were also compared to interviews conducted in 1985. An unmistakable finding was that the number of intimate relationships the average person has is on the decline.

New Homes Designed for the Dysfunctional Family

The Ledbetter family likes to spend time at home together—just not in the same room. They built a 3,600-square-foot house with special rooms for studying and sewing, separate sitting areas for each child, and a master bedroom far from the other areas. Then there's the escape room where, Mr. Ledbetter says, "Any family member can go to get away from the rest of us."

The Mercer Island, Washington, industrial designer says his 7- and 11-year-old daughters fight less, because their new house gives them so many ways to avoid each other. "It just doesn't make sense for us to do everything together all the time," he says.

After two decades of pushing the open floor plan—where domestic life revolved around a big central space and exposed kitchens gave everyone a view of half the house—major builders and top architects are walling people off. They're touting one-person Internet alcoves, locked-door away rooms and his-and-her offices on opposite ends of the house. The new floor plans offer so much seclusion, they're "good for the dysfunctional family," says Gopal Ahluwahlia, director of research for the National Association of Home Builders.

Fletcher, 2004, p. W1.

Faithfulness

I knew a man who had Alzheimer's disease for more than a decade. He was institutionalized for the last few years of his life. During those years, his wife faithfully and lovingly visited him every day. She would have hurt inside to miss a day, and his spirits were raised each time she came. She was faithful to him. **Faithfulness** means always being there for someone despite what they do in return.

I also remember highlights in our family life such as important birthdays, professions of faith, and graduations. The joy of those days was increased by family and friends dropping by, phoning, or sending a greeting. For these family members and friends, stopping to rejoice as an act of faithfulness put the brakes on their daily lives as they shared in the lives of others. Faithfulness brings blessing and healing.

There are other examples of unfaithfulness, like Peter's denials of Jesus before Jesus' death or the prodigal son's temporary friends. Christians are sometimes unfaithful to God, too. Proverbs says, "Like a bad tooth or a lame foot is reliance on the unfaithful in times of trouble" (25:19). When people are unfaithful to God, the land will mourn, and "all who live in it waste away" (Hosea 4:3). The devastating effects of various sexually transmitted diseases can be painful consequences of unfaithfulness. Unfaithfulness leads to pain and a lack of wellness.

I have wondered at times whether anyone really cares that I am here. Are people faithful to me? I have usually asked that question when I was down and discouraged about life, and I felt lonely and alienated, not well. Just imagine how Jesus felt when everyone, including his faithful Father, left him alone to die on a cross. But God is always faithful. Jesus rose from the dead because of God's faithfulness. God's faithfulness will be a "shield and rampart" (Psalm 91:4), and he offers this gift of healing. When I felt lonely and deserted it was comforting and healing to find protection in the faithfulness of a loving God and in the concerned comments of a friend. You can offer the same faithful protection to people you meet by caring in times of need and sharing the joys of a celebration. As you care for others, they experience greater wellness and so do you.

Faithfulness: Were you unfaithful in the last week? List two ways you can be more faithful to your friends, family, and God.

_____

_____

_____

_____

_____

_____

_____

That's not exactly new information. Beginning in the mid-1960s, Harvard professor Robert Putnam began describing diminished memberships in parent–teacher associations, unions, and civic clubs and organizations (Page, 2006). In his more recent book, titled *Bowling Alone*, Putnam reported drops as great as 60 percent in attendance at dinner parties, civic meetings, and family suppers; in blood and charitable donations; and even in recreational leagues such as bowling (Putnam, 2000).

Relational Coaching

Most students describe themselves as "good with people." Walters and colleagues (2006) polled more than 1,300 students who attended Christian colleges and universities. Almost universally the students rated their ability to deal effectively with other people higher than every other measure of wellness surveyed (physical fitness, body image, weight management, stress, sleeping habits, and dietary behavior).

Despite these youthful assertions, older men and women of faith reported interpersonal problems as one of their leading concerns. In one of the largest mission surveys, including 55 different North American protestant agencies, missionaries identified personal conflict with other missionaries as their number-one problem (Johnson & Penner, 2005). A whopping 40 percent of pastors around the world report that they have a major clash with another church member at least once a month (Fuller Institute of Church Growth, 1993). One new religious denomination is formed each week, and most of those emerge not from growth and expansion but as a result of contention and discord (Waldman, 1992).

In light of these facts, the remainder of this chapter discusses four suggestions targeted toward college students for increased effectiveness in relationships.

Suggestion 1: Begin at Home

The first of the Ten Commandments that deals with how humans should treat others charges children to obey and honor their parents (Deuteronomy 5:16). That commandment is the only one with a promise attached: "so that you may live long and that it may go well with you." God's promise for increased well-being is linked to how children relate to their parents. Like it or not, one aspect of life that is undeniably in God's will is the parents you have. People do not exist by random chance, but as a result of God's purpose.

Several passages describe how God either closes or opens the wombs of mothers according to his will (Genesis 20:18, 29:31, 30:22, 1 Samuel 1:5). Both the psalmist David and the prophet Isaiah acknowledge God's hand in the creation of human life (Psalm 139:13, Isaiah 44:2). You can be sure that your existence is not a blunder and your parents weren't given to you by mistake.

For many, that belief is comforting and a strong reflection of God's goodness. Others who have been abused by their parents physically, emotionally, or psychologically find that difficult to accept. How can a God of compassion place a defenseless child into a family to be neglected, harassed, and violated? Some thoughtful people have formulated responses to difficult questions like this (see Lewis, 1944; Yancey, 1997), but it's hard for a neglected or abused person to accept such a reality. No matter how difficult it is, God commands people to not only accept but also to obey and honor their parents—not the ones they wish they had, but the ones they were given.

Children, obey your parents in the Lord: for this is right. Honor your father and mother. (Ephesians 6:1–2)

Obeying parents (except when doing so violates God's authority) is no small matter to God. If severity of punishment indicates the gravity of the offense, consider the consequences in the Old Testament for disobedient children:

If a man has a stubborn and rebellious son who does not obey his father and mother and will not listen to them when they discipline him, his father and mother shall take hold of him and bring him to the elders at the gate of his town. They shall say to the elders, "This son of ours is stubborn and rebellious. He will not obey us. He is a profligate and a drunkard." Then all the men of his town shall stone him to death. (Deuteronomy 21:18–20)

Other passages make it very clear that God is serious about children obeying and honoring their parents.

The eye that mocks a father, that scorns obedience to a mother, will be pecked out by the ravens of the valley, will be eaten by the vultures. (Proverbs 30:17)

If a man curses his father or mother, his lamp will be snuffed out in pitch darkness. (Proverbs 20:20)

Cursed is the man who dishonors his father or his mother. (Deuteronomy 27:16)

Because the commands of parental obedience and honor are so close to the heart of God and essential to our well-being, Satan works overtime in creating a cultural disregard for parental authority. Gone are the days when children said "Yes, sir" and "No, ma'am" when speaking to adults. Welcome to a culture in which songs and TV shows humor young audiences with their irreverent style and disregard for parental authority. In this era, even the most heinous language directed toward parents seems acceptable to many. Eminem, the triple-platinum rapper, gained widespread popularity for his no-holds-barred defamation of authority. In his song "Cleaning Out My Closet" he raps about his mother who has been on welfare and addicted to drugs and sleeps around. His conclusion? He hopes "she burns in hell" (AZLyrics, 2006). As shocking as the lyrics are, his mother's response is even more startling. She said, "That's just artistic expression" (ABC News, 2004).

Accepting your parents as part of God's plan and obeying and honoring them despite their imperfections is the first step in moving toward relational maturity.

Suggestion 2: Connect Spiritually

You have heard that opposites attract, but experience and research indicate the opposite. Walk into any student cafeteria and you will see tables segregated by race, hobbies, and a host of other characteristics. One sociologist who conducted a nationwide survey concluded that Americans nearly always end up befriending and marrying people who are similar to them in age, race, ethnicity, socioeconomic class, and education level (Michael et al., 1994). Another study that examined more than 500,000 couples found that Caucasians are 8 times more likely to marry Caucasians than non-Caucasians, Hispanics are 12 times more likely to marry Hispanics, Asians are 55 times more likely to marry Asians, and African Americans are 365 times more likely to marry African Americans (Michael et al., 1994). When given an option, people seem to choose similarity over differences. Christians are no exception. One noted evangelical author states that within two years of conversion, the typical Christian has few if any nonbelieving friends (Stebbins, 1995).

What conclusions can be drawn from this strong bias toward like-mindedness? Actually, similarities can serve as a foundation on which differences are welcomed. Note what occurred among the early believers in the book of Acts:

> All the believers were one in heart and mind. No one claimed that any of his possessions was his own, but they shared everything they had. (Acts 4:32)

Earlier in Acts the writer describes the conversion of 3,000 individuals from many cultures and tongues who accepted the apostle Peter's plea to repent and placed their faith in Jesus. Because of their similarities in emotion (heart) and theology (mind), these new believers not only gathered with others who were vastly different, but they also shared "everything they had." Apparently, faith in Jesus overshadowed their differences in income, skin color, and language.

The ideal foundation for relationships is to have a deep spiritual connectedness. Then, like a tree that separates into hundreds of different branches, the relationship bears fruit in different locations.

To use a vocal analogy: Singing in harmony, not in unison, makes beautiful music in God's choir. In a well-trained choir, the different members sing different parts, and when all the parts come together the musical effect is more powerful than if all of them sing the same part. The same is true within Christ's kingdom. Spiritual oneness allows different people to sing the same lyrics in many different tones.

Suggestion 3: Adjust Expectations

"Lower your standards for marriage" sounds like the desperate cry of a frustrated single person, not the counsel of social scientists who study successful marriages. Dr. Paul Amato, professor of sociology, demography, and family studies at Penn State University, says there has been a significant shift in the views of marriage during the past several decades (Amato et al., 2003). Surveys of high school and college students 50 and 60 years ago report that most unmarried couples wanted to get married in order to have children and buy a home. Now couples are looking for much more. They want love, self-fulfillment, a wonderful family, intellectual stimulation, sexual fulfillment, and a soul mate (Previti & Amato, 2003).

Writer Polly Shulman (2004, pp. 33-34) aptly describes the new trend in spouse selection:

> We once prized marriage for the practical pairing of the cash-producing father and the home-building mother. Now we want it all—a partner who reflects our taste in status, who sees us for who we are, who loves us for all the "right" reasons, who helps us become the person we want to be. We've done away with the rigid social order, adopting instead an even more onerous obligation: the mandate to find a perfect match. While having a marriage that fulfills many of our needs isn't bad, the unrealistic, high expectations of marrying superwoman or superman is.

Single people unwilling to concede on any of their standards live in somewhat of a relational "hokey-pokey," with one foot "in" the relationship and the other foot "out," looking for someone more suited to their taste. "Is this all there is? Am I as happy as I should be? Would I be happier, smarter, a better person with someone else?" Those are the questions that plague single people searching for the ultimate partner.

The truth is that no spouse will, or even has the potential to, satisfy all relational needs. Believing they will ultimately satisfy all needs leads to frustration and disappointment. The concept of "happily ever after" is OK for fairy tales but will not stand the weight of a real relationship. Diane Sollee, founder of the Coalition for Marriage, Family and Couples Education, says, "Marriage is a disagreement machine" (Shulman, 2004, p. 34). She adds, "We have a highly romanticized notion that if we were with the right person, we wouldn't fight" (Shulman 2004, p. 37)." According to research by marriage and family therapist Dr. John Gottman, happily married couples disagree about as much as couples who get divorced (Gottman et al., 2006). The fundamental differences between those couples are their expectations and willingness to come to a workable compromise.

It is not just expectations for romantic relationships that can benefit from an overhaul. Friends, ministers, co-workers, politicians, employees, and bosses are human, too, and in their humanness they make mistakes, have troublesome weaknesses and irritable quirks, and sometimes even sin. Invariably, as relationships deepen through time and exposure, less desirable attributes surface. Qualities that may seem fascinating, charming, or at least tolerable in someone you occasionally see can be maddening in someone you have to live with day in and day out.

When relational problems emerge, it is easy to feel suckered by a "bait and switch" promotion like the one that happened to a woman from the state of Georgia in 2005. It is hard to imagine how excited Norreasha Gill must have been in May 2005, when she won the big "100 Grand" contest run by her local radio station, WLTO-FM. She won by listening to the station for several hours and being the 10th caller at a specified time. The night before she went to collect her prize, she promised her three young children that they were going to get a minivan, a new backyard, and lots of shopping. Imagine how she felt when the station manager explained that she won a Nestle's 100 Grand candy bar, not $100,000 (Gandelman, 2006).

Entering a relationship with high hopes for spiritual connection, intellectual stimulation, and synergistic compatibility is not necessarily bad. It is honorable to expect the "good," but it's also wise to realize that no human relationship can be perfect.

Suggestion 4: Resolve Conflict

Because of their frailties, people will experience everything from minor misunderstanding to serious strife. Contention can chafe and blister, like a rock in a shoe. Or, it has the power to build good-ness, trust, and solidarity. The fundamental factor in determining the outcome is the response to the contention. The choice is in your hands. You have the power to offer clemency or to hold captive.

On June 11, 1963, Vivian Malone, a young African American woman, was escorted by federal troops to ensure her admittance into the University of Alabama. She was hoping to become the first black student to attend the institution. Upon her arrival at school, her way was blocked by a staunch believer in racism and segregation, Governor George Wallace. The governor's blockade failed and Vivian eventually became the first African American student to graduate from the university.

Several years later, Governor Wallace regretted his actions. He was taken in his wheelchair to the Dexter Avenue Baptist Church in Montgomery, Alabama, where he formally apologized and asked the African American community to forgive him. After that service, he sought out a private meeting with Vivian to personally apologize. Vivian met with the governor and told him that she had forgiven him years earlier. In a 2003 interview, she was asked about this conversation.

"You said you'd forgiven him many years earlier?"

"Oh yes."

"And why did you do that?"

"This may sound weird. I'm a Christian, and I grew up in the church. I was taught that no other person was better than I—that we were all equal in the eyes of God. I was also taught that you forgive people, no matter what. And that was why I had to do it. I didn't feel as if I had a choice." (Nick, 2005, p. 10)

Her upbringing may have made Vivian feel like she had no choice, but she did. And her choice not only freed the governor, but it also liberated Vivian from years of anger and resentment.

The alternative to forgiveness was illustrated in the popular 1994 movie *Forrest Gump*. In this movie, Tom Hanks, who plays Forrest Gump, accomplishes the incredible despite being physically and mentally challenged.

In one scene, Forrest and his childhood friend Jenny are walking down an old gravel road shaded by hardwood trees. Jenny carries her sandals, and the walk seems pleasant until they happen upon an abandoned, weather-worn house. The sight is horrifying to Jenny. It's her childhood home, a place where Jenny had been abused by her alcoholic father.

Forrest sees the pain etched on Jenny's face as she walks ahead of him toward the abandoned house. Suddenly, Jenny throws her shoes at the house and then begins picking up rocks and furiously throwing them against the house. Years of pent-up anger are unleashed. When nothing is left to throw at the house, Jenny falls to the ground crying. Forrest sits down in the muddy driveway beside her, and says,

"Sometimes, I guess, there just aren't enough rocks" (Tisch, Finerman, & Zemeckis, 1994).

Despite the destructive consequences of unforgiveness, some remain imprisoned by unforgiveness for years. One reason for this is not knowing how to restore damaged relationships. Fortunately, Peacemakers International, a nonprofit, Christian organization that has partnered with thousands of individuals as they seek resolution, has outlined and made available for reprint the

The Peacemaker's Pledge

As people reconciled to God by the death and resurrection of Jesus Christ, we believe that we are called to respond to conflict[1] in a way that is remarkably different from the way the world deals with conflict. We also believe that conflict provides opportunities to glorify God, serve other people, and grow to be like Christ.[2] Therefore, in response to God's love and in reliance on His grace, we commit ourselves to respond to conflict according to the following principles:

1. **Glorify God**

   Instead of focusing on our own desires or dwelling on what others may do, we will seek to please and honor God—by depending on His wisdom, power, and love, by faithfully obeying His commands, and by seeking to maintain a loving, merciful, and forgiving attitude.[3]

2. **Get the Log Out of Your Own Eye**

   Instead of attacking others or dwelling on their wrongs, we will take responsibility for our own contribution to conflicts—confessing our sins, asking God to help us change any attitudes and habits that lead to conflict, and seeking to repair any harm we have caused.[4]

3. **Go and Show Your Brother His Fault**

   Instead of pretending that conflict doesn't exist or talking about others behind their backs, we will choose to overlook minor offenses and will talk directly and graciously with those whose offenses seem too serious to overlook. When a conflict with another Christian cannot be resolved

in private, we will ask others in the body of Christ to help us settle the matter in a biblical manner.[5]

4. **Go and Be Reconciled**

   Instead of accepting premature compromise or allowing relationships to wither, we will actively pursue genuine peace and reconciliation—forgiving others as God, for Christ's sake, has forgiven us, and seeking just and mutually beneficial solutions to our differences.[6]

By God's grace, we will apply these principles as a matter of stewardship, realizing that conflict is an assignment, not an accident. We will remember that success, in God's eyes, is not a matter of specific results but of faithful, dependent obedience. And we will pray that our service as peacemakers brings praise to our Lord and leads others to know His infinite love.[7]

---

[1]Matt. 5:9; Luke 6:27-36; Gal. 5:19-26
[2]Rom. 8:28-29; 1 Cor. 10:31-11:1; James 1:2-4.
[3] Ps. 37:1-6; Mark 11:25; John 14:15; Rom. 12:17-21; 1 Cor. 10:31; Phil. 4:2-9; Col. 3:1-4; James 3:17-18, 4:1-3; 1 Peter 2:12.
[4]Prov. 28:13; Matt. 7:3-5; Luke 19:8; Col. 3:5-14; I John 1:8-9.
[5] Prov. 19:11; Matt. 18:15-20; 1 Cor. 6:1-8; Gal. 6:1-2; Eph. 4:29; 2 Tim. 2:24-26; James 5:9.
[6]Matt. 5:23-24; 6:12; 7:12; Eph. 4:1-3, 32; Phil. 2:3-4.
[7]Matt. 25:14-21; John 13:34-35; Rom. 12:18; 1 Peter 2:19; 4:19.

From *The Peacemaker: A Biblical Guide to Resolving Personal Conflict* © Kenneth Sande (Baker Books, 3rd edition, 2004). Used by permission. Visit www.Peacemaker.net for additional information about biblical peacemaking.

What Americans Believe About Forgiveness

The Institute for Social Research (ISR), the world's largest academic survey and research organization, surveyed 1,423 representative American adults to determine their attitudes and behaviors related to forgiveness (Williams, 2001). Here are some of their findings:

- Three-quarters believe they have been forgiven by God for their mistakes.
- Sixty percent reported they have forgiven themselves for wrongdoings.
- Forty-three percent have gone to others to be forgiven.
- Women are more forgiving than men.
- Middle-agers and older adults are more likely to forgive others than younger adults are.

Peacemaker's Pledge. The pledge, reprinted on page 272, describes an attitude and four specific steps that can be applied to repair interpersonal conflict.

Next Steps

The self-analysis exercises at the beginning of this chapter focused on giving you a deeper understanding of yourself as well as opening up potential vistas of exploration with others. So begin with personality, values, and gifts, but move deeper into personal and cultural history, politics, and theology. Each person you meet is undiscovered territory ripe with intrigue and mystery.

Next I covered the need to search out, discover, and cultivate interpersonal relationships. Social, physical, and spiritual wholeness depend on it. A growing body of research suggests that the quality of social relationships affects every area of life.

Finally, because most people can benefit from coaching in relationships, I outlined four practical interpersonal suggestions. These suggestions are not meant to be exhaustive, but are a beginning point from which deeper growth and understanding can be realized.

Key Terms

faithfulness

Johari Window

personality

personality type

spiritual gifts

values

Review Questions

1. Identify the value God places on humans compared to the rest of creation.
2. List four characteristics the Myers-Briggs Personality Inventory measures. Identify the letters associated with each characteristic.
3. Write one-sentence descriptions of each of the following spiritual gifts:
   a. Administration
   b. Apostleship
   c. Craftsmanship
   d. Creative communication
   e. Discernment
   f. Encouragement
   g. Evangelism
   h. Faith
   i. Giving
   j. Helps
   k. Hospitality
   l. Intercession
   m. Knowledge
   n. Leadership
   o. Mercy
   p. Prophecy
   q. Shepherding
   r. Teaching
   s. Wisdom

4. Identify at least two scientific studies that suggest a connection between relational and physical well-being.

5. Identify at least three cultural shifts that make intimacy more difficult.

6. Identify four principles from the text for deepening relationships.

1. Your highest values

Values Clarification

The following is a list of 75 different values (Kise, Stark, & Hirsh, 1996). Feel free to add more of your own. Rate each value with an *A*, *B*, or *C*, according to how consistently it has affected your past choices.

Place an *A* next to values that have consistently affected your choices.

Place a *B* next to values that have occasionally affected your choices.

Place a *C* next to values that have rarely or never affected your choices.

Accuracy	____	Fortune	____	Perseverance	____
Achievement	____	Friendship	____	Personal development	____
Advancement	____	Generosity	____	Physical fitness	____
Adventure	____	Growth	____	Possessions	____
Aesthetics	____	Happiness	____	Power	____
Artistic expression	____	Health	____	Prestige	____
Authenticity	____	Helping others	____	Privacy	____
Balance	____	Honesty	____	Productivity	____
Challenge	____	Humor	____	Purpose in life	____
Character	____	Independence	____	Recognition	____
Cleanliness	____	Influence	____	Religious beliefs	____
Competition	____	Integrity	____	Responsibility	____
Conformity	____	Justice	____	Security	____
Contribution	____	Knowledge	____	Self-respect	____
Control	____	Learning	____	Service	____
Cooperation	____	Leisure	____	Solitude	____
Creativity	____	Location	____	Spirituality	____
Efficiency	____	Love	____	Spontaneity	____
Excitement	____	Loyalty	____	Stability	____
Fairness	____	Money	____	Structure	____
Faith	____	Nature	____	Success	____
Family	____	Orderliness	____	Tolerance	____
Financial security	____	Organization	____	Tradition	____
Fitness	____	Peace	____	Variety	____
Flexibility	____	People	____	Wisdom	____

From P. Walters and J. Byl, 2008, *Christian paths to health and wellness* (Champaign, IL: Human Kinetics).

Now, take all the *A* values, and put them in clusters according to which ones seem similar to you. For instance, if you placed an *A* next to Authenticity, Honesty, and Integrity, and you see those as similar, put them together in a cluster. Some of these words may stand alone, in their own cluster. Don't limit the number of clusters you have. If you have fewer than five, repeat the process with the *B* values.

If Felix, from *The Odd Couple*, were taking this test, he might make a cluster out of cleanliness, orderliness, and organization, another out of family, and one out of control, stability, and structure. Oscar would probably come up with a cluster out of flexibility, spontaneity, and variety, a second made up of adventure and excitement, and a third out of independence and leisure.

Counting a cluster as one value, write a brief phrase or sentence next to each cluster that succinctly describes what it means for you. Here are some examples:

Accuracy: Being correct, even in the tiniest details

Competition: Consistently out-performing my opponents

Happiness: Finding joy, pleasure, or satisfaction in the work I do and the relationships I have

Prestige: Being perceived as successful by my peers and associates

Security: Feeling safe and confident about my future

Finally, select the five values (clusters) that influence your choices the most. It may be difficult to narrow them down to five, so think carefully. You don't need to order them, since most likely they exert different levels of influence at different times. Identify your highest values in the following space.

_____

_____

_____

_____

_____

_____

_____

_____

_____

From P. Walters and J. Byl, 2008, *Christian paths to health and wellness* (Champaign, IL: Human Kinetics).

2. Your spiritual gifts

Spiritual Gift Inventory

As you read through the following list, mark each paragraph according to how well you believe it describes you. When you finish, try to decide which three of the paragraphs you marked describe you most accurately.

Y: Yes, it very much describes me.

S: It somewhat or slightly describes me.

N: No, it doesn't describe me.

?: I'm not sure.

___ a. Developing strategies or plans to reach identified goals; organizing people, tasks, and events; helping organizations or groups become more efficient; creating order out of organizational chaos.

___ b. Pioneering new projects; serving in another country or community; adapting to different cultures and surroundings; being culturally aware and sensitive.

___ c. Working creatively with wood, cloth, metal, paints, glass, etc.; working with different kinds of tools; making things with practical uses; designing or building things; working with your hands.

___ d. Communicating with variety and creativity; developing and using particular artistic skills (art, drama, music, photography); finding new and fresh ways to communicate ideas to others.

___ e. Distinguishing between truth and error, good and evil; accurately judging character; seeing through phoniness or deceit; helping others to see what's right and wrong in life situations.

___ f. Strengthening and reassuring troubled people; encouraging or challenging people; motivating others to grow; supporting people who need to take action.

___ g. Looking for opportunities to build relationships with nonbelievers; communicating openly and effectively about faith; talking about spiritual matters with nonbelievers.

___ h. Trusting God to answer prayer and encouraging others to do so; having confidence in God's continuing presence and ability to help, even in difficult times; moving forward in spite of opposition.

___ i. Giving liberally and joyfully to people in financial need or projects requiring support; managing money well in order to free more of it for giving.

___ j. Working behind the scenes to support the work of others; finding small things that need to be done and doing them without being asked; helping wherever needed, even with routine or mundane tasks.

___ k. Meeting new people and helping them to feel welcome; entertaining guests; opening your home to others who need a safe, supportive environment; setting people at ease in unfamiliar surroundings.

___ l. Frequently offering to pray for others; expressing amazing trust in God's ability to provide; showing confidence in the Lord's protection; spending a lot of time praying.

___ m. Carefully studying and researching subjects to understand them better; sharing knowledge and insights with others when asked; sometimes gaining information that is not attainable by natural means.

From P. Walters and J. Byl, 2008, *Christian paths to health and wellness* (Champaign, IL: Human Kinetics). Adapted, by permission, from Bruce Bugbee and Don Cousins. *The Network Curriculum Participant Guide,* © 1994, 2005 by The Willow Creek Community Chruch and Bruce Bugbee and Don Cousins. (2005) The Zondervan Corporation. For additional resources, go to www.brucebugbee.com.

_____ n. Taking responsibility for directing groups; motivating and guiding others to reach important goals; managing people and resources well; influencing others to perform to the best of their abilities.

_____ o. Empathizing with hurting people; patiently and compassionately supporting people through painful experiences; helping those generally regarded as undeserving or beyond help.

_____ p. Speaking with conviction to bring change in the lives of others; exposing cultural trends, teachings, or events that are morally wrong or harmful; boldly speaking truth even in places where it may be unpopular.

_____ q. Faithfully providing long-term support and nurture for a group of people; providing guidance for the whole person; patiently but firmly nurturing others in their development as believers.

_____ r. Studying, understanding, and communicating biblical truth; developing appropriate teaching material and presenting it effectively; communicating in ways that motivate others to change.

_____ s. Seeing simple, practical solutions in the midst of conflict or confusion; giving helpful advice to others facing complicated life situations; helping people take practical action to solve real problems.

Key to Spiritual Gifts

a. Administration

b. Apostleship

c. Craftsmanship

d. Creative communication

e. Discernment

f. Encouragement

g. Evangelism

h. Faith

i. Giving

j. Helps

k. Hospitality

l. Intercession

m. Knowledge

n. Leadership

o. Mercy

p. Prophecy

q. Shepherding

r. Teaching

s. Wisdom

From P. Walters and J. Byl, 2008, *Christian paths to health and wellness* (Champaign, IL: Human Kinetics). Adapted, by permission, from Bruce Bugbee and Don Cousins. *The Network Curriculum Participant Guide,* © 1994, 2005 by The Willow Creek Community Chruch and Bruce Bugbee and Don Cousins. (2005) The Zondervan Corporation. For additional resources, go to www.brucebugbee.com.

References

ABC News. (2004). Eminem, the boy who loved to bounce. Retrieved February 26, 2004, from www.abcnews.go.com.

Alighieri, D. (1998). *The divine comedy* (A. Mandelbaum, Trans.). New York: Oxford University Press.

Amato, P.R., Johnson, D.R., Booth, A., & Rogers, S.J. (2003). Continuity and change in marital quality between 1980 and 2000. *Journal of Marriage and Family, 65*(1): 1-22.

AZLyrics. (2006). AZLyrics.com. Retrieved September 9, 2006, from www.azlyrics.com/lyrics/eminem/cleaninoutmycloset.html.

Barna, G. (2001). *The power of team leadership.* Colorado Springs, CO: Waterbrook Press.

Berkman, L.F., & Syme, S.L. (1979). Social networks, host resistance and mortality: A nine-year follow-up study of Alameda County residents. *America Journal of Epidemiology, 128*(2): 370-380.

Bugbee, B., Cousins, D., & Hybels, B. (1994). *Network: The right people. . .in the right places. . .for the right reasons.* Grand Rapids, MI: Zondervan.

Buss, D.M. (1985). Human mate selection. *American Scientist, 73*: 47-51.

Draper, E. (1992). *Draper's book of quotations for the Christian world.* Wheaton, IL: Tyndale House.

Duin, J. (2002). Why singles boycott churches. *Breakpoint* (April): 10-15.

Eisenberger, N.I., Lieberman, M.D., & Williams, K.D. (2003). Does rejection hurt? An MRI study of social exclusion – Rejection by other people in a social situation triggers brain activity resembling that produced by physical pain. *Science, 302*(5643): 290-293.

Fields, J.S. (1996). Face: Susan Graham. *Texas Monthly* (December): 10.

Fletcher, J. (2004). The dysfunctional family house. *Wall Street Journal* (March 26): W1, W8.

Franzen, J. (1998). American notes – Imperial bedroom: The real problem with privacy is that we have too much of it. *The New Yorker* (October 12): 48-54.

Freud, S. (1953). *The standard edition of the complete psychological works of Sigmund Freud.* London: Hogarth Press and the Institute of Psycho-Analysis.

Fuller Institute of Church Growth. (1993). Fuller Institute of Church Growth. *Leadership Journal* (January): 26.

Gandelman, J. (2006). The moderate voice: Radio DJ sued by "100 Grand" joke contest "winner." Retrieved September 18, 2006, from www.themoderatevoice.com/posts/1119773729.shtml (site discontinued).

Gottman, J., Gottman, J., & Declaire, J. (2006). *Ten lessons to transform your marriage: America's love lab experts share their strategies for strengthening your relationship.* New York: Crown.

Graham, S. (2006). Susan Graham. Retrieved September 8, 2006, from www.susangraham.com/index.htm.

Heath, C. (1999). The unbearable Bradness of being. *Rolling Stone* (October 28): 26.

Johnson, C., & Penner, D. (2005). Sources of missionary conflict. Retrieved July 29, 2005, from http://tatumweb.com/pulpit/sermons/comfort-2001-12-30.html.

Keirsey, D., & Bates, M. (1984). *Please understand me* (5th ed.). Del Mar, CA: Prometheus Nemesis.

Kise, J., Stark, D., & Hirsh, S. (1996). *LifeKeys.* Minneapolis, MN: Bethany House.

Lewis, C.S. (1944). *The problem of pain.* New York: Macmillan.

Lindbergh, A.M. (1992). *Gift from the sea* (50th anniversary ed.). New York: Pantheon.

Luft, J.A.I.H. (1955). *The Johari window, a graphic model of interpersonal awareness.* Paper presented at the western training laboratory in group development, Los Angeles, UCLA.

McPherson, M., Smith-Lovin, L., & Brashears, M.E. (2006). Social isolation in America: Changes in core discussion networks over two decades. *American Sociological Review, 71*(3): 353-376.

Michael, R.T., Gagnon, J.H., Laumann, E.D., & Kolata, G. (1994). *Sex in America: A definitive survey.* Boston: Little and Brown.

Nick, S. (2005). Transition: Vivian Malone Jones. *Newsweek* (October 24): 10.

Oliver, M.A.M. (1994). *Conjugal spirituality: The primacy of mutual love and Christian tradition.* Kansas City: Sheed and Ward.

Ornish, D. (1990). *Reversing heart disease.* New York: Ballantine.

Ornish, D. (1999). *Love and survival.* New York: HarperCollins.

Page, C. (2006). You're not alone. *Chicago Tribune* (July 2): 2.

Peacemakers. (2004). The peacemaker pledge. Retrieved June 6, 2007, from www.peacemaker.net/site/c.aqKFLTOBIpH/b.1172255/apps/s/content.asp?ct=1245339.

Peterson, E. (2003). *The message: The Bible in contemporary language.* Omaha, Nebraska: Quickverse.

Previti, D., & Amato, P.R. (2003). Why stay married? Rewards, barriers, and marital stability. *Journal of Marriage and Family, 65*(3): 561-573.

Putnam, R.D. (2000). *Bowling alone: The collapse and revival of American community.* New York: Simon and Schuster.

Shulman, P. (2004). Great expectations. *Psychology Today*: 33-34, 37-38, 41-42.

Siegler, I.C., Longino, C., & Johnson, C. (1992). The Georgia Centenarian Study: Comments from friends. *The International Journal of Aging & Human Development, 34*(1): 77-82.

Simon, N. (1968). *The Odd Couple.* Retrieved February 21, 2005, from www.imdb.com/title/tt0063374.

Stebbins, T. (1995). *Friendship evangelism by the book: Applying first century principles to 21st-century relationships.* Camp Hill, PA: Christian Publications.

Thomas, G. (2000). *Sacred marriage.* Grand Rapids, MI: Zondervan.

Tisch, S., Finerman, W., & Zemeckis, R. (1994). *Forrest Gump.* Paramount Pictures.

U.S. Census Bureau. (2005a). Table A1. Marital status of people 15 years and over, by age, sex, personal earnings, race, and hispanic origin/1:2005. Retrieved September 25, 2006, from www.census.gov.

U.S. Census Bureau. (2005b). Unmarried and single Americans. Retrieved September 25, 2006, from www.census.gov/Press-Release/www/releases/archives/families_households/006840.html.

Waldman, S. (1992). Religious denominations. *The New Republic, 27*(20): 32.

Walters, P., Gustafson, J., Williams, B., & Carlson, K. (2006). *What your students are really thinking.* Paper presented at the Christian Society of Kinesiology, Sport, and Leisure, Boston, MA.

Warren, R. (2002). The purpose-driven life: What on earth am I here for? Retrieved June 7, 2007, from www.loc.gov/catdir/enhancements/fy0633/2002011471-d.html.

Williams, D. (2001). How link between forgiveness and health changes with age. Retrieved September 23, 2006, from www.umich.edu/news/index.html?Releases/2001/Dec01/r121101a.

Yancey, P. (1997). *Where is God when it hurts? A comforting healing guide for coping with hard times* (Rev. and updated; Zondervan mass market ed.). Grand Rapids, MI: Zondervan.

Suggesetd Readings

Chapman, G.D. (1995). *The five love languages: How to express heartfelt commitment to your mate.* **Chicago: Northfield.**

In this guidebook you'll learn how to identify your love language (Words of Affirmation, Quality Time, Gifts, Acts of Service, and Physical Touch) and how to speak the love language of others.

Goleman, D. (1998). Working with emotional intelligence. Retrieved August 9, 2007, from www.loc.gov/catdir/bios/random058/98018706.html.

Business leaders and outstanding performers are not defined by their IQs or even their job skills, but by their "emotional intelligence". From this premise, Goleman describes how to quantify your emotional skill.

Keirsey, D., & Bates, M. (1984). *Please understand me* **(5th ed.). Del Mar, CA: Prometheus Nemesis.**

Using the popular Myers-Briggs personality inventory, Keirsey helps people better understand themselves and others.

Kise, J., Stark, D., & Hirsh, S. (1996). *LifeKeys.* **Minneapolis, MN: Bethany House.**

This book is about discovering who you are, why you're here, and what you do best.

Matthews, G., Zeidner, M., & Roberts, R.D. (2002). *Emotional intelligence: Science and myth.* **Cambridge, MA: MIT Press.**

This book examines current thinking on the nature, components, determinants, and consequences of emotional intelligence.

Yancey, P. (1997). *Where is God when it hurts?: A comforting, healing guide for coping with hard times* **(Rev. and updated). Grand Rapids, MI: Zondervan.**

This book attempts to comfort those who feel abandoned, rejected, and isolated from a loving God.

Suggesetd Web Sites

www.fivelovelanguages.com

Five different ways people express love.

www.haygroup.com/tl/EI/Default.aspx

Test your emotional intelligence at this Web site.

www.queendom.com

If you like taking tests, Queendom offers the largest online battery of professionally developed and validated psychological assessments anywhere.

Conclusion

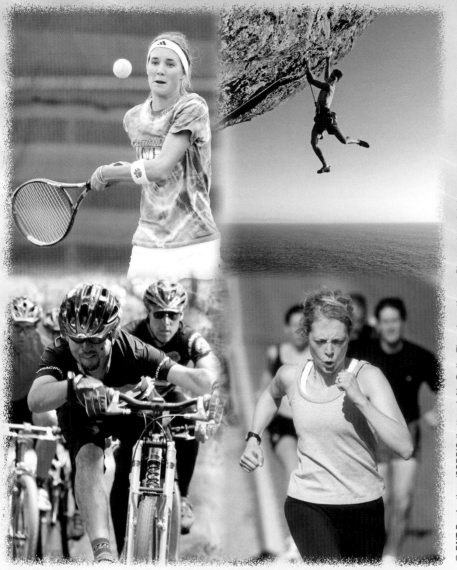

© RNT Productions/CORBIS (bottom left), © Jim Thornburg/Aurora Photos (top right)

Offering Your Life as a Living Sacrifice

John Byl

After reading this chapter, you should be able to do the following:

1. Understand how an eternal perspective shapes wellness.
2. Understand how prayer plays a positive role in wellness.
3. Review the seven steps to make wellness a reality.

We've completed a course together focusing on physical, emotional, and relational wellness. But what does it all mean? In Romans 11:36, the Bible points to what gives meaning: "For from him and through him and to him are all things. To him be the glory forever! Amen" (also restated in 1 Corinthians 8:6). To find meaning in the physical, emotional, and relational self, you need to own your past and recognize that all good things come from God, make decisions today and recognize that every breath depends on God's grace, and look to the next steps and your future and offer every part of your life as a living sacrifice to God. There is one purpose in the push for wellness: to glorify God (1 Corinthians 10:31).

Before concluding this book, I want to cover two more steps. The first step involves looking at a sense of eternity and using prayer as help in a wellness walk. The second step involves reviewing the main threads of each chapter to ensure success in improving and maintaining a high level of wellness.

Tools for Achieving Wellness

At least two steps are particularly important in achieving wellness:

1. Understand the big picture. Your existence is eternal. Seeing the big picture ought to fundamentally change many attitudes.
2. The power of prayer, a time of communication with God, has many positive benefits.

Eternity

To believe in God is to gain eternal life. **Eternal life** does not begin when you die but is a present reality. The well-known verse John 3:16 notes that everyone who believes in Jesus Christ "has eternal life." It does not say that believers *will get* it, but rather they *have* it. It has been said that "life is too short to worry about it." The Christian view is quite the opposite: Life is too long to worry about it.

Remembering that you live forever ought to change the way you think about rushing through your 70 or so years on earth. Whether a loan gets paid off in 10 years or 20, in the context of eternity, is rather inconsequential. A million years from now, as you sit drinking juice on a hillside overlooking the New Jerusalem, what do you think you will say about the big game you lost, the date that didn't work out, the exam you blew, or the business deal you just missed?

Having an attitude of life as eternal does not contradict Paul's encouragement to "press on toward the goal" (Philippians 3:14) or Jesus' declaration to use talents, not bury them (Matthew 25:14–30), or God's command to "fill the earth and subdue it" (Genesis 1:28). Ask yourself: What are you trying to build in this life? Houses or homes? Personal investments or kingdom investments? Remembering that life goes on forever ought to open people to the leading of the Holy Spirit and make them more dependent on God's providence. Resting in God will also improve wellness.

Prayer

You've probably seen little sayings like "No prayer, no peace. Know prayer, know peace," or "Why pray when you can worry and fret?" Prayer is probably one of the most powerful ways of opening up to the Holy Spirit. Several scripture passages speak powerfully about the authority of prayer: "Is any one of you in trouble? He should pray" (James 5:13). "Cast all your anxiety on him because he cares for you" (1 Peter 5:7). "Do not be anxious about anything, but in everything, by prayer and petition, with thanksgiving, present your requests to God. And the peace of God, which transcends all understanding, will guard your hearts and your minds in Christ Jesus" (Philippians 4:6–7; see also 1 Timothy 2:1–2).

You wouldn't talk to a friend or lover only to get things. Rather, you talk to them because you want to share in their lives. God wants us to do the same through **prayer**. Some academics would suggest that the effect of prayer is experienced more individually than empirically (Duckro & Magaletta, 1994), but others suggest that "religiosity and prayer contribute without question to one's quality of life and perceptions of well-being" (Poloma & Pendleton, 1991, p. 81). Speak often with God.

Seven Steps to Wellness

Throughout this text we have encouraged you to not walk aimlessly through life, but to walk with purpose and direction as you are led by God. It's important to have a realistic and positive view of who you are; to anticipate major obstacles and strategize how to move beyond them; and to celebrate God, who you are, and what you are able to achieve. Life was meant to be abundant. Here's a review of seven steps towards successful wellness in life. The assignment on page 287 asks you to do one last review of your specific goals, obstacles to success, intervention strategies, and measures of success—so you know when and what to celebrate!

Step 1: State the Goal

In Paul's letter to the Ephesians he said that a person oriented to God will not be tossed around in life like inner tubes in a water slide, but will grow up to be a solid Christian (Ephesians 4:14–15).

In chapter 1, we included Paul's exhortation "to offer your bodies as living sacrifices, holy and pleasing to God—this is your spiritual act of worship" (Romans 12:1). Furthermore, in Christ's call to be perfect (Matthew 5:48), an overarching goal is to show God through the body.

Making life changes (as spiritual worship, as seeking godly perfection) is a difficult task and one that takes a lifetime. Writing down goals provides accountability in accomplishing them. The saying that Rome was not built in a day is a good reminder to always keep the big picture in mind and to paint positive strokes for today.

Step 2: Assess Your Present Lifestyle

A second step we suggested is to know yourself, especially in relation to God. Remember the uniqueness of each fingerprint, and the uniqueness of each personality, the past, present, and future. It is important to know yourself in relation to God and others. It is good to remember that God values you (Luke 12:23–25).

Consider Paul's reminder to value living in relation with others:

Love must be sincere. Hate what is evil; cling to what is good. Be devoted to one another in brotherly love. Honor one another above yourselves. Never be lacking in zeal, but keep your spiritual fervor, serving the Lord. Be joyful in hope, patient in affliction, faithful in prayer. Share with God's people who are in need. Practice hospitality. Bless those who persecute you; bless and do not curse. Rejoice with those who rejoice; mourn with those who mourn. Live in harmony with one another. Do not be proud, but be willing to associate with people of low position. Do not be conceited. Do not repay anyone evil for evil. Be careful to do what is right in the eyes of everybody. If it is possible, as far as it depends on you, live at peace with everyone. (Romans 12:9–18)

Step 3: Design a Specific Plan

A third step we covered was to set goals that are realistic, specific, measurable, and concrete. Setting goals in this manner best helps achieve them. Do not count on good intentions along to motivate you. Having concrete goals helps us direct our lives and gives us specific accomplishments to celebrate.

Step 4: Predict Obstacles

Predict obstacles that might keep you from achieving your goals for healthy living. The Lord's Prayer recognizes these with the request, "And lead us not into temptation, but deliver us from the evil one" (Mathew 6:13). It is good to remember that temptations are not unique to you nor are they so powerful that they will inevitably overtake you. Paul said that the temptations each person experiences are not unique and that God "will not let you be tempted beyond what you can bear. But when you are tempted, he will also provide a way out so that you can stand up under it" (1 Corinthians 10:13).

Challenges in life bring growth. Paul writes that trials develop perseverance, and perseverance leads to maturity (James 1:2–4). Don't be beaten by obstacles, but rise to their challenges in God's strength and grow through them to become more than you are today.

Step 5: Plan Intervention Strategies

Step 5 involves formulating intervention strategies to help in complying with the plan. It's important to identify weaknesses and strengths and develop strategies to move forward. Remember that you don't need to go purely on your own strength. As Paul said: "I can do everything through him who gives me strength" (Philippians 4:13). We need to know ahead of time the likely obstacles to our goals to healthy living. We also need to know how we can avoid these obstacles or how we can successfully pass through these tough places without being derailed.

Step 6: Assess Compliance With the Plan

In step 6, you determined how you would evaluate how well you were sticking to your plan. Looking back at yesterday's successes and challenges helps plan a more effective tomorrow. We've set concrete goals, but when do we know when we've crossed another bridge on the road to successful living? We need to know when we've crossed this bridge and how long we have kept ourselves from crossing back over again to unhealthy practices. We need to know how we are succeeding.

Step 7: Assess Progress of Your Overall Goal

Step 7 is to plan celebrations along the way to encourage progress in achieving your goals. Physical, emotional, and relational wellness is an opportunity to enjoy and glorify God. As you enjoy God you give him glory, and as you glorify God you give him enjoyment. Open your life and experience God's blessing of physical, emotional, and relational wellness. Feel God's healing touch through this benediction:

> The Lord bless you and keep you;
>
> the Lord make his face shine upon you
>
> and be gracious to you;
>
> the Lord turn his face toward you
>
> and give you peace.

(Numbers 6:24–26)

Next Steps

You've completed this course, so you won't have it to support you from here. However, you should have interventions built in so you are accountable and supported by others and by God. Pursue joyful and purposeful life with God that brings Him glory and is of service to others, through maintaining and enhancing your wellness.

Key Terms

eternal life

prayer

Review Questions

1. How does the realization that you live forever affect your wellness?

2. How do your conversations with God through prayer affect your wellness?

Application Activities

1. In each chapter we ask you to think about how you maintain a healthy fitness level or how you need to change your life to make permanent lifestyle alterations. The following assignment has you develop comprehensive and refined goals to achieve and maintain a total healthy lifestyle.

Assignment—Putting It All Together

Your name: _____

Today's date: _____

In the first column on the left side of the box, write your specific mission statement and your eight goals. Next, write the major obstacles that you foresee impeding the realization of your goals. Then write the key intervention strategies you will put in place to overcome the potential obstacles. Finally, note what will you accomplish, and when, so you can celebrate when you reach your goals.

Goal	Obstacles	Interventions	Success?
Mission statement			What? When?
Body image			What? When?
Strength			What? When?
Cardio			What? When?
Flexibility			What? When?
Nutrition			What? When?
Stress			What? When?
Sleep			What? When?
Relationships			What? When?

From P. Walters and J. Byl, 2008, *Christian paths to health and wellness* (Champaign, IL: Human Kinetics).

References

Duckro, P., & Magaletta, P. (1994). The effect of prayer on physical health: Experimental evidence. *Journal of Religion and Health, 33*(3): 211-219.

Poloma, M., & Pendleton, B. (1991). The effects of prayer and prayer experiences on measures of general well-being. *Journal of Psychology and Theology, 19*(1): 71-83.

Suggested Readings

Nouwen, H. (1998). *Making all things new* **(reissue). San Francisco: Harper.**

The book is about more than prayer, but truly points to wellness.

Suggested Web Sites

www.sacredspace.ie

Sacred Space is a helpful Web site to help you spend 10 minutes praying as you sit at your computer. It has on-screen guidance and scripture chosen special every day. It is available in more than 20 languages. There is also a guide to physical positioning, breathing exercises, listening tools, and the use of poems and pictures to assist your prayer life. The site is operated by Irish Jesuits.

Appendix A

Guide for Family and Friends
of a Person With Food and Weight Problems

When first approaching a friend or family member, understand that she may not welcome your concern and may even react with anger or denial. She will discuss the eating disorder with someone when she feels ready. She will probably feel more able to do so if she knows that you are concerned but are not going to force her into anything before she's ready. You may need to make an exception if the condition constitutes a medical emergency. Be prepared for the possibility that a discussion about the eating problems might not lead to any change in attitude or behavior. Again, this is because the person may have very good reason for not giving up the eating disorder as a coping strategy.

Here are a few other suggestions:

- Focus on feelings and relationships, not on weight and food.

- Convey concern for the person's health while still respecting his privacy. Eating disorders are often a cry for help, and the person will appreciate knowing that someone is concerned.

- A family should not allow their own lives and habits to be hindered by a dieting child.

- A family should set caring and reasonable but firm limits in a consistent manner. This may come up when the person affected wants to skip meals or eat alone or gets angry when someone eats her "special" food.

- Avoid commenting on appearance; the person is already overly focused on this. Comments about weight or appearance, even if the intent is complimentary, will only perpetuate the obsession with body image.

- Demanding change or berating the person for eating habits will not work. Avoid power struggles around eating. Eating disorders are often expressions of a need for control or a substitution for lack of control that the person feels in other areas of his life. Trying to trick or force someone to eat can make things worse.

- Realize that the person will go at her own pace in getting better. By gently giving her information and being supportive, you are enabling her to see and consider alternatives to the present situation.

- Examine your own attitudes about food, weight, body image, and body size to ensure you do not convey any prejudice or exacerbate the desire to be thin. If the person expresses feeling fat or wanting to lose weight, instead of saying, "You're not fat," suggest he explore his fears about being fat and what he thinks he can achieve by being thin. Encourage reflection on the pressures in society to look a certain way and how this negatively affects his self-esteem. Think about the way you personally are affected by body image pressures, and share these with the person in a supportive manner.

- Seeing someone you love struggling with an eating disorder might make you feel very scared, angry, frustrated, and helpless. However, be careful not to blame her for her struggle. Try to understand that eating problems as a coping strategy for dealing with painful emotions or experiences. Despite the grief the eating disorder causes people and those around them, it may be hard to let go.

- Finally, it is important that you do not take on the role of the therapist. Do only what you feel capable of. It is often helpful for family members or friends to get some support for themselves. You need take care of yourself while dealing with your friend or family member.

From P. Walters and J. Byl, 2008, *Christian paths to health and wellness* (Champaign, IL: Human Kinetics). Reprinted with permission from the National Eating Disorder Information Centre, Toronto, Ontario.

Appendix B

Questionnaires on Eating Behaviors

The following two tests do not formally diagnose an eating disorder. The questions presented involve thoughts, behaviors, and feelings that are common in someone with an eating disorder. Therefore it will provide you with some insight on your present attitudes about eating.

If you answer yes to three or more questions on questionnaire #1, it could be a sign that you have an eating disorder or the beginning of one. You may want to consider seeing a therapist or talking to someone at an eating disorder clinic about this matter.

Table B.1 Questionnaire #1

Instructions: Please answer yes or no to the following questions.	Yes or No
1. Do you starve yourself regularly?	
2. Do you binge and then make yourself vomit?	
3. Do you feel out of control when you eat?	
4. Do you feel powerful and in control when you are able to abstain from eating?	
5. Do you binge on food when you are experiencing negative feelings (e.g., anger, sadness, loneliness)?	
6. Do you feel that you do not deserve to eat?	
7. Do you know the calorie contents in the food that you eat?	
8. Do you feel the only control you have in your life is in the areas of food and weight?	
9. Do you believe that you are fat, even though people tell you otherwise?	
10. Do you feel that you have to be perfect in everything you do?	
11. Do you use laxatives, diet pills, or diuretics as a method of weight control?	
12. Do you exercise to burn calories, rather than to stay fit?	
13. Are you secretive about your eating habits?	
14. Do you feel anger toward anyone that questions your eating habits?	
15. Do you feel guilty after you eat?	
16. Do you hear negative messages in your head (e.g., saying that you are fat, ugly, worthless, etc.)?	

From P. Walters and J. Byl, 2008, *Christian paths to health and wellness* (Champaign, IL: Human Kinetics). Adapted from Thompson & Comeau, 2000.

(continued)

Table B.1 *(continued)*

Instructions: Please answer yes or no to the following questions.	Yes or No
17. Do you avoid social events because there will be food present?	
18. Do you think about food constantly?	
19. Do you have an intense fear of gaining weight?	
20. Do you feel ashamed of your eating behaviors?	
21. Do you feel that no matter what you do you will never be good enough?	
22. Do you think you may have an eating disorder?	

From P. Walters and J. Byl, 2008, *Christian paths to health and wellness* (Champaign, IL: Human Kinetics). Adapted from Thompson & Comeau, 2000.

Table B.2   Questionnaire #2

Instructions: Please circle the word or number that best represents your answer to the question. Eating disorders are potentially life-threatening, but they can be overcome with proper information, support, and counseling. The earlier you seek help, the better, although it is never too late to start on the road to recovery.

1. I have eating habits that are different from those of my family and friends.	1 - Often	2 - Sometimes	3 - Rarely	4 - Never
2. I find myself panicking if I cannot exercise as I planned because I am afraid I will gain weight if I don't.	1 - Often	2 - Sometimes	3 - Rarely	4 - Never
3. My friends tell me I am thin, but I don't believe them because I feel fat.	1 - Often	2 - Sometimes	3 - Rarely	4 - Never
4. (Females only) My menstrual period has stopped or become irregular due to no known medical reasons.	1 - True	2 - False		
5. I have become obsessed with food to the point that I cannot go through a day without worrying about what I will or will not eat.	1 - Almost always	2 - Sometimes	3 - Rarely	4 - Never
6. I have lost more than 15 percent of what is considered a healthy weight for my height and currently weigh that or weigh less (please see appendix C).	1 - True	2 - False		
7. I would panic if I got on the scale tomorrow and found out that I had gained 2 pounds (4.5 kg).	1 - Almost always	2 - Sometimes	3 - Rarely	4 - Never
8. I find that I prefer to eat alone or when I am sure no one will see me, so I make excuses so I can eat less and less with friends and family.	1 - Almost always	2 - Sometimes	3 - Rarely	4 - Never

From P. Walters and J. Byl, 2008, *Christian paths to health and wellness* (Champaign, IL: Human Kinetics).

9. I find myself going on uncontrollable eating binges during which I consume large amounts of food to the point that I feel sick and make myself vomit.	1 - Never	2 - Less than 1 time per week	3 - 1 to 6 times per week	4 - 1 or more times per day

Only answer the rest if your answer to #9 was 1; otherwise leave blank.

10. I find myself compulsively eating more than I want to while feeling out of control or unaware of what I am doing.	1 - Never	2 - Less than 1 time per week	3 - 1 to 6 times per week	4 - 1 or more times per day
11. I use laxatives or diuretics as a means of weight control.	1 - Never	2 - Rarely	3 - Sometimes	4 - Regularly
12. I find myself cutting up my food into small pieces or hiding food so people will think I ate it, chewing it and spitting it out without swallowing it, or making certain foods off-limits.	1 - Often	2 - Sometimes	3 - Rarely	4 - Never
13. People around me have become very interested in what I eat, and I get angry at them for pushing me to eat more.	1- Often	2- Sometimes	3 - Rarely	4 - Never
14. I have felt more depressed and irritable recently than I used to or have been spending an increasing amount of time alone.	1 -True	2 - False		
15. I keep a lot of my fears about food and eating to myself because I am afraid no one would understand.	1 - Often	2 - Sometimes	3 - Rarely	4 - Never
16. I enjoy making gourmet or high-calorie meals for others as long as I don't have to eat any myself.	1 - Often	2 - Sometimes	3 - Rarely	4 - Never
17. The most powerful fear in my life is the fear of gaining weight or becoming fat.	1 - Often	2 - Sometimes	3 - Rarely	4 - Never
18. I exercise a lot (more than four times per week and more than four hours per week) as a means of weight control.	1 - True	2 - False		
19. I find myself totally absorbed when reading books or magazines about dieting, exercise, and calorie counting to the point I spend hours studying them.	1 - Often	2 - Sometimes	3 - Rarely	4 - Never
20. I tend to be a perfectionist and am not satisfied with myself unless I do things perfectly.	1 - Almost always	2 - Sometimes	3 - Rarely	4 - Never
21. I go through long periods of time without eating or when eating very little as a means of weight control.	1 - Often	2 - Sometimes	3 - Rarely	4 - Never
22. It is important to me to try to be thinner than all of my friends.	1 - Almost always	2 - Sometimes	3 - Rarely	4 - Never

Add up the numbers on this questionnaire to get a total score.

From P. Walters and J. Byl, 2008, *Christian paths to health and wellness* (Champaign, IL: Human Kinetics).

Table B.3 Scoring Key for Questionnaire #2

Score	Response	Recommendations
38 or less	Strong tendencies toward anorexia nervosa	If you scored below 50 it would be wise for you to seek more information about anorexia nervosa and bulimia nervosa. Contact a counselor, pastor, teacher, or physician to find out if you have an eating disorder. If you do, talk about what kind of assistance would be best for you.
39 – 50	Strong tendencies toward bulimia nervosa	See previous recommendations
50 – 60	Weight conscious; may or may not have tendencies toward an eating disorder; not likely to have anorexia or bulimia; may have tendencies toward compulsive eating or obesity	If you scored between 50 and 60, it would be a good idea for you to talk to a counselor, pastor, teacher, or physician to determine if you have an eating disorder and if you do to learn how to get some help.
Over 60	Unlikely to have anorexia or bulimia; however, scoring 60 does not rule out tendencies toward compulsive eating or obesity.	If you scored over 60 but have questions and concerns about the way you eat or your weight, it would be a good idea for you to talk to a counselor, pastor, teacher, or physician to determine if you have an eating disorder; if you do to learn how to get some help.

From P. Walters and J. Byl, 2008, *Christian paths to health and wellness* (Champaign, IL: Human Kinetics); Reiff & Reiff, 1999.

Appendix C

Strength-Training Program

Phase I: day 1	Sets/effort 1/85-100%	Repetitions 12-15	Repetition speed 2/0/2	Rest between sets 60-90 s
Seated leg extension	Wt 50 Reps 12	Notes		
Lat pull-down	Wt Reps	Notes		
Seated back extension	Wt Reps	Notes		
Abdominal crunch	Wt Reps	Notes		
Chest press	Wt Reps	Notes		
Lateral raise	Wt Reps	Notes		

(continued)

From P. Walters and J. Byl, 2008, *Christian paths to health and wellness* (Champaign, IL: Human Kinetics).

(continued)

Phase I: day 1	Sets/effort 1/85-100%	Repetitions 12-15		Repetition speed 2/0/2	Rest between sets 60-90 s
Arm extension	Wt	Notes			
	Reps				
Arm curl	Wt	Notes			
	Reps				

Phase I strength-training program

Weeks 1-2	WEEK 1			WEEK 2		
	Day 1	Day 2	Day 3	Day 1	Day 2	Day 3
Seated leg extension	Wt	Wt	Wt	Wt	Wt	Wt
	50	50	50	50	60	60
	Reps	Reps	Reps	Reps	Reps	Reps
	12	13	14	15	12	13
Lat pull-down	Wt	Wt	Wt	Wt	Wt	Wt
	Reps	Reps	Reps	Reps	Reps	Reps
Seated back extension	Wt	Wt	Wt	Wt	Wt	Wt
	Reps	Reps	Reps	Reps	Reps	Reps
Abdominal crunch	Wt	Wt	Wt	Wt	Wt	Wt
	Reps	Reps	Reps	Reps	Reps	Reps
Chest press	Wt	Wt	Wt	Wt	Wt	Wt
	Reps	Reps	Reps	Reps	Reps	Reps

Weeks 1-2	WEEK 1			WEEK 2		
	Day 1	Day 2	Day 3	Day 1	Day 2	Day 3
Lateral raise	Wt	Wt	Wt	Wt	Wt	Wt
	Reps	Reps	Reps	Reps	Reps	Reps
Arm extension	Wt	Wt	Wt	Wt	Wt	Wt
	Reps	Reps	Reps	Reps	Reps	Reps
Arm curl	Wt	Wt	Wt	Wt	Wt	Wt
	Reps	Reps	Reps	Reps	Reps	Reps

Phase II: day 1	Sets/effort	Repetitions	Repetition speed	Rest between sets
	1/85-100%	9-12	2/0/2	60-90 s
45-degree leg press	Wt	Notes		
	Reps			
Leg curl	Wt	Notes		
	Reps			
Low row	Wt	Notes		
	Reps			
Incline back extension	Wt	Notes		
	Reps			
Torso rotation	Wt	Notes		
	Reps			
Reverse crunch	Wt	Notes		
	Reps			
Chest fly	Wt	Notes		
	Reps			

(continued)

From P. Walters and J. Byl, 2008, *Christian paths to health and wellness* (Champaign, IL: Human Kinetics).

(continued)

Phase II: day 1	Sets/effort	Repetitions	Repetition speed	Rest between sets
	1/85-100%	9-12	2/0/2	60-90 s
Bent-over rear cable raise	Wt	Notes		
	Reps			
Standing dumbbell curl	Wt	Notes		
	Reps			
Triceps push-down	Wt	Notes		
	Reps			

Phase II strength-training program

Weeks 3-4	WEEK 3			WEEK 4		
	Day 1	Day 2	Day 3	Day 1	Day 2	Day 3
45-degree leg press	Wt	Wt	Wt	Wt	Wt	Wt
	Reps	Reps	Reps	Reps	Reps	Reps
Leg curl	Wt	Wt	Wt	Wt	Wt	Wt
	Reps	Reps	Reps	Reps	Reps	Reps
Low row	Wt.	Wt.	Wt.	Wt.	Wt.	Wt.
	Reps	Reps	Reps	Reps	Reps	Reps

From P. Walters and J. Byl, 2008, *Christian paths to health and wellness* (Champaign, IL: Human Kinetics).

Weeks 3-4	WEEK 3			WEEK 4		
	Day 1	Day 2	Day 3	Day 1	Day 2	Day 3
Incline back extensions	Wt.	Wt.	Wt.	Wt.	Wt.	Wt.
	Reps	Reps	Reps	Reps	Reps	Reps
Torso rotation	Wt.	Wt.	Wt.	Wt.	Wt.	Wt.
	Reps	Reps	Reps	Reps	Reps	Reps
Reverse crunches	Wt.	Wt.	Wt.	Wt.	Wt.	Wt.
	Reps	Reps	Reps	Reps	Reps	Reps
Chest fly	Wt.	Wt.	Wt.	Wt.	Wt.	Wt.
	Reps	Reps	Reps	Reps	Reps	Reps
Bent-over rear cable raises	Wt.	Wt.	Wt.	Wt.	Wt.	Wt.
	Reps	Reps	Reps	Reps	Reps	Reps
Standing dumbell curl	Wt.	Wt.	Wt.	Wt.	Wt.	Wt.
	Reps	Reps	Reps	Reps	Reps	Reps
Tricep push down	Wt.	Wt.	Wt.	Wt.	Wt.	Wt.
	Reps	Reps	Reps	Reps	Reps	Reps

From P. Walters and J. Byl, 2008, *Christian paths to health and wellness* (Champaign, IL: Human Kinetics).

Phase III: day 1	Sets/effort	Repetitions	Repetition speed	Rest between sets
	1/85-100%	6-9	2/0/2	60-90 s
Box squat	Wt	Notes		
	Reps			
Leg adduction	Wt	Notes		
	Reps			
One-arm dumbbell row	Wt	Notes		
	Reps			
Hanging leg raise/stability ball sit-up	Wt	Notes		
	Reps			
Bench press	Wt	Notes		
	Reps			
Seated press	Wt	Notes		
	Reps			

(continued)

From P. Walters and J. Byl, 2008, *Christian paths to health and wellness* (Champaign, IL: Human Kinetics).

(continued)

Phase III: day 1	Sets/effort	Repetitions		Repetition speed	Rest between sets
	1/85-100%	6-9		2/0/2	60-90 s
Seated alternating dumbbell curl	Wt	Notes			
	Reps				
Seated two-arm dumbbell triceps press	Wt	Notes			
	Reps				

Phase III **strength-training program**

Weeks 5-6	WEEK 5			WEEK 6		
	Day 1	Day 2	Day 3	Day 1	Day 2	Day 3
Box squat	Wt	Wt	Wt	Wt	Wt	Wt
	Reps	Reps	Reps	Reps	Reps	Reps
Leg adduction	Wt	Wt	Wt	Wt	Wt	Wt
	Reps	Reps	Reps	Reps	Reps	Reps

Weeks 5-6	WEEK 5			WEEK 6		
	Day 1	Day 2	Day 3	Day 1	Day 2	Day 3
One-arm dumbell row	Wt	Wt	Wt	Wt	Wt	Wt
	Reps	Reps	Reps	Reps	Reps	Reps

From P. Walters and J. Byl, 2008, *Christian paths to health and wellness* (Champaign, IL: Human Kinetics).

Hanging leg raise/stability ball sit-up	Wt	Wt	Wt	Wt	Wt	Wt
	Reps	Reps	Reps	Reps	Reps	Reps
Bench press	Wt	Wt	Wt	Wt	Wt	Wt
	Reps	Reps	Reps	Reps	Reps	Reps
Seated press	Wt	Wt	Wt	Wt	Wt	Wt
	Reps	Reps	Reps	Reps	Reps	Reps
Seated alternating dumbell curl	Wt	Wt	Wt	Wt	Wt	Wt
	Reps	Reps	Reps	Reps	Reps	Reps
Seated two-arm dumbell triceps press	Wt	Wt	Wt	Wt	Wt	Wt
	Reps	Reps	Reps	Reps	Reps	Reps

Glossary

actin—A protein filament inside of the myofibril that combines with myosin to generate force.

activating event, or stressor—Any event or condition that triggers a stress response.

adenosine triphosphate (ATP)—The body's most readily available source of energy. ATP is composed of one adenosine molecule and three phosphate groups.

aerobic capacity—The maximum ability to take in, transport, and use oxygen.

aerobic endurance—The body's ability to sustain prolonged physical activity that uses the cardiorespiratory system.

aerobic exercise—Activities that predominantly use the oxidative energy system.

aesthetician—One who studies aesthetics; one who studies the nature of beauty.

alimentary canal—The large, muscular tube in the digestive system through which food passes from the mouth to the anus.

all-or-nothing thinking—Looking at things in absolute, black and white categories.

amenorrhea—The absence of menstruation.

amino acids—The essential building blocks of proteins.

anaerobic—Activities that predominantly use the phosphagen and glycolytic systems and do not require oxygen for metabolic work.

anorexia athletica—Exercising compulsively in an effort to control weight and in a misguided attempt to gain a sense of power, control, and self-respect.

anorexia nervosa—An eating disorder characterized by an intense fear of becoming obese, a distorted body image, and extreme weight loss. A form of self-starvation.

antagonist—The muscle or group of muscles that can either slow down or stop a particular movement.

antioxidants—A chemical that reduces the rate of oxidation reactions in a specific context. These substances found in food help prevent cell damage.

arousal—A physiological and psychological state of increased activation, alertness, and readiness to respond.

ascetic—One who holds a view that through renunciation of worldly pleasures it is possible to achieve a higher spiritual or intellectual state.

asceticism—A view that through renunciation of worldly pleasures it is possible to achieve a high spiritual or intellectual state.

Atkins diet—A diet high in protein and saturated fat and that avoids all forms of carbohydrate.

atrophy—A decrease in the muscle mass.

attribution—Term used to represent the underlying meaning one places on the events or circumstances of their lives.

ballistic flexibility—The ability to move through a range of motion with bobbing, bouncing movements.

barbell collar—The protective clamps that secure plates on a weightlifting bar.

behavior shaping—The modification of situations or behavior consistent with your plan.

behavior substitution—When you substitute an undesirable behavior with a healthy behavior. For example, instead of having coffee and a cigarette after dinner, you go for a brisk walk.

binge eating disorder—An eating disorder characterized by recurrent episodes of binge eating. There is a sense of lack of control over eating during the episode; of eating faster than normal; eating until feeling uncomfortably full; and feeling disgusted with oneself, depressed, or guilty after overeating.

bingeing—Characterized by eating, in a discrete period of time, an amount of food that is definitely larger than most people would eat in a similar period of time under similar circumstances.

blood volume—The volume of blood (both red blood cells and plasma) in a person's circulatory system. A typical adult male has approximately 5 liters of blood.

body composition—A measure of the distribution of fat and lean body mass in the human body. This measure is most often expressed in percent body fat. For example, 17 percent body fat means that 17 percent of an individual's body weight is made up of fat; the other 83 percent is lean body mass.

body dysmorphic disorder (BDD)—Reverse anorexia, when individuals, typically men, become obsessed with the perception that they are not muscular enough.

body image—Composed of the following: a perceptual component that relates how accurately a person estimates his body size; a subjective component that involves feelings, thoughts, and attitudes toward the body; and a behavioral component that refers to repetitive checking and the tendency to avoid situations where the person might feel uncomfortable about his body.

bolus—The term used for any fairly large quantity of matter. In the context of chapter 8, it refers to food making its way through the digestive tract.

brain waves—The rhythmic waves of voltage arising from electrical activity within brain tissue.

bulimia nervosa—An eating disorder characterized by episodes of binge eating followed by fasting, self-induced vomiting, or the use of diuretics or laxatives.

calorie—A measurement of energy. One calorie is the amount of energy used to raise 1 kilogram of water 1 degree Celsius.

capilarization—The process of increasing the density of the smallest blood vessels in the body where oxygen and carbon dioxide are exchanged.

carbohydrate—Organic compounds (starches, sugars) that provide energy to the body.

cardiac muscle—A type of striated muscle found exclusively within the heart.

cardiac output—Amount of blood pumped by the heart in one minute. Cardiac output is the product of stroke volume and heart rate.

cardiorespiratory assessment—Evaluating the working capacity of the cardiorespiratory system.

cardiorespiratory endurance—The ability to sustain prolonged physical activity that uses the cardiorespiratory system.

cardiorespiratory fitness—The body's ability to sustain prolonged physical activity that uses the cardiorespiratory system.

cholesterol—A sterol and a lipid found in the cell membranes of all body tissues. An excessive level of cholesterol in the blood is a primary risk factor for heart disease. Most physicians consider blood cholesterol below 200 mg/dl as normal.

chyme—The term used to describe the substance remaining after the bolus has been digested in the stomach.

circadian rhythm—The term *circadian* comes from the Latin *circa*, "around," and *dias*, "day," meaning "around a day." This 24-hour cycle was first described by Franz Halberg.

clinical depression—A condition identified by clusters of symptoms such as sadness, hopelessness, motivation, too much or too little sleep, restlessness or inability to sit still, feelings of worthlessness, and thoughts of death or suicide.

cognitive–behavioral therapy—A kind of psychotherapy that involves recognizing unhelpful or destructive patterns of thinking and reacting, then modifying or replacing them with more realistic or helpful ones.

cognitive restructuring, or reframing—The process of learning to refute cognitive distortions, or fundamental faulty thinking, with the goal of replacing irrational beliefs with more accurate and beneficial ones.

complete proteins—The term used to describe foods that contain the nine essential amino acids (examples are meat, egg, dairy products).

complex carbohydrate—Multiple molecules of sugar that bond together to form starch and fiber (examples are bread, pasta, and cereal).

creation—The story about a personal God who walked in the garden with Adam and Eve and everything he made.

creeping obesity—A gradual increase of weight year after year, which eventually makes a person excessively overweight.

deep breathing—The act of breathing deep into the lungs by flexing the diaphragm, rather than breathing shallowly by extending the rib cage.

delta brain waves—Electromagnetic oscillations in the frequency range of 2 Hz or less, characteristic of the deepest stages of sleep.

depression—A state of sadness, loss of pleasure, or low mood.

dieting—A process of restrictive eating usually caused by body dissatisfaction, preoccupation with thinness, and the false belief that self-worth is dependent on body size. Dieting creates a physiologically driven preoccupation with food and can have devastating results such as eating disorders or even suicide.

digestive system—A series of connected organs whose purpose is to break down, or digest, food.

disaccharides—A carbohydrate composed of two sugar molecules.

discernment—The ability to show godly and wise judgment.

discretionary calories—Additional calories allotted to individuals following the low fat and sugar recommendations on the new food guide pyramid.

disordered eating—Behaviors resemble anorexia nervosa or bulimia nervosa but the person who has the disorder is not clinically anorexic or bulimic because such people may continue to menstruate, or, for example, are individuals who regularly purge but do not binge eat, or who binge eat less than twice weekly.

drive theory—Within the context of stress management, this theory suggests a linear relationship between stress and performance exists. In other words, as stress increases, so does performance.

duodenum—The first part of the small intestine. It is a hollow, jointed tube connecting the stomach to the jejunum.

dynamic flexibility—The ability to move slowly and rhythmically through a full range of motion.

easy cycle—Cycling at an intensity at which your heart rate is 60 percent to 75 percent of your maximum.

easy run—Running at an intensity at which your heart rate is 60 percent to 75 percent of your maximum.

easy swim—Swimming at an intensity at which your heart rate is 60 percent to 75 percent of your maximum.

easy walk—Walking at an intensity at which your heart rate is 60 percent to 75 percent of your maximum.

eating disorders not otherwise specified (EDNOS)—Eating disorders characterized by individuals engaging in unhealthy dieting practices, such as skipping meals, fasting, or using diet pills or laxatives.

electrical impedance devices—These devices send small currents through the body to estimate body fat. They measure the amount of water in the body. Elements of the body such as blood and muscle have a lot of water. Elements of the body such as fat and bone are highly resistive. The higher the resistance to the small currents, the more fat one has.

electroencephalography (EEG)—Tests by a device developed in the 1920s that allows measurement of the electrical activity of the brain.

emotional reasoning—Reasoning based on how you feel. "I feel lousy; therefore those people are lousy" is a statement based on emotional reasoning.

endomysium—Connective tissue located inside of the fascicle that surrounds individual muscle cells.

endorphins—Chemicals produced by the brain that increase feelings of well-being and decrease pain.

energy metabolism—A series of chemical reactions that break down food particles to produce energy.

epimysium—The outermost connective tissue surrounding individual muscle fibers.

esophageal sphincter—A circular muscle that separates the esophagus and stomach. It relaxes during swallowing, forming an opening through which the food can pass.

esophagus—The organ in the digestive tract that connects the mouth to the stomach.

eternal life—Life that does not begin when we die, but is the present reality.

evolutionist—One who believes that people were formed through an impersonal process of time and chance.

faithfulness—Always being there for someone despite what he or she does in return.

fall—Refers to Adam and Eve's sin in the Garden of Eden, precipitating people's universal and pervasive disposition to turn their backs on God.

fascicles—Fibrous connective tissue surrounding and separating muscle bundles.

fat—Lipids in foods or in the body, composed mostly of triglycerides.

female athlete triad syndrome—The combination of three interrelated conditions that are associated with athletic training: disordered eating, amenorrhea, and osteoporosis.

fiber—The nonstarch polysaccharides that are not digested by human digestive enzymes.

fight-or-flight response—First described by Walter Cannon in 1929. His theory states that humans react to threats with an urge to either fight or flee.

FITT principle—Acronym representing four exercise prescription variables: frequency, intensity, time, and type.

flexibility—Generally defined as the range of motion (ROM) that is possible in a joint or group of joints.

free radicals—A molecule with one or more unpaired electrons that causes cellular damage by its effort to stabilize by regaining an electron.

frequency—The number of training sessions per week.

fructose—A type of monosaccharide.

fulfillment—God's honoring his promise that all things will be made new, and there will be an eternal "new heaven and a new earth" (Revelation 1:1).

functional capacity—The ability of the human body to perform physical activity, which is influenced by muscular strength.

galactose—A type of monosaccharide.

general adaptation syndrome (GAS)—Describes the body's short-term and long-term reaction to stress. Alarm reaction, resistance, and exhaustion are the three stages in this classic model first described by Dr. Hans Selye.

gentleness—An attitude that does not produce anxiety precipitated by fear, but recovery nurtured by love.

glucose—A type of monosaccharide, a simple sugar. It is one of the most important forms of carbohydrate.

glycemic—The presence of glucose (sugar) in the blood.

glycemic index—Rating of the potential foods to raise levels of blood glucose.

glycemic load—The amount of total carbohydrate in a particular food multiplied by the glycemic index (of that food), then divided by 100.

glycogen—Stored form of glucose in the liver, muscles, and kidneys.

glycolysis—The chemical breakdown of glucose in which ATP is produced.

glycolytic energy system—Term used to describe the physiological process of glycolysis.

goals—Specific targets as you move toward fulfilling your mission statement.

Golgi tendon organs—Located in tendons, they are stimulated by high tension that is created in tendons when the related muscles contract with sufficient force. The reflex reaction is relaxation of the contracting muscle.

goodness—To act justly and to love mercy and to walk humbly with your God.

happiness—Feeling pleasure, contentment, or joy. Feeling satisfied that something is right or has been done right.

heart rate—Frequency of cardiac contractions, typically inferred from pulse.

heart rate monitor—A device used to accurately measure heart rate.

Helicobactor pylori—Bacteria in the stomach that cause inflammation and ulcers.

hydrochloric acid (HCL)—A powerful acid secreted from thousands of gastric glands lining the stomach that serves to destroy harmful bacteria. As people age, the amount of HCL produced decreases.

hydrostatic weighing—Involves immersing a client in a tub of water and weighing the person. The more dense and muscular the person is, the more he or she is inclined to sink and be heavier on the scales. The more fat a person has, the more the person is inclined to float and the lighter he or she would be on the scales. This method is generally considered the best measure of body fat.

hypermobility—Excessive range of motion (ROM) in joints.

hypertrophy—Enlargement of muscle tissue. This can be done for a brief period of time via blood profusion during exercise or more permanently through overload adaptation to muscle fibers.

hyponatremia—A condition that occurs when the body's sodium level falls below normal as a result of salt loss from sweat.

ileum—The last part of the small intestine. It absorbs vitamins from the chyme.

individualized zones of optimal functioning (IZOF)—A stress/performance model in which optimal zones of stress can vary from person to person and according to the task required.

insoluble fiber—Fiber that does not dissolve in water. It prevents constipation by making feces bulkier and softer so they pass more quickly and easily through intestine.

insomnia—A sleep disorder in which a person has difficultly falling asleep or staying asleep.

inverted-U theory—This model of stress purports a positive linear relationship of stress and performance up to a certain point, after which increased levels of stress result in decreased performance.

isokinetic—Resistance training in which the rate and speed of movement is controlled or held constant.

isometric—Resistance training in which contractions are made with no accompanying movement (an example is standing in a doorway and pushing against the frame).

isotonic—Resistance training in which the load (weight) is constant throughout the exercise.

jejunum—The middle part of the small intestines. The tissue on the inside of it absorbs nutrients.

Johari Window—A model for describing four areas of self-knowledge.

joy—The ability to respond to God's triumphs; seeing, feeling, and expressing celebration in God's victories.

kilocalorie—The amount of energy necessary to raise a liter of water by 1 degree Celsius. Please note this term is what is generally called a *calorie* when discussing nutrition and exercise.

kindness—To focus on knowing another's need and helping to fulfill it, particularly to relatives, guests, and those that are in some way dependent on you.

labeling—Identifying with your shortcomings. Instead of saying, "I made a mistake," a person says, "I'm a jerk, a fool, a loser."

lactate—A fatiguing metabolite produced during glycolysis; also called lactic acid.

lactose—A disaccharide consisting of galactose and glucose connected together.

laxity—Greater than normal range of motion (ROM) in joints.

lean body mass (LBM)—The weight of the body minus fat. This includes muscle, all other organs, bones, and connective tissue.

love—Commitment to care for others.

lower and upper limit—The minimum and maximum prescribed threshold of intensity, typically expressed in percent of maximum heart rate.

macronutrients—Nutrients required by the human body in large amounts (water, carbohydrate, protein, and fat).

maltose—A disaccharide and an important component of sugar.

maximal oxygen consumption ($\dot{V}O_2$max)—Largest amount of oxygen the body can consume at work. Typically expressed in milliliters of oxygen per kilogram of body weight per minute. $\dot{V}O_2$max is the abbreviated notation.

mental filtering—Dwelling on the negatives and ignoring the positives.

metabolism—Series of chemical reactions that break down food particles to produce energy.

micronutrients—Nutrients that humans need only in very small amounts (vitamins and minerals).

milliliters of oxygen per kilogram of body weight per minute—A measure associated with maximum oxygen testing that quantifies the amount of oxygen used in one minute by the body weight of the subject.

minerals—Substances formed naturally that are needed in small amounts to help the body function normally.

mission statement—A big-picture, inspirational, and precise statement of where you want your life to go.

mitochondria—A structure found in all cells that increases the body's ability to use oxygen to produce work.

moderate cycle—Cycling at an intensity at which your heart rate is 70 percent to 85 percent of your maximum.

moderate run—Running at an intensity at which your heart rate is 70 percent to 85 percent of your maximum.

moderate swim—Swimming at an intensity at which your heart rate is 70 percent to 85 percent of your maximum.

moderate walk—Walking at an intensity at which your heart rate is 70 percent to 85 percent of your maximum.

monosaccharides—The simplest form of carbohydrate. They consist of one sugar molecule.

monounsaturated fat—Fatty acids that have only one double-bonded carbon molecule (electrons hold it together), which results in lowered blood cholesterol levels compared to polyunsaturated fats.

motor neurons—Neurons in the spinal cord and brain stem that combine with muscle fibers to create muscular contractions, or movement.

motor unit—A single motor neuron; groups of motor units coordinate the contraction of a single muscle.

muscle dysmorphia—Classified as a subcategory of body dysmorphic disorder. A disorder that straddles both anxiety disorders and eating disorders, it is characterized by chronic pre-occupation with body shape, which occurs in conjunction with changes in eating and exercise practices.

muscle spindles—Sensors scattered among muscle cells and fibers and stimulated by the extent and speed of muscle stretch. The reflex reaction is a contraction of the stretched muscle.

muscular endurance—The ability of a muscle or muscle group to sustain repeated contractions.

muscular strength—The maximal force that a muscle or muscle group can produce. This is generally expressed as any one-repetition maximum (1RM).

myofibril—The parallel alignment of protein filaments within a muscle cell that interacts and slides by one another during muscle contraction.

myofilament—The filament of myofibrils constructed from proteins. Myofilaments consist of two types, thick and thin. Thin filaments consist primarily of the protein actin; thick filaments consist primarily of the protein myosin.

myoglobin—An oxygen-binding pigment in muscle, similar to hemoglobin in the blood. It acts as an oxygen store and aids in the diffusion of oxygen.

myosin—A protein filament inside of the myofibril that combines with actin to generate force.

naloxone—An intravenously injected drug used to counter the effects of narcotic drugs used during surgery or to treat pain. It is administered in hospital settings. It is also used by athletes to block the euphoric feeling created by endorphins during exercise.

net carbohydrate—The total grams of carbohydrate per serving minus the grams of sugar alcohols and fermentable fiber.

non-rapid-eye movement (NREM)—The majority of sleep is spent in this phase. There are four stages of NREM.

nutrient density—The amount of nutrients available in a single item of food.

nutrition—The science of how eating affects the body. A broader definition includes the social, economic, cultural, and psychological aspects of eating.

obesity—Having excessive fat (over 30 points on a BMI calculation).

one-repetition maximum (1RM)—The maximum amount of weight an individual can lift for one successful repetition.

Ornish diet—A diet that relies largely on carbohydrate and includes only minimal amounts of animal protein.

osteoblast—The building of skeletal tissue.

osteoclast—Erosion of skeletal tissue.

osteoporosis—A skeletal disease in which bone mineral density is gradually diminished, making bones more vulnerable to compression and shear fractures.

overload principle—The assumption that for training adaptation to occur, a physiological system must be exercised at a level beyond that to which it is presently accustomed.

oxidative energy system—Term used to describe oxidative, or aerobic, metabolism.

oxidative metabolism—Chemical process in which oxygen is used in the production of energy.

pace cycle—Cycling at an intensity at which heart rate is above 85 percent of maximum.

pace run—Running at an intensity at which heart rate is above 85 percent of maximum.

pace swim—Swimming at an intensity at which heart rate is above 85 percent of maximum.

pandemic—The outbreak of disease that affects people over a large geographic area.

patience—The ability to be long-suffering.

peace—To live in harmony with God and others and to experience personal wellness within.

pepsin—A digestive enzyme that is released in the stomach to break apart food protein into particles.

perimysium—The layer of connective tissue (inside of the epimysium) that holds the fascicles together.

peristalsis—Smooth muscular contractions that propel the food bolus through the esophagus to the stomach.

personality—A dynamic and organized set of characteristics possessed by a person that uniquely influences his or her cognitions, motivations, and behaviors in various situations.

personality type—The psychological classification of people according to particular personality traits, such as extroversion and introversion.

phosphagen system—An anaerobic energy system in which ATP is manufactured when phosphocreatine is broken down. The system represents the most rapidly available source of energy in the body.

polysaccharides—Carbohydrate that contain long chains of molecules bonded together.

polyunsaturated fat—Fatty acids that have more than one double-bonded carbon molecule.

post-traumatic stress disorder (PTSD)—Certain psychological consequences of exposure to, or confrontation with, highly traumatic stressful experiences.

prayer—Talking to God as to friends and lovers for the purpose of sharing in their lives.

protein—A substance made up primarily of amino acids. Protein is an essential nutrient, but not a major source of energy.

providence—God's loving care and protection.

psychoneuroimmunology (PNI)—A specialized field of research that studies the interactions between behavior, the brain, and the immune system of the body.

purging—A method of ridding the body of food through self-induced vomiting or the use of diuretics, laxatives, or enemas.

pyloric sphincter—A hard ring of smooth muscle that separates the stomach and the small intestine. It lets food pass from the stomach to the duodenum (small intestine).

range of motion (ROM)—The flexibility around a joint.

rapid-eye movement (REM)—This stage of sleep is characterized by rapid movements of the eyes. During this period, the body is paralyzed and dreams are more frequent than at any other stage of sleep. This accounts for about 25 percent of sleep time.

rational-emotive therapy—A method of treatment, originally developed by Albert Ellis, that focuses on actively attempting to resolve cognitive, emotional, and behavioral problems.

rectum—The organ in the digestive process that temporarily stores fecal matter before it is excreted through the anus.

redemption—To make all things new in Christ.

repetitions—A quantity that represents the number of times a muscle or muscle group completes a predetermined movement pattern.

repetition speed—The length of time that it takes to complete one repetition. The three specific phases of repetition speed are concentric phase, eccentric phase, and the interval in between.

resistance training—Lifting weights of various size in order to develop increased muscular tone and strength.

rest interval—The length of rest between sets.

resting heart rate—The heart rate of someone who must not have eaten or exercised in the previous three hours and must lie in a prone position for at least 20 minutes before testing.

resting metabolic rate (RMR)—The rate at which energy is used by a body at complete rest.

runner's high—A heightened condition or state of euphoria reported by individuals during or after aerobic exercise, generally associated with elevated level of endorphins.

sarcomeres—The basic building blocks of myofibrils. Sarcomeres are connected one to another in skeletal muscle, giving it a striated appearance.

saturated fat—Forms of fat that are normally solid at room temperature (e.g., butter).

self-controlled—To let God be in charge of your life.

set—In strength training a set is a predetermined number of repetitions. For example, two sets of 12 repetitions means that an individual completed 12 repetitions, rested, then completed 12 more.

simple carbohydrate—Single molecules of sugar that provide the body with glucose.

skeletal muscle—Muscle attached to the skeleton that is used to facilitate movement by applying force (via contraction) to bones and joints.

skinfold measurements—Measures the fat beneath the skin with calipers at several key spots. There are more than 100 different equations and ways of doing this, showing that this type of measurement has potential but is also problematic.

sleep apnea—A sleep disorder characterized by loud snoring and pauses in breathing during sleep. These episodes, called apneas (without breath), generally cause disruptive sleep.

sleep cycle—Term used to describe the process of going through all five stages of sleep. Generally, it takes approximately 90 minutes to transverse all fives stages of sleep.

sleep debt—The cumulative effect of not getting enough sleep.

sleep deprivation—A general lack of necessary sleep.

sleep hygiene—A general term used to collectively describe one's behavioral habits surrounding sleep.

sleep spindles—Bursts of brain activity during stage 2 sleep that consists of 12 to 16 Hz waves that occur for 0.5 to 1.5 seconds.

sleep stages—Term used to describe the various phases, or periods, of sleep. Most experts agree that there are five distinct stages of sleep. *Stage one:* light stage of sleep in which a transition from wakefulness is made; *stage two:* lighter stage of sleep in which consciousness to an external stimuli is decreased; *stage three:* the first phase of deep sleep, which primarily functions as a transition into stage four sleep; *stage four:* the deepest sleep of all, this stage of sleep along with stage three sleep is primarily associated with physical restoration; *stage five or REM sleep:* characterized by rapid eye movements (REM), mental restoration, and dreams.

smooth muscle—A type of nonstriated muscle found in the walls of organs, blood vessels, gastrointestinal tract, and elsewhere in the body. Most smooth muscle contracts involuntarily.

soluble fiber—Fiber that dissolves in water to form a gel. Some people think it lowers blood cholesterol and controls blood sugar.

spiritual gifts—Special abilities or capacities given by God for the edification of other people.

static flexibility—The ability to hold a stretched position.

stomach—A primary organ in the digestive system where food is broken down before passing into the small intestine.

stress—Any specific or nonspecific response of the body to any demand made on it.

stress hardy—Surviving and even thriving during unfavorable conditions.

stroke volume—The amount of blood being pumped in the heart by the cardiac muscle during exercise. As the heart becomes stronger, it becomes more efficient at pumping blood, and stroke volume increases.

sucrose—A disaccharide commonly known as table sugar.

suicide—The act of deliberately killing oneself.

target heart rate zone—Prescribed upper and lower limit of aerobic intensity.

theta brain waves—Electromagnetic oscillations in the frequency range of 4 to 8 Hz, describing transitory or lighter phases of sleep.

trace minerals—Dietary minerals needed by the human body in extremely small quantities.

values—Accepted principles or standards embraced by an individual or group.

variable resistance—Resistance training method in which the load (weight) changes during the exercise.

variety—Being varied or diverse in the selection of food.

villi and microvilli—Tiny, fingerlike projections that line the inner walls of the small intestine. Even smaller projections on the surface of the villi are called microvilli. These structures enhance the surface of the small intestine by approximately 150 times.

vitamins—Essential organic substances used by the body for metabolism, protection, and development.

weight preoccupation—An excessive concern with one's body weight.

weight restoration—Particularly for those who have anorexia, restoring weight through diet is one of the first steps in the process toward recovery.

Index

Note: The italicized *f* and *t* following page numbers refer to figures and tables, respectively.

A

abdominal crunch 125*f*, 126*f*, 296
abdominal fat, effect of sit-ups on 110
Abkhasians 266
Abraham 200
academic work, stress of 196
academic workload, as sleep thief 231-23
acne, and steroids 34
actin 116, 307
activating events 196-198, 307
activism, frenzy of 235
activity
    building into lifestyle 68
    importance of 67
    in MyPyramid 178
Adam and Eve 5-6
adenosine triphosphate 80, 81*t*, 307
adolescents, and eating disorders 41
Adrenaline and Stress (Hart) 223
advertising industry, and body image 44
aerobic capacity 87, 307
aerobic endurance 88, 307
aerobic exercise 79, 85, 87, 307
aerobic exercise prescription 83-89
aestheticians 5, 307
affluence, and depression 14
age, and sleep needs 237
Agras, S. 46
Ahluwahlia, Gopal 267
Alice's Adventures in Wonderland (Carroll) 14
Alighieri, Dante 257
alimentary canal 162, 307
all-or-nothing thinking 199-200, 307
alpha brain waves 246*f*
Alter, M.J. 145-146, 147
alternative stretching exercises 151
Amato, Paul 270
amenorrhea 39, 307
American College of Sports Medicine
    aerobic exercise intensity level 85
    aerobic exercise time recommendation 87
    flexibility test recommendations 147
    high-risk stretching exercises 151
    stretching recommendations 149-150
amino acids 166, 307
anaerobic 80, 307
Anderson, Paul 106
anger 7. *See also* seven deadly sins
anorexia athletica 39, 47*t*, 307. *See also* eating disorders not otherwise specified (EDNOS)
anorexia nervosa
    about 38, 307
    Heather's story 32-33
    physical complications of 47*t*

risk factors 40
    treatment goals for 50*t*
antagonist muscles 149, 307
antidepressants, side effects of 60
antioxidants 173, 307
apathy 7
appetite 60, 65
apple-shaped people 62*f*, 63. *See also* pear-shaped people
application activities
    bench press one-repetition maximum test 138-139
    gift assessment 52
    grip test 135
    leg press one-repetition maximum test 139-140
    life's mission 26-28
    1.5 mile run test 101
    one-minute push-up test 135-136, 137*f*
    one-minute sit-up test 136-137, 138*f*
    reflections on body 52
    resting heart rate 99
    sleep/alertness log 252
    spiritual gift inventory 53-54, 277-278
    stress assessment test 224
    three-minute step test 99-101
    to-do list 223
    12-minute walk/run test 101-102
    values clarifications 275-276
Aqua Fit (Katz) 89
arm curl 125*f*, 126*f*, 296, 297
arm extension 125*f*, 126*f*, 296, 297
Armstrong, Lance 81
arousal 200, 201, 307
ascetic 9, 177, 307
asceticism 188, 307
atherosclerosis 64
Atkins diet 64, 307
Atlas, Charles 120
atrophy 108, 307
attribution 213, 307
avarice 7

B

bad cholesterol 78
Baechle, Thomas 124
ballistic flexibility 144, 307
ballistic stretching 148-149, 151
barbell collars 120, 307
barriers 22*t*, 24*t*
Bartoli, Cecilia 265
basal metabolic rate, and dieting 36
Basarion 158
beds 249
bedtime ritual 249
behavior contract 23
behavior shaping 24
behavior substitution 24, 307
beliefs, stress of 198-199
Bell, G. 145, 151

bench press 130*f*, 132*f*, 303*f*, 305*f*
bench press one-repetition maximum test 113, 138-139
bent-over rear cable raise 128*f*, 129*f*, 300, 301
Berger, Roy 113
Berkouwer, G.C. 5
beta brain waves 246*f*
biking. *See* cycling
binge eating disorder. *See also* eating disorders not otherwise specified (EDNOS)
    about 39, 307
    physical complications of 47*t*
    risk factors 40
    treatment goals for 50*t*
bingeing 36, 38, 307
The Biology of Human Starvation (Keys) 187
biotin 170*t*, 172*t*
Blonna, Richard 206
blood volume 82, 307
body
    dissatisfaction with 43
    God's providence for 9
    as God's temple 8-9
    as house of God's spirit 48
    obsession with appearance 34
    personal views of 4
    reflections on 52
    respecting 38
    resurrection of 9
    shaping with strength training 108-109
    stewardship of 77
    during transition periods 38
body composition 108-109, 110, 308
body dysmorphic disorder 39, 41, 308. *See also* eating disorders not otherwise specified (EDNOS)
body fat, cutting 65
body image
    about 35-36, 308
    causes of concerns 36
    dealing with negative image 37-38
    ideal for 43*f*, 44
    North American cultural ideals 36-37
    peer pressure 37
    puberty 37
body mass index
    about 61
    calculating 62
    guidelines 61*t*
    increases with sleep deprivation 65
bolus 160, 308
bone mineral density 112*f*
bones, and resistance training 112
bone structure, and flexibility 144
boredom, and sleepiness 236
Borg, Gunnar 86-87
bottled water 173

Bowling Alone (Putnam) 14, 268
box squat 130*f*, 131*f*, 303*f*, 304*f*
Bradberry, Travis 194
brain
    brain waves 245-246, 308
    communication within 212*f*
    stimulation in walking 66
breathing technique, in weightlifting 133
Briggs, Kathryn 259
Buchanan, Mark 186
bulimia nervosa
    about 38-39, 308
    physical complications of 47*t*
    risk factors 40
    treatment goals for 50*t*
Burns, D. 199
Buss, David 262

C
calcium 174*t*, 185*t*
calories
    about 162-163, 308
    discretionary calories 183
    empty calories 163
    and healthy sustainability 63-64
    input and output 63
Canada
    Canadian Food Guide 183-184
    obesity in 60
    stress management studies 204
Canadian trunk forward flexion test 147
Cannon, Walter 200
canola oil 64
capilarization 82, 308
carbohydrate
    about 308
    categories and functions 166*t*
    functions of 162*t*
    terminology 164-166
cardiac muscle 115, 308
cardiac output 83, 308
cardiorespiratory assessment 83, 308
cardiorespiratory endurance
    about 76, 308
    evaluating 81, 83
    and sleep deprivation 242
cardiorespiratory exercise, benefiting from 77-79
cardiorespiratory fitness 90-96, 308
cardiorespiratory training 82, 84*f*
Celebration of Discipline (Foster) 186
celibacy, or marriage 264
challenge 209
change, barriers to 24*t*
Chariots of Fire (Hudson) 244
chemical imbalances, and depression 211
chest fly 128*f*, 129*f*, 299, 301
chest press 125*f*, 126*f*, 296
children 248*t*, 269-270
chloride 174*t*
choices, determined by biblical principles 15-16
cholesterol 77-78, 170, 308
Christian counseling 214
Christian Paths to Health and Wellness (Walters and Byl)
    features viii-ix
    purpose vii
    structure viii

chromium 175*t*
chronic stress 202
chyme 161, 308
circadian rhythms 237, 308
"Cleaning Out My Closet" (Eminem) 269-270
clinical depression 209, 210, 308
Clinton, Bill 247
Cockburn, Bruce 18
cognitive-behavioral therapy 214, 308
cognitive impairment, and sleep deprivation 241
cognitive restructuring 199, 308
college students
    academic rigor for Christian college students 232
    better grades with more sleep 241
    with depression 194, 210*f*
    eating disorders 41-42
    eating habits 159
    feeling overwhelmed 195*f*
    happiness survey 220
    hours of sleep per night 233*f*
    intensity of common stressful events 198*t*
    with natural sleep rhythm 247
    relational abilities 194
    and sleep deprivation 231-233
    valuable traits of romantic partner 262
    working harder 232
commitment 208
complete proteins 166, 308
complex carbohydrate 164, 166*t*, 308
computers, taking breaks from 66, 68
conflict, resolving 271-273
consequences, of stress 200
control 208-209
Cook, K.V. 42
Coolidge, Calvin 247
copper 175*t*
Corbin, C.B. 151
Cornelison, Floyd 231, 239, 240
counseling, for depression 214
Cousins, Norman 206
Covey, Steven 15
creation 5-6, 256, 308
creeping obesity 60-61, 111, 308
Cronkite, R. 78
cross-country skiing 89
cultural ideals 36-37
cultural isolation 266-268
cycles 230
cycling
    beginning program 96*t*
    benefits of 67
    as cardiorespiratory exercise 95-96
    guidelines 95-96
    as motivator 68

D
Daehlie, Bjorn 89
daily activity, and barriers 22*t*
daily planning 209
Dante 257
David 207
death
    by dehydration 176
    obesity-related 60
    and sleep deprivation 243, 245
    transition at 10
decision making 260-261

deep breathing 205, 308
deep sleep 247
dehydration, death by 176
delta brain waves 246, 308
depression
    about 209, 309
    and affluence 14
    on campus 210*f*
    causes 210-211, 213
    college students with 194
    and eating disorders 44
    exercise as treatment for 78
    and nutritional deprivation 187
    steps to take 215-216
    struggling with 32
    and suicide 216
    symptoms 210
    treatment 213-214
desolate creation 6
Diagnostic and Statistical Manual of Mental Disorders (American Psychological Association) 38
diary, keeping 24
DiClemente, C.C. 19, 21
dietary fat 162*t*, 168, 170
Dietary Guidelines for Americans 2005 (U.S. Department of Health and Human Services) 168, 177
dietary regimen, in Jesus' time 187
dieting
    about 35, 309
    approaches to 64
    facts about 36
    low-carbohydrate diets 164-166
digestive system
    about 159-162, 309
    and food choices 158
    illustrated 161*f*
disaccharides 164, 309
discernment 14, 309
discretionary calories 183, 309
disordered eating 39, 309
distorted thinking 199-200
Divine Comedy (Alighieri) 257
Dodson, J.D. 201
Doyle, Paddy 114
dreams 237, 247
drive theory 201, 309
driving, while drowsy 241
duodenum 161, 309
dynamic flexibility 144, 309
dynamic stretching 148
dysfunctional families, homes for 267

E
Earle, Roger 124
easy cycle 96*t*, 309
easy run 93-94*t*, 309
easy swim 95*t*, 309
easy walk 91*t*, 309
eating
    changing habits 67
    college students' habits 159
    moderation in 181
    reasonable portions 68
    speed eating 162
    30-day pizza experiment 160
eating behavior questionnaires 291-294*t*
eating disorders
    about 38
    anorexia nervosa 38

biological influences 45
bulimia nervosa 38-39
case study, anorexia nervosa 32-33
causes of 42
and dieting 36
differences between men and
    women 46
family influences 45-46
helping those with food and weight
    problems 289
physical complications of 47*t*
prevalence of 41-42
psychological influences 44-45
recovery from 50-51
risk factors 40
sociocultural influences 42-44
specific treatment goals for 50*t*
*Eating Disorders in Women and
    Children* (Lewis) 50
eating disorders not otherwise
    specified (EDNOS)
    about 309
    anorexia athletica 39
    binge eating disorder 39
    body dysmorphic disorder 39, 41
    female athlete triad syndrome 39
Edison, Thomas 247
EDNOS. *See* eating disorders not
    otherwise specified (EDNOS)
education 24*t*, 218
Einstein, Albert 247
Eisenhower, Dwight D. 176-177
electrical impedance devices 61, 309
electroencephalography 245, 309
Eliot, T.S. 209
elliptical machines 89
Ellis, Albert 196, 199
Eminem 269-270
Emotional Intelligence (Golemar) 194
emotional irritability, and sleep
    deprivation 241
emotional quotient 194
emotional reasoning 199, 200, 309
emotions, as building blocks of
    personality 44
empty calories 163
endomysium 115, 309
endorphins 78, 309
endurance
    enabling with weight training 113
    feats of 79
    moving beyond 88
    muscular endurance 113
Endurance (Lansing) 76
endurance training, body composition
    changes from 110*t*
energy metabolism 171*t*, 309
energy systems 80, 81*t*
envy 6-7. *See also* seven deadly sins
epimysium 115, 309
eptin 65
erector spinae muscles 118*f*
esophageal sphincter 160, 309
esophagus 160, 309
estimated maximum heart rate 85
eternal life 284, 309
evolutionist 5, 309
exercise. *See also* aerobic exercise;
    strength training
    body image improved by 38
    daily participation in 64

obsession with 32, 34, 39
and sleeping behaviors 248-249
and stress 206
tranquilizing effect of 78
exercises
    abdominal crunch 125*f*, 126*f*, 296
    arm curl 125*f*, 126*f*, 296, 297
    arm extension 125*f*, 126*f*, 296, 297
    bench press 130*f*, 132*f*, 303*f*, 305*f*
    bent-over rear cable raise 128*f*,
        129*f*, 300, 301
    box squat 130*f*, 131*f*, 303*f*, 304*f*
    chest fly 128*f*, 129*f*, 299, 301
    chest press 125*f*, 126*f*, 296
    45-degree leg press 127*f*, 128*f*, 299,
        300
    hanging leg raise/stability ball sit-
        up 130*f*, 131*f*, 303*f*, 305*f*
    incline back extension 119*f*, 127*f*,
        129*f*, 299, 301
    lateral raise 125*f*, 126*f*, 296, 297
    lat pull-down 125*f*, 126*f*, 296
    leg adduction 130*f*, 131*f*, 303*f*, 304*f*
    leg curl 127*f*, 128*f*, 299, 300
    low row 127*f*, 129*f*, 299, 300
    one-arm dumbbell row 130*f*, 131*f*,
        303*f*, 304*f*
    reverse crunch 127*f*, 129*f*, 299, 301
    seated alternating dumbbell curl
        131*f*, 132*f*, 304*f*, 305*f*
    seated back extension 119*f*, 125*f*,
        126*f*, 296
    seated leg extension 122*f*, 123*f*,
        125*f*, 126*f*, 296
    seated press 130*f*, 132*f*, 303*f*, 305*f*
    seated two-arm dumbbell triceps
        press 131*f*, 132*f*, 304*f*, 305*f*
    standing dumbbell curl 128*f*, 129*f*,
        300, 301
    torso rotation 127*f*, 129*f*, 299, 301
    triceps push-down 128*f*, 129*f*, 300,
        301
expectations, adjusting 270-271
Extraordinary Swimming for Everyone
    (Laughlin) 95
extrovert type 260*t*

F
faith 214
faithfulness 268, 309
fall 6, 309
family
    eating disorders influences of 45-46
    helping those with food and weight
        problems 289
    role in feelings and thoughts 45*f*
    support from 215
fascicles 115, 309
fasting 186-187
fat 309. *See also* body fat; dietary fat
fat burners 34
fat-burning metabolism 110-111
fatigue, and sleep deprivation 240-241
fatty acids 168
Feeling Good (Burns) 199
feeling type 261*t*
fellowship offerings 49
female athlete triad syndrome. *See
    also* eating disorders not
    otherwise specified (EDNOS)
    about 39, 310
    physical complications of 47*t*

risk factors 40
treatment goals for 50*t*
fiber 166, 166*t*, 310
Fields, Jamie 265
fight-or-flight response 200, 310
financial matters, stress of 197
fitness, in fun ways 66
Fitnessgram 148
FITT principle
    about 83, 310
    alternatives to 89
    frequency 83-84
    intensity 84-87
    time 87
    type 87-89
Flegal, K.M. 60
flexibility
    about 144, 310
    amount for health 147
    assessing 147-148
    factors affecting 144-145
    importance of 145-147
    improving and maintaining 148-151
    making time for exercises 144
    testing 147-148
fluoride 175*t*
focus 14, 15-16
Fogelholm, M. 67
folate 170*t*, 172*t*
food
    food group information 182*f*
    food labels 168-169
    glycemic index and load for various
        foods 165*t*
    as God's gift 64
    helping those with food and weight
        problems 289
    portion size changes from 1985 to
        2005 180*t*
    preparing own 66
    variety in 178, 181
    vegetable categories 182-183
    whole grains 182
"Food for Fitness" 177, 179*f*
Food Guide Pyramid 177, 179*f*
forgiveness 271, 273
Forrest Gump 271-272
45-degree leg press 127*f*, 128*f*, 299, 300
Foster, Richard 186
Francis, Bev 108*f*
Frankl, Victor 208
Franklin, Benjamin 248
Franzen, Jonathan 266-267
free radicals 173, 310
free weights 120-121
frequency, FITT principle 83-84, 310
Freud, Sigmund 256
friends
    having 14
    helping those with food and weight
        problems 289
    peer pressure 16
    support from 215
fructose 164, 310
fulfillment 9-11, 310
functional capacity 113, 310
future concerns, stress of 196

G
Gabriel, M. 146
galactose 164, 310
Gardner, Randy 240

gastric ulcers 161
general adaptation syndrome 202, 310
genetics, and depression 211
genetic variation, and flexibility 147
gentleness 242, 310
gherlin 65
Gift by the Sea (Lindbergh) 256
Gill, Norreasha 271
Gledhill, N. 146
glucose 80, 164, 310
gluttony 7, 158. *See also* seven deadly
    sins
glycemic 310
glycemic index 164, 310
glycemic load 64, 165, 310
glycogen 80, 310
glycolysis 80, 310
glycolytic energy system 80, 81*t*, 310
goals
    application activities 26-28
    assessing progress of 25, 286
    Christian paths to 19
    defined 310
    for lifestyle change plan 21-22
    realism in establishing 21-22
    setting 19, 21, 285
    for weight control 63-65
God
    balanced passion for glory of 251
    beauty defined by 37
    communication with 97
    counting his blessings 207
    and creation 5-6
    in creation of human life 269
    discerning will of 18
    discipline for good 88
    enduring nature of plans of 79
    evaluation of people as very good
        32
    expanding limits of his children 88
    faithfulness of 268
    glorifying 272
    goodness of 107
    his wants for people 47-48
    keeping central in life 215
    kindness of 97
    love of 20
    mission of 15
    modesty of 256
    orientation to 285
    patience of 150
    peace granted by 49
    providence for body 9
    receiving his gifts 158-159
    resting on seventh day 243-244
    Sabbath blessed by 244
    and self-acceptance 33
    showing through body 285
    as strength of heart 134
    supportive prayer with 215*f*
godly difference, making 18
Golemar, Daniel 194
Golgi tendon organs 149, 310
good cholesterol 78
goodness 106, 107, 310
Goodwin, Fred 202-203
Gottman, John 271
Graham, Billy 244
Graham, Susan 265
Grant, Ulysses S. 244
greed 7. *See also* seven deadly sins

Grenier, S.G. 145
grip strength 114, 136*t*
grip test 113, 135
Grou, Jean Nicholas 257

H
Hales, Dianne 78
Hammer, L. 46
hand dynamometer 132
hanging leg raise/stability ball sit-up
    130*f*, 131*f*, 303*f*, 305*f*
Hanks, Tom 271
happiness
    defined 310
    and life satisfaction 217
    source of 219-220
    survey responses 220*f*
    your major sources of 222*t*
happiness myths
    education 218
    money 217-218
    weather 219
    youth 218-219
Harris, A.H.S. 78
Hart, Archibald 223
healing, as opposite of sinning 8-9
healthy bodies 266
healthy relationships 266
healthy sustainability 63-64
heart disease 36, 77-78
heart rate 83, 310. *See also* estimated
        maximum heart rate; maximum
        heart rate; resting heart rate
heart rate monitor 86, 99, 310
Hedge, Alan 250
Helicobacter pylori 161, 310
Hem, Erlend 89
Hemingway, Ernest 218
Henderson, Joe 92
Herbert, R.D. 146
Herman, C.P. 45, 46
Higdon, Hal 92
high-density lipoproteins 77-78
high-risk stretching exercises 151
Hill, R.H. 146
Hirofumi, Hanaka 85
Hoeger, S.A. 145
Hoeger, W.W.K. 145
holiness, as physical act 8
Holmes, Thomas 196
Holy Spirit
    love through power of 20
    opening up to 284
    vignettes on fruit of viii-ix
homes, for dysfunctional families 267
Homme, Martha 37
hormones 124, 200
human body. *See* body
human physiology, and nutrition 158
humor 206
hunter-gatherer diet 64
hurdler's stretch 151*f*
husbands, annual hours of work 234*f*
hydrochloric acid 160-161, 310
hydrostatic weighing 61, 310
hypermobility 144, 310
hypertrophy 108, 310
hyponatremia 176, 310

I
ignorance, as sleep thief 235-236
Iknoian, Therese 91

ileum 161, 311
image 5
immune function, enhancing 78-79
"Imperial Bedroom" (Franzen) 266-267
inadequate social support, and
        depression 211
incline back extension 119*f*, 127*f*, 129*f*,
        299, 301
individualized zones of optimal
        functioning 201, 202*f*, 311
indoor stationary cycling 96
Ingham, Harry 257
injury
    reduction with stretching 146
    susceptibility by gender 124
    and weight gain 60
in-line skating 89
insoluble fiber 166, 311
insomnia 237, 311
instant gratification 24*t*
intensity, FITT principle 84-87
interpersonal relationships, stress of
        197
intervention strategies, planning 23-
        25, 27, 285
intimacy, damaged 6
introvert type 260*t*
intuitive type 260*t*
inverted-U theory 201, 202*f*, 311
iodine 174*t*
iron 174*t*, 185*t*
Ironman Triathlon 79
Ironmind Enterprises 114
irrational thoughts, and depression
        211, 213
isokinetic 120, 311
isometric 120, 311
isotonic 120, 311

J
Japanese college students, and sleep
        deprivation 231-233
jejunem 161, 311
Jesus
    acceptance of displays of love 235
    bearing one another's burdens 215
    disciples' secure position 114
    against evil 107
    fasting 186-187
    focus on 47
    inner peace of 203
    and John the Baptist 200
    and joy 207
    living like 47
    mission of 15
    Peter's denials of 268
    and redemption 7
    and Sabbath laws 244-245
    and worry 203-204
Job 217
jogging 89, 92
Johari Window 257, 311
Johnson, Spencer 209
John the Baptist 200
joint restriction 145
journal, keeping 24
joy 207, 311
Joy, Richard 114
judging type 261*t*
Jung, Carl 259

K

Karren, Keith 206
Katch, Frank 110
Katz, Jane 89
Kell, R.T. 145, 151
Keys, Ancel 187
kilocalorie 163, 311
kindness 97-98, 311
Knight, Jean 133
Knowing God (Packer) 97
Kobasa, Susan 206, 208-209
Kobayashi, Takeru 162
Kraus, H. 145
Kukkoken-Harjula, K. 67
Kushida, Clete 250

L

labeling 199, 200, 311
lactate 80, 311
lacto-ovo-vegetarian 184*t*, 185*f*
lactose 164, 311
lacto-vegetarian 184*t*
Lansing, Alfred 76
lateral raise 125*f*, 126*f*, 296, 297
lat pull-down 125*f*, 126*f*, 296
Laughlin, Terry 95
laughter 206
"Laughter" (Cockburn) 18
laxity 144, 311
Lazarus, Richard 196
laziness 7. *See also* seven deadly sins
lean body mass 110, 311
lean protein 64
Ledbetter family 267
leg adduction 130*f*, 131*f*, 303*f*, 304*f*
leg curl 127*f*, 128*f*, 299, 300
leg press one-repetition maximum test 113, 139-140
Lemmon, Jack 258
Levine, M.P. 46
Liddell, Eric 244
life expectancy 60
life structuring 261
lifestyle. *See also* permanent lifestyle change
    assessing 26, 65, 67, 285
    building activity into 68
    and hunter-gatherer diet fundamentals 64
    infusing movement into 76
    small, positive changes 64
lifting form 132-133
ligament strength 144-145
Lindbergh, Anne Morrow 256
Lindsey, R. 151
lipoproteins 77-78
Lochstampfor, Brandon 111*f*
Lombardi, Vince 88
loneliness 266-268
Longfellow, Henry Wadsworth 244
long-range planning 209
love
    about 20, 311
    biblical view of 20
    healing power of 266
Love and Survival (Ornish) 266
low-carbohydrate diets 164-166
low-density lipoproteins 77-78
lower and upper limit 311
lower-back pain 117-118, 145, 250
lower limit, target heart rate zone 84-85

low row 127*f*, 129*f*, 299, 300
Luft, Joseph 257
lust 7. *See also* seven deadly sins
Lynch, Paul 114

M

macronutrients 162, 311
magnesium 174*t*
major life changes, avoiding 215
Malone, Vivian 271
maltose 164, 311
Man: The Image of God (Berkouwer) 5
manganese 175*t*
Man's Search for Meaning (Frankl) 208
Marcel, Gabriel 4
marriage, or celibacy 264
Marx, John 114
mass media 16-17, 42-44
materialism 7
Matthau, Walter 258
mattresses 249-250
maximal oxygen consumption (VO$_2$max)
    defined 311
    formulas for 100
    in milliliters of oxygen per kilogram of body weight per minute 83
    standards for 101*t*
    testing 81
maximal ventilation 82
maximum heart rate, estimation in older adults 85
Mayer, John 194
McCheyne, Robert Murray 250-251
McCullough, Michael 220
McGill, S.M. 145, 151
McNicolas, F. 46
meat eater 185*f*
medication, for depression 214
meditation 97
men
    body image causes of concern 36-37
    eating disorders differences with women 46
    eating disorders risk 41
    flexibility of 147
    media shaping views of 43
    recovery from eating disorders 50
mental filtering 199, 200, 311
Merton, Thomas 235
The Message (Peterson) 264
metabolism 60, 110-111, 311
micronutrients 162, 311
microvilli 161
milliliters of oxygen per kilogram of body weight per minute 83, 308
Milo of Croton 106, 116, 134
mind-body connection 194-195
minerals
    about 173, 311
    major and trace minerals 174-175*t*
    primary functions of 162*t*
mission statement
    about 17, 311
    application activities 26
    beginning with central theme 17
    building excitement 18-19
    inspiring action 18-19
    love as part of 20

making visible 19
    others' input on 19
    putting it all together 287
    refining 18
    revisiting and evaluating 19
    writing 17-18
mitochondria 82, 311
moderate cycle 93*t*, 96*t*, 311
moderate run 93-94*t*, 311
moderate swim 95*t*, 311
moderate walk 91*t*, 92*t*, 312
moderation, in eating 181
modified hurdler's stretch 151*f*
molybdenum 175*t*
money, and happiness 217-218
monosaccharides 164, 312
monounsaturated fat 64, 168, 312
mood, survey on improving 221*f*
mood swings, and steroids 34
Moos, R. 78
Moriarty, Dick 42
mortality rate, of Abkhasians 266
mothers, role in eating disorders 46
Mother Teresa 251
motor neurons 115, 312
motor unit 115, 312
muscle anatomy 115-116
muscle dysmorphia
    about 41, 312
    physical complications of 47*t*
    risk factors 40
    treatment goals for 50*t*
muscle elongation 145
muscle spindles 148-149, 312
muscular endurance 113, 312
muscular strength
    about 113, 312
    assessing 113
    drive for 34, 37
    increasing with weight training 113
    and sleep deprivation 242
Myers, David 14
Myers, Isabel 259
Myers-Briggs model 259-261
myofibrils 115, 312
myofilaments 116, 312
myoglobin 82, 312
myosin 116, 312
MyPyramid
    food group information 182*f*
    home page 181*f*
    illustrated 180*f*
    personalizing 181-183
    principles of 178, 181
    vegetarian diet modifications 186*t*

N

naloxone 78, 312
narcolepsy 237
National Eating Disorder Information Centre 35
National Health and Nutrition Examination Survey 182
National Sleep Foundation 234-235, 236, 238-239, 241
Natural Killer cells 79
negative reinforcements 23
negative thoughts, and depression 211, 213
net carbohydrate 165, 312
Network (Bugbee, Cousins, and Hybels) 265

neurons, anatomy of 212*f*
neurotransmitters 213
New Food Guide 178
niacin (vitamin B3) 170*t*, 172*t*
Nicholas, Stephen 91
Nieman, David C. 83
non-rapid eye movement 245, 246-247, 312
Norcross, J.C. 19, 21
Norris, Bob 111*f*
nutrient density 163, 312
nutrients 162-164
nutrition. *See also* vegetarian diet
   about 158, 312
   biblical principles 158
   biblical references to fasting 186-187
   Canadian Food Guide 183-184
   defined 159
   food labels 168-169
   guidelines and principles 176-178
   MyPyramid 178, 180*f*, 181
   personalizing MyPyramid 181-183
nutritional deprivation study 187
nutritional supplements 34
nuts, and cholesterol 170

O
obesity
   in Canada 60
   costs in United States 61
   creeping obesity 60-61
   deaths attributable to 60
   defined 312
   facts about 60
   pandemic in North America 60
obsession, with food 44-45
obsessive-compulsive behavior 33
obstacles
   Paul's warning 48
   predicting 23, 27, 285
   in weight control 67
The Odd Couple (Simon) 258
oil 183
older adults, maximum heart rate estimation 85
olive oil 64
Olympic Games 106
omega-3 fatty acids 64
one-arm dumbbell row 130*f*, 131*f*, 303*f*, 304*f*
1.5 mile run test 101
one-minute push-up test 113, 135-136, 137*f*
one-minute sit-up test 113, 136-137, 138*f*
one-repetition maximum 113, 312
open window theory 79
Ornish, Dean 266
Ornish diet 64, 312
Ornstein, R. 206
osteoblast 112, 312
osteoclast 112, 312
osteoporosis 39, 64, 112, 312
overindulgence 7
overload principle 116, 312
overweight 60
ovo-vegetarian 184*t*
oxidative energy system 80, 81*t*, 312
oxidative metabolism 80, 312
oxygen consumption, physiological changes to increase 82

P
pace cycle 96*t*, 312
pace run 93-94*t*, 312
pace swim 95*t*, 312
Packer, J.I. 97
pandemic, defined 312
panothenic acid 170*t*, 172*t*
parental obedience 269-270
parents, influence on children's weight concerns 37
The Passion of the Christ 256
patience 150, 313
Patton, George 203
Paul
   on celibacy 264
   on creation 5, 6
   on daily pressures 204
   on enslavement by law 245
   on gluttony 158
   guarding against extremes 188
   on kindness 97-98
   living in relation with others 285
   on obstacles 48
   offering body as living sacrifice 8, 14, 25, 285
   paradoxical state of holy and unholy intentions 199
   on perseverance 285
   pressing on toward goal 284
   on reconciliation 8
   rejoicing in God 207
   on Sabbath 245
   on temptations 285
peace 48-49, 313
Peacemaker International 272-273
Peacemaker's Pledge 272, 273
peace offerings 49
pear-shaped people 62*f*, 63. *See also* apple-shaped people
Peck, Robert Scott 217
pedometer 89
peer pressure 16, 37
pepsin 160, 313
perceiving type 261*t*
perceptions, stress of 198-199
perfectionism 44
performance, relationship with stress 201*f*
perimysium 115, 313
peristalsis 160, 313
permanent lifestyle change
   assessing present lifestyle 22
   compliance assessment 25
   designing plan for 21-23
   implementing 23-25
perseverance 88
personality
   about 258, 313
   classifications as artificial 259
   early establishment of 259
   fallibility of classifications 259
   "Odd Couple" example 258-259
personality type
   about 259, 313
   decision making 260-261
   energizing factors 259-260
   life structuring 261
   receiving information 260
Peterson, Eugene 264
Peter the Great 114
phosphagen system 80, 313

phosphorus 174*t*
physical activity, for weight loss 63
physical appearance, body image 35-36
physical illness, and stress 194
physical impairment, and sleep deprivation 241-242
physical wellness vii, ix
phytochemicals 164
Pipher, Mary 43
Pitt, Brad 258
Plato 4
Plowman, S.A. 145
Polivy, J. 45, 46
Polycarp of Smyrna 206, 208
polysaccharide 164, 166, 313
polyunsaturated fat 64, 168, 313
positive attitude 215
positive reinforcements 23
post-traumatic stress disorder 196, 313
potassium 174*t*
prayer 206, 215, 216, 284, 313
President's Council for Physical Fitness and Sports 177
pressures 16-17, 235
pride 6. *See also* seven deadly sins
Prochaska, J.O. 19, 21
procrastination 24*t*
productivity 208-209
proportionality, in food 181
proprioceptive neuromuscular facilitation 148, 149
Protas, E.J. 147
protein
   about 166, 168, 313
   athletes' needs 167
   functions of 162*t*
   lean protein 64
protein supplements 34
providence 9, 313
psychoneuroimmunology 194, 313
psychosis, and sleep deprivation 242
psychosocial endurance 88
puberty, and body image 37
pulmonary diffusion 82
pulse, measuring 86, 99*f*
purging 38, 313
purpose 15-16
Putnam, Robert 14, 268
pyloric sphincter 161, 313

Q
quick stress test 195
Quinney, A. 145, 146, 151

R
Raab, W. 145
Rahe, Richard 196
range of motion 144, 313
rapid eye movement (REM) 245, 313
rating of perceived exertion 86-87
rational-emotive therapy 214, 313
reaction time, decrease with sleeplessness 243*f*
reality checks 205
receptors 213
reconciliation 272
rectum 162, 313
redemption 7-8, 313
refocusing 205
reframing 199
Reiley, K.L. 42

rejection 267
relational abilities 194
relational coaching 268-273
relationships, value of 256
REM. *See* rapid eye movement (REM)
REM sleep 247
repetitions 116, 313
repetition speed 121, 313
repetitive strain injury 68
research, filtered through eyes of
    Christian faith vii
residual lung volume 82
resistance machines 120-121
resistance training 108, 112, 313
resting heart rate
    application activity 99
    defined 313
    standards 100*t*
    test for 81
resting metabolic rate 110, 313
rest intervals 116, 313
results, charting or graphing 24-25
resurrection 9-11
reverse crunch 127*f*, 129*f*, 299, 301
Reviving Ophelia (Pipher) 43
Riboflavin (vitamin B2) 170*t*, 171*t*
righteous worry 203-204
The Road Less Traveled (Peck) 217
Romanowski, William 16-17
romantic partners, valuable traits 262,
    263*t*
romantic relationships, expectations
    for 271
Ross, John 240
runner's high 78, 206, 313
running
    as cardiorespiratory exercise 92
    5-K run 12-week plan 93-94*t*
    guidelines 92
    with hand or ankle weights 91
Russell, C. 145

S
Sabbath 243-245
safety helmets 95
Saint Ascepsimas 158
sanctity of life 217
Sarah 200
sarcomere 116*f*, 313
saturated fat 168, 313
Schermer, F. 46
Schweitzer, Albert 244
seated alternating dumbbell curl 131*f*,
    132*f*, 304*f*, 305*f*
seated back extension 119*f*, 125*f*, 126*f*, 296
seated leg extension 122*f*, 123*f*, 125*f*,
    126*f*, 296
seated press 130*f*, 132*f*, 303*f*, 305*f*
seated two-arm dumbbell triceps
    press 131*f*, 132*f*, 304*f*, 305*f*
Seeing Yourself in God's Image
    (Homme) 37
Seerveld, Calvin 5
selenium 175*t*
self-acceptance 265
self-confidence, and body image 35
self-controlled 177, 313
self-denial 158
self-destructive thinking 199
self-esteem
    and body image 35
    and eating disorders 45

lowered by dieting 36
    physical appearance link to 35
    struggling with 32
self-exploration 257
self-insight 257
self-knowledge, areas of 257*f*
self-understanding 256
Seligman, Martin 217
Selye, Hans 194, 202, 204-205
sensing type 260*t*
Serious Strength Training (Bompa, Di
    Pasquale, and Cornachia) 124
serotonin 213
sets 116, 313-314
seven deadly sins 6-7
SHAPE 265-266
sheets 249-250
shoulder flexibility test 148
Shrier, I. 146
Shulman, Polly 270
Simon the Stylite 158
simple carbohydrate 164, 166*t*, 314
Simplify Your Life (St. James) 209
sin, and depression 211
sinful desire 7
sinning, healing as opposite of 8-9
sit-and-reach test 145, 147
skeletal muscle 115, 116*f*, 314
skinfold measurements 61, 314
sleep
    alarm clock usage by adults 238*f*
    American adults hours per night
        233*f*
    architecture of 245-247
    average hours per night of
        Americans 232*f*
    bed and accessories 249
    children's changing requirements
        248*t*
    chronic sleep deprivation 231
    college students' hours per night
        233*f*
    consistent schedule for 248
    electroencephalograph images
        246*f*
    personal sleep needs 247
    quality sleeping environment 249
    sleeping like a log 248-249
    wakeathon of Tripp 231, 239-240
    workers with eight or more hours
        per night 235*f*
sleep/alertness log 252
sleep apnea 237, 314
sleep cycle 247, 314
sleep debt 237, 314
sleep deprivation
    chronic sleep deprivation 231
    cognitive impairment 241
    death 243, 245
    defined 314
    effects of 240
    emotional irritability 241
    general fatigue 240-241
    and increased body mass index 65
    physical impairment 241-242
    psychosis 242
    sleep deprivation quiz 238-239
sleep disorders 237
sleep hygiene 248, 314
sleep I.Q. test 236-237
sleep spindles 246, 314

sleep stages 245, 314
sleep thieves
    about 231
    academic workload 231-233
    ignorance 235-236
    pain of humanity 235
    work 234
sloth 7. *See also* seven deadly sins
Smolak, L. 46
smooth muscle 115, 314
Sobel, D. 206
social rejection 267
social relationships, and happiness
    220
social support, inadequate 211
Socrates 4
sodium 174*t*
Sollee, Diane 271
soluble fiber 166, 314
specific warm-up 124
Spinning 96
spiritual faith 220
spiritual gift inventory 53-54, 277-278
spiritual gifts 264-265, 314
spirituality, as physical act 8
spiritually connecting 270
spiritual matters, stress of 196-197
spot reduction theory 110
spouse selection 270-271
sprain 144
Spurlock, Morgan 160
St. James, Elaine 209
stair-climbing 89
stairs, using 66
standing dumbbell curl 128*f*, 129*f*, 300,
    301
Stanford University Center for the
    Diagnosis and Treatment of
    Sleep Disorders 238
static flexibility 144, 314
static stretching 148
"Steps to a Healthier You" 181
steroids 34-35
Stice, E. 44
stomach 160, 314
Stott, John 188
strength
    grip strength 114
    possibilities 113-115
    world records 113-114
    world's strongest man 106
strength training
    about 106-107
    benefits of 108-113
    body composition changes from
        110*t*
    concepts 116
    and lower-back pain 117-118
    muscles targeted during 117*f*
    safety in 132-133
    types of 119-121
    women's goals 124
strength-training program
    about 121
    combining free weights and
        machines 127
    completion of exercises 123
    different workouts concept 123
    exercise substitution 123
    first day 121
    one hard set principle 122

strength-training program *(continued)*
    phase I, day 1 125*f*, 295-296
    phase I, weeks 1-2 122*f*, 123*f*, 126*f*, 296-297
    phase II, day 1 127-128*f*, 299-300
    phase II, weeks 3-4 128-129*f*, 300-301
    phase III, day 1 130-131*f*
    phase III, weeks 5-6 131-132*f*
    progression speed 122-123
    repeating phases 123-124
    starting weight 121-122
    warm-up 124
    workout card 122
stress
    ABCs of 195-200
    activating events 196-198
    and college students 198*t*
    consequences 200
    defined 195, 314
    and depression 211
    intensity of common stressful events 197*t*
    managing 204-206
    and mind–body connection 194-195
    pros and cons 200-201
    quick stress test 195
    serious stress management 206, 208-209
    turning ugly 202-203
    as weight-control obstacle 67
stress assessment test 224
stress hardy 206, 208-209, 314
stressors 196-198
stress-related hormones 200
stretches 68
stretching, benefits of 146
stroke volume 82, 83, 314
strong social relationships 220
subjective well-being
    bottom ten countries 219*f*
    top ten countries 218*f*
success or failure attitude 24*t*
sucrose 164, 314
sugar 167
suicide 216-217, 314
Super-Size Me (Spurlock) 160
support group 23
suppressor cells 79
swimming 92, 95*t*
Swindoll, Charles 230

T
Takaha, Michael 91
target heart rate zone 84-86, 314
tendon elongation 145
testosterone, levels for men and women 108*f*
tetanus 230
T helper cells 79
theta brain waves 246, 314
thiamin (vitamin B1) 170*t*, 171*t*
thinking type 261*t*
Thomas Aquinas, on gluttony 158
three-minute step test 99-101
Three Steps Forward, Two Steps Back (Swindoll) 230
time, FITT principle 87
time management 208-209
to-do list 209, 223
torso rotation 127*f*, 129*f*, 299, 301
trace minerals 173, 314

trans fats 64
Transtheoretical Model of Stages of Change 21*t*
trauma, and depression 211
triceps push-down 128*f*, 129*f*, 300, 301
Tripp, Peter 231, 239-240
twelve-minute walk/run test 101-102
type, FITT principle 87-89

U
ulcers 161
understatement 256
upper limit, target heart rate zone 84-85
urine, checking color of 173
U.S. Army Challenge for Body-Weight Exercises 114-115
U.S. Department of Agriculture, dietary guidelines 177

V
Valsalva maneuver 133
values 262, 264, 314
values clarifications 275-276
Vansittart, Charles 114
variable resistance 120, 314
variety, in food 178, 181, 314
vegan 184*t*, 185*f*
vegetarian diet 184-185, 186*t*
villi 161, 314
vitamins
    about 170, 314
    biotin 170*t*, 172*t*
    essential 170*t*
    fat-soluble and water-soluble 171-172*t*
    folate 170, 172*t*
    functions of 162*t*
    panothenic acid 170*t*, 172*t*
    vitamin A 170*t*, 171*t*
    vitamin B1 (thiamin) 170*t*, 171*t*
    vitamin B2 (riboflavin) 170*t*, 171*t*
    vitamin B3 (niacin) 170*t*, 172*t*
    vitamin B6 170*t*, 172*t*
    vitamin B12 170, 172*t*, 185*t*
    vitamin C 170, 172*t*
    vitamin D 170*t*, 171*t*, 185*t*
    vitamin E 170*t*, 171*t*
    vitamin K 170*t*, 171*t*
$\dot{V}O_2$max. *See* maximal oxygen consumption ($\dot{V}O_2$max)
voluntary neuromuscular contraction 115-116

W
waist-to-hip ratio 63
wakeathon of Tripp 231, 239-240
walking
    beginning program 91*t*
    benefits of 66, 67
    as cardiorespiratory exercise 88-89, 90-91
    guidelines for 91
    with hand or ankle weights 91
    with pedometer 89
Walking Fast (Iknoian) 91
walk/jog program 92*t*
Wallace, George 271
Walters, Corrie 109*f*
Walters, P. 268
Warburton, D.E.R. 146
warm-up 124, 132
water

about 173
in diet 64
drinking too much of 176
effects of water loss 176
functions of 162*t*
water workout 89
weather, and happiness 219
weighing methods 61, 69
weight control
    assessing compliance with plan 69
    goal setting 63-65
    helping those with food and weight problems 289
    intervention strategies 67-68
    overall goal assessment 69
    predicting obstacles 67
    present lifestyle assessment 65, 67
    specific plan design 67
weightlifting safety 132-133
weight loss 36
weight-loss strategy, best 63
weight preoccupation 33, 35, 314
weight restoration 51, 314
weight training 113
Weldon, S.M. 146
Welk, G. 151
well-being. *See* subjective well-being
wellness
    assessing present lifestyle 285
    intervention strategies 285
    physical wellness vii, ix
    plan compliance assessment 286
    predicting obstacles 285
    progress assessment of goals 286
    seven steps to 284-286
    specific plan design 285
    stating goal 285
    tools for achieving 284
West, Louis 231, 239
Weston, Edward 91
whole grains 182
Who Moved My Cheese? (Johnson) 209
wives, annual hours of work 234*f*
women
    body composition of 108-109
    body dissatisfaction 43
    body image causes of concern 36-37
    eating concerns of 42
    eating disorders differences with men 46
    eating disorders prevalence 41
    flexibility of 147
    obesity levels in Canada 60
    recovery from eating disorders 50
    strength-training goals 124
Woods, Tiger 232
Woodson, Elizabeth 109*f*
work, as sleep thief 234-235
work-life conflict 204
world happiness 217
worry, defined 204
Wright, Wilbur 244

Y
Yerkes, R.M. 201
YMCA sit-and-reach test 147-148, 149*t*
youth, and happiness 218-219

Z
Zatorski, Jack 113
zinc 174*t*, 185*t*

About the Editors

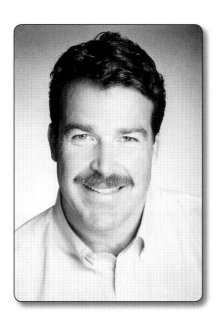

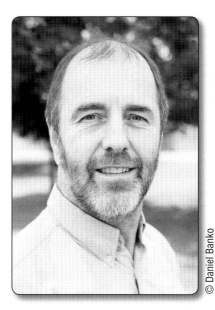

© Daniel Banko

Peter Walters, PhD, is an associate professor of Applied Health Science at Wheaton College, a private coeducational interdenominational Christian college in Illinois. Since 1996, he has directed the wellness program at the university level. During that time he has evaluated the health and wellness behavior of more than 5,000 college students. Prior to his career in academics, Dr. Walters was actively involved in several parachurch organizations, including Campus Crusade for Christ, the Navigators, and the Fellowship of Christian Athletes. In addition to these ministry opportunities, he served as director of student ministries in three local churches.

Dr. Walters has presented and published his wellness research at several national conferences and in peer-reviewed journals. He also participates competitively in weightlifting and bodybuilding to ensure that he stays grounded in practical applications and not merely theoretical constructs.

Dr. Walters is certified as an educational trainer from the American Council on Exercise, the National Strength and Conditioning Association (NSCA), and the American College of Sports Medicine (ACSM). He is also a member of the NSCA, the ACSM, and the Christian Society of Kinesiology and Leisure Studies (CSKLS). In his spare time, Dr.

Walters enjoys weightlifting, cycling, and participating in triathlons.

John Byl, PhD, is a professor of Physical Education at Redeemer University College in Ancaster, Ontario, Canada, where he has taught a wellness course for several years.

Dr. Byl is a member of CSKLS and is the host of their listserv. He is also a host of the listserv for Church Sport and Recreation Ministries, an organization that connects church recreation and sport.

Dr. Byl has been a professor since 1986, and has received numerous awards. In June 2006, he was given the Literary Award, which honors current members of CSKLS who have demonstrated the integration of faith writing into one of the disciplines represented in the society. He also received the Presidential Award, which recognizes those who have displayed actions compatible with the mission of CSKLS.

Dr. Byl has edited, authored, or coauthored 15 books, including *Physical Education, Sports, and Wellness: Looking to God as We Look at Ourselves.*

About the Contributors

Dianne E. Moroz, MS, is an adjunct professor at Redeemer University College in Ancaster, Ontario, Canada, and teaches a course in wellness. Her mission statement is to respect, love, and honor all of God's creation. To act on this, she will work to grow emotionally, socially, and intellectually for the purpose of being a better steward and contributing to the well-being of all of God's children and creation.

Doug Needham, PhD, is a professor at Redeemer University College in Ancaster, Ontario, Canada. He also currently serves as the dean of Sciences and Social Sciences. His teaching interests include introductory psychology, adolescent development, cognitive psychology, health psychology, and creativity. Dr. Needham's research interests include the following: the role of incubation (taking a break) in problem-solving, analogical transfer in problem-solving tasks (i.e., using one problem to help solve another), and an examination of morality and values in adolescents. Dr. Needham hopes that his contributions to this book will provide useful information to students on how to prevent stress and depression, how to cope with them, and how to help others who are dealing with them. Above all, he hopes that readers understand that these conditions are treatable, that no one needs to experience them for long, and that a person's relationship with God can sustain and heal.

Heather Strong, MS, is a PhD candidate in the Department of Kinesiology at McMaster University in Hamilton, Ontario, Canada. Her dissertation research is focused on how exercise can help improve body image concerns among women. She loves to go for long walks with her two Boston terriers, her husband, and her two-year-old daughter Lauren. She feels passionate about helping those suffering from body image concerns and eating disorders.

Bob Weathers, PhD, is a professor of Physical Education and Exercise Science at Seattle Pacific University. His view of wellness involves all things working together for good: Wellness-nurturing behaviors are those that simultaneously express love for God, self, others, and the rest of the created order. He believes that a life of love-motivated behavior is not a burden; rather, it can be expected to produce the joy, peace, and other traits identified in Galatians 5:22–23. Such a life, he believes, is made possible by the grace of God, who loves all people despite their imperfections and empowers everyone with his spirit to love him in return and to accept themselves and others as well. Bob celebrates the gift of physical activity and especially enjoys active adventures in and on the water.

Bud Williams, PhD, is an associate professor of Applied Health Science at Wheaton College. He feels most fulfilled in his calling when introducing students to wellness and health science concepts so that they can be better stewards of their lives and more effective in serving God in their respective callings. He is refreshed by participating in a variety of outdoor activities with family and friends.